D0222154

ATI TEAS® Study Manual

FOR THE TEST OF ESSENTIAL ACADEMIC SKILLS

CONTENT AUTHORS/ REVIEWERS

Alejandra Dashe, PhD in Anthropology

Alicia Sussman, M.Ed. Secondary Mathematics Education

Amanda Clark, PhD Science Education

Angela Broaddus, PhD Curriculum &Instruction

Arunsudha Raghubalan, MS Science Biochemistry

Benjamin Morgan Feltham, "MS Medieval History, BA Modern History"

Bonnie C. Walter, M.Ed Secondary Education

Carol M. Hollar-Zwick, Master of Arts

Charlotte Waters, MS Science Education

Deidre Meyer, MS Instructional Design

Derek Prater, MS Journalism

Dr. Naureen Qasim, M.B.B.S.

Elizabeth Rubio, Bachelor of Science, Genetics

Gayle Pearson, Bachelor of Science, English

George Christoph, M.Ed. Mathematics, NBCT

Jennifer Emrick, Master of Professional Writing

Joe Meyer, BS Mathematics, NBCT

Karen Lee Banks, EdD Educational Technology & E-Learning

Kenneth W. Stewart, "Bachelor of Science in Chemistry, Physics, Mathematics, Honors Bachelor of Education"

Kris Shaw, MS Education

L Charles Biehl, MS Education Administration

Lydia Bjornlund, Master of Education

Mandy B. Hockenbrock, MA Leadership in Teaching

Matthew R. Leach CAGS Mathematics Education

Melissa O'Connor, MS English Education

Nancy Geldermann, MS Curriculum & Instruction, NBCT

Pamela Wagner, M.Ed. Science Education, NBCT

Shauna Hedgepeth, MS Science Education

Susan Keiffer-Barone, Ed.D Curriculum & Instruction, NBCT

Suzanne Myers, MS Curriculum & Instruction

Todd A. Wells, Ph. D., PhD in Chemistry

Vidya Rajan, PhD Genetics

Reprinted December 2022

Manager of content development: Ron Watson, Integra Software Services

Project management: Joanne Manning, Integra Software Services

Copy editing: Kelly Von Lunen, Kya Rodgers, Rebecca Her, Marlo Bennett, Randa Tantawi, Kevin Jackson-Mead

Layout: Bethany Phillips, Ascend Learning

Illustrations: Randi Hardy, Ascend Learning

Online media: Brant Stacy, Ron Hanson, Britney Fuller, Trevor Lund

Cover design: Jason Buck, Ascend Learning

Interior book design: Bethany Phillips, Ascend Learning

Important Notice to the Reader

Introduction

Welcome to the ATI TEAS® Study Manual, your guide to successful preparation for the Test of Essential Academic Skills (TEAS). This book provides you with an overview of the content and skills included on the TEAS along with suggestions for effectively preparing for the test. First, this guide will outline the parts of the test. The TEAS covers a broad range of essential skills in reading, math, science, and English and language usage that you have developed over the course of your academic career. Next, this guide will help you create a study plan for success in each subject area. Finally, this study guide provides lessons covering each objective of the TEAS test plan. Lessons include examples, diagrams, and graphic organizers to help you review key ideas. Each lesson ends with practice questions similar to those you will encounter on the TEAS. A detailed explanation of the correct answer for each question is also included to ensure you understand key concepts that will appear on the TEAS.

TEAS SUBJECT AREAS

The TEAS test was developed for health science schools to evaluate the academic preparedness of prospective students. Questions on the TEAS assess student knowledge of 64 ¬objectives that address topics presented in grades¬ 7 to 12. The objectives describe skills and concepts that health science educators believe are most important for success in health science programs. The objectives cover the academic subject areas of:

- Reading
- Math
- Science
- English and Language Usage

The 64 lessons in this manual provide instruction for each of the 64 objectives of the TEAS. Keep in mind that the examples provided in the manual are not comprehensive. They do not include all the possible content appropriate for that objective. The chapters do, however, provide a clear overview of the content and skills you will encounter on the TEAS.

TEAS QUESTIONS

The TEAS is composed of 170 items that include 20 unscored pretest items, the majority of which are four-option, multiple-choice questions. With the introduction of the TEAS VII test plan in 2022, alternate item types will start to be incorporated into the test. These include:

- Multiple select (select all that apply)
- Supply answer (fill-in-the-blank numeric response)
- Ordering (put options in the correct sequence)
- Hot spot (select an area of an image)

The test is available in both paper-and-pencil (multiple-choice questions only) and computer-administered formats. Questions from the four subject areas are grouped in separate sections, and each has a separate, individual time limit. The following table provides the number of questions and time limits for each section of the TEAS, listed in order of administration.

Subject Area	Number of Questions	Time Limit
Reading	45 questions (6 pretest)	55 min
Mathematics	38 questions (4 pretest)	57 min
Science	50 questions (6 pretest)	60 min
English and language usage	37 questions (4 pretest)	37 min

Total	170 questions (20 pretest)	209 min

Questions in each subject area are organized by the key topics being assessed. There are a set number of questions for each key topic. The following table shows the number of scored questions for each key topic.

Subject Areas and Key Topics	Scored Items
Reading	*39*
Key ideas and details	15
Craft and structure	9
Integration of knowledge and ideas	15
Math	*34*
Numbers and algebra	18
Measurement and data	16
Science	*44*
Human anatomy and physiology	18
Biology	9
Chemistry	8
Scientific reasoning	9
English and language usage	*33*
Conventions of standard English	12
Knowledge of language	11
Using language and vocabulary to express ideas in writing	10

TAKING THE TEAS

The TEAS is administered in a standardized environment overseen by a proctor. The proctor will ensure that all testing protocols are strictly enforced.

For the most updated information about registering for and taking the TEAS, visit atitesting.com/teas/register. This is the best source for current information based on the mode of administration that you will be using.

WHAT TO BRING

- Photo ID: To be admitted to your testing session, you will need to present proper photo identification, such as a driver's license, passport, or green card. You will not be admitted or be able to take the test if your ID does not meet the following requirements: government-issued, current photograph, examinee signature, and permanent address. A credit card photo or a student ID does not meet the criteria.

- Writing instrument: Be sure to bring two sharpened No. 2 pencils with attached erasers. No other writing instruments are allowed.

- ATI log-in information: If you are taking the online version of the test, you will need to create a student account at www.atitesting.com prior to your test day and remember to bring your log-in information with you.

WHAT NOT TO BRING

Plan ahead and leave the following items at home or in your car because they are not permitted in the exam room:

- No additional apparel is allowed, including but not limited to jackets, coats, hats, and sunglasses. Discretionary allowances are made for religious apparel. All apparel is subject to inspection by a proctor.

- No personal items of any sort are allowed, including but not limited to purses, computer bags, backpacks, and duffel bags.

- No electronics of any kind are allowed, including but not limited to cell phones, smartphones, beepers/pagers, digital watches, and smartwatches.

- No food or drink is allowed, unless it is documented as a medical necessity.

WHAT TO EXPECT

- Testing staff will check your photo ID, admit you to your test room, and direct you to a seat.

- Proctors in the room will monitor any odd or disruptive behavior. This should not include you, but if it does, you will be dismissed, and your exam will not be scored.

- A four-function calculator will be provided by the testing center. Personal calculators will not be allowed. Calculators provided do not have built-in functionalities or other special features.

- The proctor will provide scratch paper for use during the test. Scratch paper cannot be used before the exam or during breaks. All paper, in its entirety, must be returned to the proctor at the end of the testing session.

- After the mathematics section, you may take a 10-minute break. During the break, do not access any of your personal items.

- If you need to leave your seat at any time other than during the break, raise your hand and the proctor will guide you. Note that timing for that section of the exam will not stop, and any time lost as a result cannot be made up.

- During the exam, if you have a technical issue with your computer or need the proctor for any other reason, raise your hand for assistance.

- Any challenges that arise during testing or any testing room complaints should be reported to the proctor before leaving the room on the day of your exam.

THE TEAS STUDY GUIDE

This guide is organized to help target your studies in preparation for your success on the exam.

- There is a unit for each subject area and a chapter for each objective.

- Each chapter provides an overview of an objective that includes an outline of important concepts along with examples of the specific knowledge and skills that pertain. Chapters also include key terms and definitions, practice questions, and study exercises.

- An answer key for the practice questions is provided at the end of each key topic section. Both answers and explanations are provided so that it is clear why the correct answer is right and why the incorrect answers are wrong. This will help you develop a deeper understanding of test-taking skills and provide thoughtful strategies to use when taking the actual test.

- There is a quiz at the end of each section that matches the number of scored items in the test plan. The quizzes provide an excellent practice opportunity because they have been developed using the same guidelines as the TEAS itself.

- A key with detailed explanations of the correct answers to each question immediately follows after each quiz.

Using this study manual to familiarize yourself with each of the TEAS objectives, to practice answering TEAS-style questions, and to guide study of the additional concepts covered on the test will pave the way to your success on the TEAS. Keep in mind, though, that this is a study guide; it should not be the only resource you use in your preparations. The TEAS covers a broad range of knowledge, and this study manual does not detail every concept that could possibly covered on the exam itself.

ONLINE PRACTICE TEAS

Two online practice versions of the TEAS are available for purchase. These practice versions were developed using the same test plan used for the actual proctored versions. They provide an opportunity for additional practice answering TEAS-style questions and also for assessing readiness for success on the TEAS. Each of these tests contains 150 items, all of which are scored. The testing interface is similar to that of the online proctored version, except that a rationale for each question and answer is provided to further your learning and understanding. On completion of the online practice test, a score report will appear with both your results and a list of topics for review. The list of topics for review will correspond to the objectives in the test plan and study manual and will indicate the areas in which you should focus additional study.

TEAS SCORING

The online version of the test is scored on completion. Your TEAS score report will be posted immediately and can be viewed at that time. Paper-and-pencil versions of the TEAS will be scored by ATI within 48 hours of their receipt from the testing site. The score report will include both the total overall score and the individual content area scores. In addition, the report will identify any specific topic areas deemed challenging for you along with references to specific places in the study manual where content can be reviewed to improve your skills.

Your ATI TEAS score report can be accessed at any time through your ATI account under My Results. In that same area, next to the score report, there is an option to create a Focused Review. A Focused Review is an online e-tool that aligns missed question topics with relevant study guide pages that will be helpful for your review.

You can also submit your TEAS score to your health science program. If you tested on-site at the program you are applying to, your TEAS transcript will already be available to them. If you want to send your transcript to a different program, visit atitesting.com/teas/ati-teas-transcript to purchase and send an official TEAS transcript to the program of your choice.

Preparation Strategies

PREPARING FOR THE TEST

When should you start studying for the test? Evidence shows that studying should begin well ahead of the time you will take the test so that by continuously reviewing the material, you will be able to store new information in your long-term rather than your short-term memory.[1] Planning to review your notes, writing mock exams, and developing concept maps are just a few strategic ways to ensure effective study time.[2] Research suggests that plans containing clear study goals, repeated study over time, and self-regulated learning (keeping track of what you do) result in improved performance[3] on exams. Studying collaboratively with peers and asking questions such as, "How could I explain this to someone else?" or "How does this apply to my life or something else that I have learned?" can also help you learn and understand the material.[4]

Time Management

One of the most effective ways to study for a test is to create a personal time-management system. Like an athlete or a musician, you need to set aside "practice time." Start taking control by doing an assessment of what actual free time you have. Plot it out. You may be surprised how a few small changes to eliminate minor distractions that steal your time will open up more time that you can then set aside for studying. With a little planning, you will find that within what appears to be a very busy day, week, or month, there is almost always a way to find a time for practice.

Tips

- Set your priorities. Decide how much time you will need for each part of the test. Review each section and think about which subjects need more of your attention. Plan to spend more time on those that you need to learn and less on those that just need your review.

- Make a schedule. Use a weekly planning tool, something you are already comfortable with, and set up a schedule. First, list things that are constant, such as work, sleep, and social obligations, and then look for blocks of time you can reserve for studying. These blocks should be planned for the time of day when you are most alert and able to concentrate rather than times when you are tired or easily distracted.

Goal Setting

Once you have organized your time, you will need to decide how to use it effectively. Use your priority list to determine what you will need to do to guarantee success in each subject area and how much time that will take. Make a list of what is required for each so you can check off both major and minor goals as they are reached.

Tips

- Be realistic. Set goals that are achievable. Do not expect to complete a challenging section of review in the same amount of time it will take for some subject with which you are more familiar.

- Be consistent. Once you have set your goals and your schedule, go to work and follow your plan. Planning ahead, setting goals, and consequently reaching them will give you confidence to achieve the success you are aiming for on the exam.

[1] Kornell, 2009; Kitsantas, 2002; Terry 2006
[2] Tinnesz, Ahun, & Kiener, 2006
[3] Kistantas, 2002
[4] van Blerkom, van Blerkom, & Bertsch, 2006; Roberts, 2008; Weinstein, Ridley, Dahl, & Weber, 1988

Reality Checks on Progress

Assign a specific time in your weekly schedule for review and reflection. Did you meet your weekly goal? If not, what adjustments can you make for the next week? Be objective and honest about what worked and what did not. Revise accordingly, check off your accomplishments, and then congratulate yourself!

Avoiding Test Anxiety

Sometimes, even with the best organization and planning, underling stress and apprehension can lead to test anxiety. Worrying about what-ifs can get in the way of success during test preparation and when actually taking the exam. Being prepared is the best way to alleviate test anxiety. Organizing your time, setting goals, and checking off your progress are the best ways to build confidence and to avoid unnecessary tension that may pop up and get in the way of your success.

Tips

- Balance your schedule. When creating your study schedule, build in regular times for leisure activities, exercise, eating, and socialization along with your plans for learning.

- Maintain a positive attitude. Be optimistic about your success. Develop a method of reassuring yourself with a slogan or a saying, even a gesture or a song, to avoid any naysaying and to reinforce an affirmative outlook.

- Get plenty of rest. The more rested you are, the more you will be able to focus on your work and accomplish both your long- and short-term goals.

- Be flexible. Even the best made plans can change. If something unexpected interrupts your schedule, be flexible. Adjust accordingly and get back on track the next day.

- Talk to others. Do not keep everything to yourself. Talk to your friends, family, and fellow test takers about what you are experiencing as you prepare for the test. Sharing your feelings with others may be a way to relieve the stress and help build your confidence.

Where and When to Study

Different people prefer different places and times to study. You might prefer a quiet library, the comfort of your own home, or perhaps a bustling coffee shop. In addition to choosing a place that is comfortable, it is equally important to choose a study site that is effective. A balance between preference and practicality must be struck when deciding where to study. A similar balance should be considered when deciding when to study. Select a time when you are most alert and least distractable.

Tips

- Check the lighting. Adequate lighting will prevent you from struggling and straining while you read and will also help you stay awake and focused.

- Check the temperature. Your study environment should not be too hot or too cold, although a cooler room is preferable to one that is excessively warm. Warm temperatures can make you sleepy.

- Check your posture. Find a place with a supportive chair and working surface that encourages you to sit upright and attentive rather than slouching or too relaxed.

- Have plenty of space. Your study area should allow you to spread everything out in an orderly manner. Materials should be organized so that they can be accessed without a great deal of maneuvering. A plus would be to have a dedicated space where you could leave your things arranged safely and protective over time.

- Avoid distractions. Choose a study area in a place with few distractions. The more focused you are when studying, the more productive and effective the studying will be.

- Study during your alert times. If you are a morning person, schedule your studying early in the day. If you are an evening person, study at night. In either case, be sure to schedule your study time in a way that does not interfere with your sleep.

Using Reading Strategies

Developing strategies for reading texts is the key to test preparation. It is especially important in using this study manual because of the large amount of information you will be reviewing. To retain more information, research suggests it is helpful to connect new content to prior information[5] as you read. Research also suggests that scanning for key words and taking notes will add to overall retention.[6] The more organized your study plan is, the more successful you will be at remembering what you have read.

Tips

- Preview the text. Before delving into the reading, read the introduction, summary, key terms and definitions, and any stated learning objectives.

- Outline the text. Outlining the text on a separate sheet of paper as you read keeps you focused on the content, helps you synthesize and internalize the material, and encourages your anticipation of what will come next in the text.

- Underline topic sentences. This will help you focus while you are reading and also identify key concepts to revisit when you go back through each section for review.

- Annotate in the margin. Note vocabulary words, key concepts, and your comments and questions in the margin of the text as you read. Interactive annotating keeps you engaged, helps you remember, and allows you to highlight key concepts and ideas as they are identified.

Test-Taking Strategies for Multiple-Choice

Remember that the TEAS is predominantly a multiple-choice test. There are specific test-taking strategies that can be used to improve your score on multiple-choice questions by helping to eliminate incorrect response choices.[7] For example, if a question has four potential answer options (i.e., A, B, C, or D), and only one of them is correct, there is an automatic 25% chance for you to select the right one. If you can eliminate one of those options, your chance of being right increases to 33%. If you can eliminate two wrong choices, your chance of being right increases to 50%.

Tips

- Rule out wrong answers. Use existing knowledge and what is presented in the text to identify obvious incorrect answers. Eliminate those and focus on those that remain.

- Cover up the choices and answer the question yourself. Given choices sometimes causes you to second-guess yourself. If you read the question first, there is a chance you might be able to answer it without looking at the answer choices. If that happens, when you do read the choices, you will be able to choose the option closest to your answer without being put off by the distractors, which are purposely included to meant to mislead you.

- Recognize opposite response options. Often, when two response choices oppose each other, it is an indication that one of them is probably the correct answer. Watch for these.

---

[5] Raphael & Au, 2005
[6] Peverly et al., 2007; Raphael & Au, 2005; Terry, 2006; Titsworth & Kiewra, 2004; Williams & Eggert, 2002
[7] Paris et al., 1991

- Look for absolute words. Look for words that tend to make statements incorrect (e.g., "always," "never," "all," "only," "must," and "will"). Answer choices containing absolute or definitive words tend to be incorrect because they are limited and can only apply in specific situations or under certain circumstances.

- Make educated guesses. If you cannot decide which response choice is best, make an educated guess based on background knowledge, logic, and reasoning.

- Work backward. Sometimes, it helps to look at the answer options first and then read the question to see if any of the answers makes sense. This technique is especially useful for math questions.

Alternate Item Types

With the introduction of the TEAS VII test plan in 2022, alternate item types will start to be incorporated into the test when administered via computer. Here are some considerations to keep in mind when you encounter these questions.

- Multiple-select questions – These are questions that prompt you to "select all that apply". Typically, these questions have four to six options. They may look like standard multiple-choice questions, but each option is essentially its own true-false question. You need to select all the options that are correct and none of the options that are incorrect based on the question posed. No partial credit is awarded for these questions.

- Supply answer – These questions will require you to enter a numeric response based on the question posed (typically requiring a calculation). The characters you enter into the response field must precisely match those for the correct answer in the system, so be sure to carefully read any parenthetical direction provided with the question stem (e.g., "Round to the tenth decimal place"). You will only be entering numeric characters, not units of measurement (e.g., "mg").

- Ordering – These questions will require you to put options in the correct sequence. For example, you may be presented with the steps for accomplishing a task, but the steps will be out of order. You will be prompted to reorder the steps (by dragging and dropping, for example) and then submit your response. Each step must be in the correct sequence, and no partial credit is awarded.

- Hot spot – These questions require you to select (typically by clicking) an area of an image based on the question posed. There are typically two to five clickable areas, and only one is correct. It may be helpful to follow the same tips as for multiple-choice questions, since the only real difference is that you'll be selecting part of an image instead of a text response.

Starting in 2022, you'll find examples of these question types in the study manual, as well as within the TEAS SmartPrep and on TEAS Online Practice tests. In some cases, the functionality may differ somewhat from how these function on the proctored TEAS exam. For example, an ordering question may use drag and drop in one product and matching/numbering in another. The concept, however, will be the same.

IMPROVING YOUR SCORE

Did you achieve the score you wanted on the practice test? If so, congratulations! If not, reevaluate your study approach and test-taking strategies. Which ones worked? Which ones did not? Research suggests that the more active strategies you incorporate into your studying, the better your performance will be in the long term.[8] Consider the following hands-on strategy tips to improve your study habits or your test score.

Tips

- Implement new study strategies immediately. If you are unhappy with your results, try a new study strategy right away.

- Join a study group. If you normally study alone, consider studying with others. Collaboration helps everyone.

- If you are in a study group, assess how the group uses the study time. Is the group mainly on task, or are there distractions, interruptions, or side conversations?

- Seek other sources, including non-text sources. If you need greater insight into a specific topic, seek out additional information online, consult with a tutor, or find supplemental texts to enhance your understanding.

- Ask yourself questions that reinforce your learning. For example, "If I had to teach this concept to another individual, how would I explain it?" or "If someone asked me to summarize this concept, what would I say?"

- Consult an academic advisor if you are experiencing test anxiety and cannot manage it. If you are experiencing extra tension or stress as a result of your time dedicated to test preparation, an advisor might be able to provide you with some extra tips to alleviate it.

- Reevaluate your work and extracurricular schedule. If you work or have extracurricular activities that interfere with your study schedule, consider reducing or rearranging your hours focused on these activities so that you can spend more time studying. Alternatively, try looking for additional opportunities to add studying time such as during a long commute, in place of watching television, or on a weekend afternoon when you have nothing else planned.

---

[8] Gettinger & Seibert, 2002

STUDY PREPARATION WORKSHEET

Use the following worksheet to help prepare for the test. Adapt it to meet your individual needs.

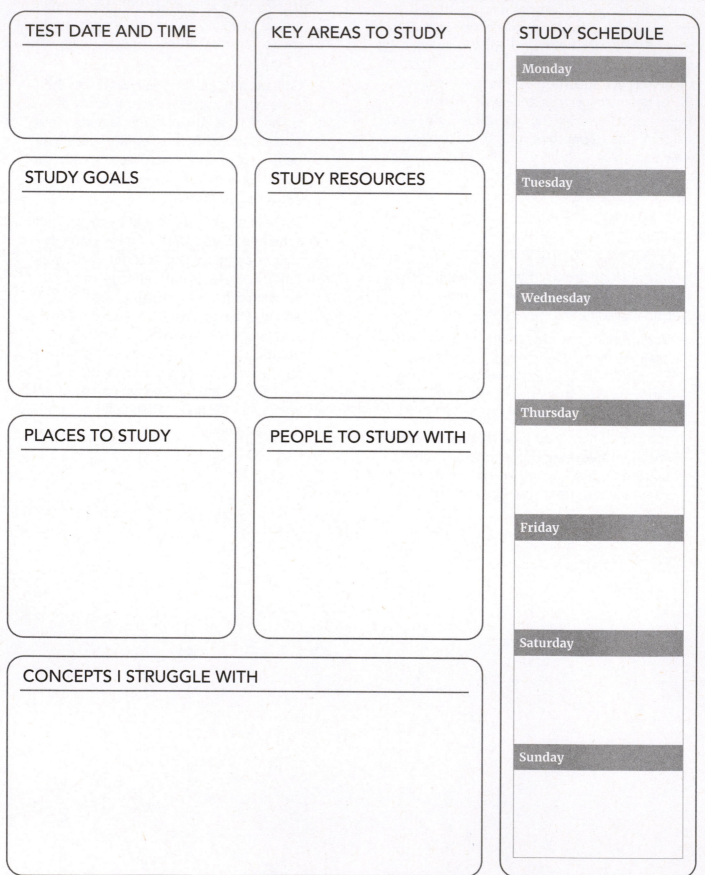

TEST DATE AND TIME

KEY AREAS TO STUDY

STUDY SCHEDULE

Monday

Tuesday

Wednesday

Thursday

Friday

Saturday

Sunday

STUDY GOALS

STUDY RESOURCES

PLACES TO STUDY

PEOPLE TO STUDY WITH

CONCEPTS I STRUGGLE WITH

Table of Contents

UNIT 2: MATHEMATICS

Unit 1: Reading

The 14 lessons in this unit cover the tasks from the ATI TEAS test plan for the Reading section. These are focused on assessment of functional literacy skills and are organized into three chapters:

- Key ideas and details
- Craft and structure
- Integration of knowledge and ideas

The Reading unit tests your knowledge of reading concepts and your ability to apply those concepts. You will be required to read various types of reading passages—including fiction, nonfiction, informational, and graphical—and those passages will be of various lengths. Some passages will have as many as seven questions based on them. Your ability to synthesize the information you have read and to think critically will be essential to your success on the Reading section of the ATI TEAS.

Each lesson introduces knowledge, skills, and abilities relevant to the corresponding Reading test plan task and provides an overview of some essential topics, along with specific examples to highlight important concepts. Practice questions at the end of each chapter will allow you to test your knowledge of select concepts. In addition, there are key terms included at the end of the chapter followed by a practice Reading quiz. This quiz includes the same number of questions as the Reading section on the ATI TEAS and matches the test plan allocations (shown below). The quiz will give you a good idea of the number and types of sources you will encounter and the questions that will accompany those sources. Keep in mind that these lessons are a great starting point and guide to your studies, but they are not an exhaustive review of all concepts that might be tested in the Reading section of the ATI TEAS. You should use other sources (textbooks, online resources, etc.) for additional study and practice in areas that you have not mastered.

There are 39 scored Reading items on the TEAS. These are divided as shown below. In addition, there will be six unscored pretest items that can be in any of these categories.

Section	Number of scored questions
Key ideas and details	15
Craft and structure	9
Integration of knowledge and ideas	15

Key Ideas and Details

R.1.1 — Summarize a multi-paragraph text

Reading **comprehension** is a vital skill in all subject areas, and the ability to summarize a multi-paragraph text is an important way to demonstrate comprehension. To summarize a text, first **identify** the **topic** and determine the author's **main idea**. The author's main idea for the text will be stated in the introduction as a **claim**, thesis, or message about the topic. Next, identify the topic sentence in each paragraph. The topic sentence states the main idea of the individual paragraph, which in turn relates to the main idea—the claim, thesis, or message of the text. Finally, evaluate the **key points** and **details** that **support** each paragraph's main idea and, likewise, function to support the overall claim, thesis, or message about the topic.

To succeed on this TEAS task, you must get used to asking yourself, "What is the topic, and what is the author's main idea (claim, thesis, or message) about the topic?" Then, examine the key points and supporting details provided by the author to determine how they relate to the main idea of each paragraph and to the main idea of the text.

Objectives

This objective includes, but is not limited to, the following examples of knowledge, skills, and abilities.

- Identify the main idea and supporting details in a single paragraph of the text.
- Identify the topic of the text.
- Identify the main idea(s) of the text.
- Identify the key points in the text.
- Explain how details support the main idea in the text.
- Paraphrase key points in the text to demonstrate an understanding of the relationship of ideas in the text.
- Distinguish between relevant and irrelevant ideas in a text needed to compose an objective summary of a multiple-paragraph text.

IDENTIFYING THE TOPIC AND MAIN IDEA

The topic of a multi-paragraph text is the subject of the entire piece of writing. The topic of a passage is often found at the beginning of the text in the title, the introduction, or a topic sentence. Examples of topics in a nursing text might include blood poisoning, body organs, or blood pressure. A good piece of writing will be clear about what topic it addresses.

Once you have identified the topic, you can then identify the main idea—the thesis, claim, or message—of the passage. To do this, answer the questions "What is the writer saying about the topic?" "What is important to know about the topic?" and "What is the author's message or claim about the topic?" For example, if the topic of a text is blood pressure, the main idea of the text could be how to measure blood pressure or that people should pay more attention to the importance of monitoring their heart rate.

comprehension. Ability to understand.

identify. Distinguish a particular idea.

topic. Subject of a text.

main idea. The thesis, claim, or message that an author states or expresses about the topic of a text; the central point in each paragraph.

claim. A statement made in an argument that something about a topic is true.

key points. Ideas that elaborate on and support the main idea about a topic in each paragraph.

details. Facts, descriptions, and other types of information that support key points.

support. Lend credibility to an idea.

IDENTIFYING KEY POINTS

In addition, the author will include key points, which elaborate on the main idea of each individual paragraph. Key points are supported by details, which provide *evidence* such as *facts*, descriptions, or other information. Working together, key points and details support the main idea of each paragraph, which in turn supports the author's main idea—the claim, thesis, or message of the text. For example, if the main idea is that people should learn how to measure their heart rate, the key points will be steps or explanations for how or why to do it. Steps would include how to check your pulse at the wrist and how to count the beats. Explanations would include why it is good for people to take their own blood pressure, and each key point would likely have supporting details with even more information given for each step or explanation.

EXPLAINING HOW DETAILS SUPPORT A MAIN IDEA

Key points and supporting details provide more information about the main idea of a text. Supporting details work to explain, elaborate, or clarify the main idea of each paragraph of a text. Explanatory details provide evidence and *reasoning* to support the key points and main idea of each paragraph. Elaborative details explore the key points and main idea of each paragraph in greater depth and explain implications. Clarifying details explain what the author means when they use specific terms.

Supporting details are not all equally important for a summary. A summary should identify which details are most important for providing evidence, clarity, and elaboration about the key points and main idea. To evaluate the importance of a supporting detail, answer these questions: "Which details explain or develop a key point or the main idea?" (major details; belong in a summary) and "Which details are related to other supporting details?" (minor details; do not belong in a summary).

For instance, in the following paragraph, statements that are *irrelevant* to a summary are in bold.

> NICU nurses provide specialized care for either premature infants or newborns who are critically ill. These compassionate and specially-trained nurses provide both required medical attention and comfort for these tiny patients. **Some nurses can choose to work instead with children or teens.** However, NICU nurses who desire to work with these newborns, the most vulnerable patient population, must earn additional certifications. **Still other nurses can choose to work in labor and delivery with pregnant patients to help bring newborns into the world.**

---

evidence. Proof, such as facts, descriptions, and examples, that an author uses to support their ideas and reasoning.

fact. Statement or data that can be proven or verified through a reputable source.

reasoning. A method or structure used to build a valid argument in a persuasive text.

irrelevant. Not applicable to the idea.

PARAPHRASING KEY POINTS

Once you have identified the topic, main idea (thesis, claim, or message), and key points, it is important to put those ideas into your own words. This will help you understand and remember what you have read. Practice reading a multi-paragraph text and rephrasing its topic, main idea, and key points in a single paragraph of four to eight sentences. By rephrasing the topic, main idea, and key points in a shorter form, you are summarizing a multi-paragraph text. For questions on this TEAS task, you will use this strategy to summarize a multi-paragraph text.

SUMMARIZING A MULTI-PARAGRAPH TEXT

Read the following passage. Think about the topic, main idea, key points, and supporting details you would need to identify and explain when summarizing the text.

> (1) In the United States, about 1.7 million adults develop sepsis yearly. Of those patients, about 270,000 die. Nurses must be educated in the early identification of sepsis to increase the standard of patient care.
>
> (2) Sepsis occurs as a result of prolonged infection. Most cases of sepsis begin as bacterial infections. When the body is fighting an infection, it releases chemicals into the bloodstream. If the body's response to these chemicals is unbalanced, sepsis can occur because the body's response to the infection begins to damage tissue. Sepsis is a potentially life-threatening condition because multiple organs can sustain damage, including the heart, lungs, kidneys, and brain. People most at risk include infants, older adults, and people with chronic medical conditions or weakened immune systems.
>
> (3) A further concern is the progression of sepsis into septic shock. Septic shock occurs when there is a dramatic drop in blood pressure and a buildup of lactic acid in the blood. This condition affects the ability of cells to function properly and produce energy. Septic shock increases the risk of death in patients. About 40% of patients with septic shock die. Survivors are at risk for future infections.

First, identify the topic and main idea—the thesis, claim, or message. Because the topic is the general subject of a passage, it helps to practice asking the following question about the topic sentence: "What am I reading about?" The following box shows how the topic can be retrieved by asking this question.

Question	Topic
What am I reading about?	Sepsis

Next, ask: "What does the author want me to know or think about the topic?"

Question	Main Idea (Thesis, Claim, or Message)
What is important to know about the topic?	Nurses must be educated in the early identification of sepsis to increase the standard of patient care.

Once a reader has identified the topic and main idea, it is essential to be able to identify and **rephrase** the key point in each paragraph and the supporting details. A vital question to ask is, "What are the most important things to know about this topic?"

The main ideas and key points in the passage illustrate the topic by explaining what sepsis is, elaborating on why it is so dangerous, and clarifying why the urgent treatment of sepsis is a priority.

---

rephrase. To explain an idea in different words.

Next, a reader must be able to identify the key points about the topic and then notice the details about those key points.

Main Ideas/Key Points	Supporting Details
Sepsis results from a prolonged infection.	Body's improper response to an infection Causes tissue and organ damage Life-threatening Infants, older adults, and people with chronic medical conditions or weakened immune systems most at risk
Sepsis can progress into septic shock.	Drop in blood pressure Buildup of lactic acid in the blood Affects proper cell function Increases risk of death
Certain groups are most at risk from sepsis.	Infants Seniors People with chronic medical conditions People with weakened immune systems

Finally, it is time to put these ideas together into a summary of a multi-paragraph text. Here is an example of such a summary.

> In the United States, sepsis is a common and potentially serious condition. For this reason, nurses must learn to recognize the conditions that lead to sepsis so that it can be treated early. Sepsis results from damage to organs and tissues after a long infection. If sepsis is not detected and treated early, it can lead to septic shock. Septic shock is when blood pressure drops and lactic acid builds up in the blood. Septic shock increases the risk of death. The groups most at risk from sepsis are older adults, infants, and people with chronic conditions or weakened immune systems.

Practice Problems

Read the passage and answer the following questions.

(1) By 2018, the obesity rate in the United States was about 43%. Nurses play a vital role in helping patients learn to control their weight and thus their risks for heart disease.

(2) Regular exercise provides numerous benefits for optimal heart health. Among these are lower blood pressure, reduced inflammation in the body, and a healthier body weight. Most importantly, a lifestyle that includes regular, consistent exercise can help reduce the chance of cardiac events. For instance, exercise helps blood circulate more effectively so the heart does not need to work as hard to pump blood to the muscles. To keep the heart healthy, the most effective exercise routine should include both aerobic activities and resistance training with moderate weights.

(3) Another way to control weight is through diet. A heart-healthy diet includes eating an appropriate portion of each of the following food categories: fruits and vegetables, whole grains, and low-fat proteins. Patients should lower their intake of unhealthy fats and salt. An occasional treat is acceptable as long as the core diet remains true to these standards. One way to achieve this eating style is to plan ahead. By planning meals, patients are able to ensure that their homes contain the ingredients they need to prepare heart-healthy meals.

1. Which of the following is the topic of the passage?

   A. Heart-healthy foods

   B. Rising obesity rates

   C. Taking care of the heart

   D. Exercise techniques

2. Which of the following is the main idea of the passage?

   A. Exercise routines should always include both aerobics and resistance training.

   B. Exercise and healthy eating should be encouraged to prevent heart disease.

   C. Planning ahead can lead to easier dietary changes.

   D. Exercise helps blood circulate more easily through the body.

3. Which of the following is a key point in paragraph 2?

   A. "Among these are lower blood pressure, reduced inflammation in the body, and a healthier body weight."

   B. "For instance, exercise helps blood circulate more effectively so the heart does not need to work as hard."

   C. "Another way to control weight is through diet."

   D. "Regular exercise provides numerous benefits for optimal heart health."

4. Which of the following is the most important supporting detail in paragraph 3?

   A. "A heart-healthy diet includes eating an appropriate portion of each of the following food categories: fruits and vegetables, whole grains, and low-fat proteins."

   B. "An occasional treat is acceptable as long as the core diet remains true to these standards."

   C. "One way to achieve this eating style is to plan ahead."

   D. "By planning meals, patients are able to ensure that their homes contain the ingredients they need to prepare heart-healthy meals."

5. In four to eight sentences, write a summary of the multi-paragraph text above.

R.1.2 — Make inferences and draw conclusions about a text's purpose and meaning

Whether you are reading an informational text, **procedure**, news article, or story, having the ability to make **inferences** and draw **conclusions** about a text's purpose and meaning by combining your own knowledge and experiences with what you have read is a true test of your comprehension. To prepare for this TEAS task, you will need to identify and evaluate evidence about the topic and events described. Then practice asking yourself, "What can I infer or conclude about the topic based on what I have just read?"

WHAT ARE INFERENCES AND CONCLUSIONS?

To fully understand a text's purpose and meaning, readers need to examine and evaluate the evidence, or information, provided by the author. The reader must observe facts, **delineate arguments**, and discern **valid** information. Strong readers also use individual knowledge and experiences, in addition to the text, to construct meaning. An inference is a logical **assumption** or guess that can be made about a topic based on evidence and reasoning, and it is similar to reading between the lines. Many readers assume that making an inference and drawing a conclusion are the same. It is true that each activity demands that a reader fill in some blanks. However, there is a subtle difference between the two. While an inference is an assumption that fills in a gap in the text based on details and evidence, a conclusion takes the information in the text to the next **logical** step or level based on details and evidence.

Objectives

This objective includes, but is not limited to, the following examples of knowledge, skills, and abilities.

- Identify evidence used in a text to support conclusions.

- Distinguish between explicit and implicit evidence given to describe conclusions.

- Explain how explicit and implicit evidence supports logical conclusions.

---

procedure. Ordered steps to follow in a set of written directions to complete a task safely, efficiently, and effectively.

inference. A logical assumption, or guess, that can be made about a topic based on evidence, reasoning, and personal experience or knowledge.

conclusion. A deduction made by a reader that takes the details, evidence, and assumptions presented in a text to the next logical step.

delineate. Describe precisely or set forth accurately in detail.

argument. A type of text consisting of a claim on a debatable issue, background information, reasoning and evidence, rhetorical appeals, counterclaims, and responses to counterclaims.

valid. Proven as true.

assumption. Supposition of an unstated idea.

logic. The framework of reasoning used to understand ideas and make sound assumptions, predictions, and conclusions.

EXPLICIT AND IMPLICIT EVIDENCE

Texts often contain both **explicit** and **implicit** information that can be used as the basis of inferences and conclusions, and both types of evidence are useful. Explicit information is directly stated in the text. There is no confusion about what it means. Implicit information refers to ideas that are suggested or **implied**. The information is not stated directly in the text. Take the following example:

> *In the past, hospital nurses could check patient vital signs only by hand, which required precision and more frequent checks. Today, however, there are a variety of monitors that can help nurses ensure that patients are stable constantly. Technology may have improved, but nurses are still as busy as they ever were.*

The author clearly states that previously, nurses had to perform procedures on hospital patients more often to check vital signs, and that today, technology ensures patients' stability "constantly." The author implies that this new technology has failed to improve nurses' lives in any truly significant way. Readers can infer, based on the explicit text evidence "still as busy as they ever were" and observations of nurses at work during regular doctor visits, that nurses have more to do than monitor vital signs. Readers can conclude that one purpose of the text is to point out that technology cannot take the place of human nurses. By combining explicit and implicit evidence with personal knowledge and experience, readers can come to understand the meaning of a text and the author's reason for writing it.

DRAWING LOGICAL CONCLUSIONS

Following is an example of using explicit and implicit evidence to draw a logical conclusion.

> *The boxer stood in her corner, trying to catch her breath while the crowd roared and her tenacious opponent snarled with confidence from across the ring. As she waited for the sound of the bell to signal the final round, sweat stung her eyes, and her muscles tensed.*

Based on any experience that you have with boxing matches, you can draw some conclusions and make some inferences.

Conclusions: The explicit details of "the bell to signal the final round" and the boxer's tensed muscles allow you to conclude that the boxer is in the final round of a difficult match. You can also logically conclude, based on the evidence of "the roaring crowd," that this match is exciting.

Inferences: You can also make some inferences about the characters. You can infer that the boxer's opponent is tough and angry because of the author's explicit description: "tenacious" and "snarled." You can also infer that the opponent is winning, and the boxer is losing, based on the implicit evidence in the paragraph: the boxer is trying to catch her breath while her opponent is snarling with confidence. It is a reasonable assumption to make that the character in the corner is losing the match or just barely keeping up the fight.

---

explicit. Describes information that is directly stated in a text.

implicit. Describes ideas that are suggested rather than stated directly in a text.

imply. Indicate an idea subtly without specifically stating it.

Practice Problems

Read the passage and answer the following questions.

After graduating from high school, Danielle decided to become a neonatal nurse. Her grandmother had been a pioneer in caring for premature babies. She had developed many of the procedures used in neonatal care. Danielle enrolled in her community college's associate degree in nursing program. She worked hard and completed the program in four semesters. As Danielle approached her graduation date, she learned about the nursing residency program at a nearby hospital. Danielle was especially intrigued by the "transition to practice" philosophy of the nursing residency program. This would allow her to find out if nursing was what she really wanted to do with her life. The next enrollment period for the program would begin soon after graduation. This meant she would be eligible to apply. However, she would also need to complete cardiopulmonary resuscitation (CPR) and basic life support (BLS) training as another requirement for joining the program. As she applied for the program, she reviewed the list of specialized areas of nursing offered. She dreamed of the day she could become a nurse in neonatal intensive care.

1. Which of the following best supports the inference that Danielle has a lot of determination?

    A. She decides to become a nurse like her grandmother.

    B. She enrolls in a nursing program in a community college.

    C. She completes the program in four semesters.

    D. She is interested in various areas of specialization.

2. Which of the following details from the passage is implicit evidence?

    A. Danielle decides to become a nurse after high school.

    B. Danielle is eligible to apply for the nursing residency program.

    C. Danielle considers various areas of specialization.

    D. Danielle wants to follow in her grandmother's foot-steps.

3. Which of the following can be concluded about the "transition to practice" program based on evidence from the passage? (Select all that apply.)

    A. It is a program specializing in neonatal care.

    B. Nursing students can begin hands-on training soon after the program ends.

    C. Nursing students can gain experience while learning about nursing.

    D. It can lead to a job in the same hospital if the student does well in the program.

    E. Students in the program would work at a nearby hospital.

4. Which of the following patients would Danielle care for as a neonatal intensive care nurse?

    A. Elderly men and women

    B. Premature or critically ill newborn infants

    C. Adults requiring surgery

    D. Children with severe burns or missing limbs

5. Using both explicit and implicit evidence from the passage, make an inference about how Danielle thought or felt about her grandmother. Then explain the evidence used to make this inference.

R.1.3 — Demonstrate comprehension of written directions

Readers and writers encounter procedural documents, or written directions, in all areas of learning. Procedural documents are **sequential**, and they involve step-by-step guidance for the completion of certain tasks. For example, engineering students read procedural programs, nursing students read pain management procedures, and biology students read laboratory procedures. All readers should be prepared to read and properly follow written directions. Procedures can be found in any text, from recipes to vehicle manuals to do–it–yourself articles. This **genre** of sequential written directions offers readers the ability to safely, efficiently, and effectively complete activities. For the TEAS, you will need to demonstrate the ability to follow directions by identifying important terms, the main idea, and key details of a procedure. You will also need to recognize the relationships among delineated tasks.

IDENTIFYING WORDS AND PHRASES THAT SIGNIFY ORDER AND RELATIONSHIP

Procedural texts are composed of specific language, features, and **structures**. These conventions help create an organizational structure that enhances comprehension. The language features include simple, **objective** language and signal words that assist the reader in recognizing the relationship among steps. Objective language is impartial, nonjudgmental, nonpersonal, and nonemotional.

Objectives

This objective includes, but is not limited to, the following examples of knowledge, skills, and abilities.

- Identify words and phrases that signify order.

- Identify contradictions between and among steps.

- Identify priorities in a set of directions.

- Identify the relationship among steps in a procedure.

- Identify missing information needed to complete a set of directions, process, or procedure.

- Determine a logical conclusion for performing a set of directions based on information provided in those directions.

For instance, if you decide to pursue a nursing degree, you will have to follow certain steps in a specific order to get enrolled in a nursing program. The following words are terms that indicate order and **sequence**.

Procedural Signal Words			
first	third	next	last
then	finally	while	before
second	now	when	after

---

sequential. Following a set order.

genre. A group of related writings or other media.

structures. Ways of logically organizing ideas to enhance comprehension.

objective. Describes language that is nonjudgmental, impartial, nonpersonal, and unemotional.

sequence. Logical order or pattern of organization in writing or texts.

Read the following paragraph. Words that signify order appear in bold.

> *When you consider enrolling in a nursing program, your **first** step is to conduct some research into which schools offer nursing degrees. You might also research nursing specializations of interest to you. **Next,** you might contact a few of the schools to ask questions and get clarification before applying to the programs of your choice. **While** filling out program applications, you might also fill out your Free Application for Federal Student Aid (FAFSA). **Then,** you would wait for responses from each school where you filed an application. **Finally,** you would make a choice about which school to attend.*

IDENTIFYING PRIORITIES IN A SET OF DIRECTIONS

Directions often use lists to indicate the priority of the steps involved. These lists can be numbered or bulleted, which makes each step clear and indicates which step takes priority over another. However, this presentation is not always the case. If a set of directions is not written as a list, signal words showing order can be used to determine *priorities*.

Whether directions are written as a list or in paragraph form, they can include signal words that show steps of high or low priority, such as "important" (high priority) or "optional" (low priority).

In the directions that follow, determine the priority based on the order of the steps and the signal words in bold.

> *To make perfect scrambled eggs:*
>
> (1) *Crack two eggs into a small bowl and discard the shells.*
> (2) *Add a teaspoon of butter or olive oil.*
> (3) *Optional: Add a tablespoon of milk.*
> (4) *Beat eggs with a fork until they are uniformly mixed.*
> (5) *Optional: Add salt or pepper to taste.*
> (6) *In a small pan, cook eggs over low heat for 3 to 5 minutes, until they are just firm. **Important!** Take the pan off the heat as soon as desired firmness is achieved to avoid scorching.*
> (7) *Serve immediately.*

---

priorities. In written directions, the hierarchy or sequence of which steps must be followed in what order; often indicated by the use of signal words.

IDENTIFY MISSING INFORMATION AND CONTRADICTION & DETERMINE A LOGICAL CONCLUSION

Ideally, a set of directions includes all the information needed to perform the task being described, and that information is both consistent and logical. However, mistakes can happen—perhaps the directions were written by someone who was not completely familiar with the procedure, or perhaps the reader is missing a page. Sometimes, directions can seem contradictory even though there are not any mistakes. This happens when directions give you "either/or" options, such as use either a butter knife or a three-pronged fork, or alternatives, such as using a particular glue unless you used synthetic wood originally. Thus, readers must be able to identify missing or contradictory information and determine a logical conclusion based on a series of actions or steps.

For example, read this set of directions and identify a missing step and a **contradiction**. Then, determine what logical conclusions you can make for how to perform the task being described in the directions.

> (1) *Place all pieces on the game board.*
>
> (2) *White-piece player goes first.*
>
> (3) *Take turns moving pieces one at a time. A turn ends when the active player removes their hand from their game piece.*
>
> (4) *If a player reconsiders their move, they should tell their opponent they are returning the piece to its original position before moving it back.*
>
> (5) *Play continues until checkmate is reached.*

In this list of steps, a step is missing between Steps 1 and 2 that describes how to set up the pieces on the game board. Steps are missing between Steps 2 and 3 that describe how to move the pieces. Step 4 contradicts Step 3—Step 3 says a player's turn ends when they remove their hand from their game piece, but Step 4 says that a player can reconsider their move and return the piece to its original position. Based on these written directions, it is logical to conclude that the player who achieves checkmate is the winner and that further information is needed to play the game.

When steps in a procedure are missing or contradictory, the reader may need to consult a second source to determine the proper sequence of steps. It is important to never assume any step is optional, even if it contradicts another step, unless the directions state that the step is optional.

---

contradiction. A statement, assertion, or instruction in a text that conflicts with information provided elsewhere in the same text.

Practice Problems

Read the passage and answer the following questions.

(1) *First, explain the intravenous (IV) catheter insertion procedure to the patient.*

(2) *Next, determine if the patient has needle phobia, and if so, keep the needle out of sight until the last minute.*

(3) *While using a soothing tone, encourage the patient not to watch the procedure.*

(4) *Before inserting the IV catheter, follow infection control protocol by wearing gloves and swabbing the injection site with an alcohol pad.*

(5) *When preparing to insert the catheter, look for a suitable vein in the patient's nondominant hand.*

(6) *If a vein is not immediately visible, carefully use your fingers to locate a suitable vein.*

(7) *Swab the injection site with an alcohol pad and then don gloves.*

(8) *Finally, upon successful insertion of the IV catheter, secure it with medical tape.*

1. Which of the following procedures is described in the passage?

   A. Infection control protocol

   B. IV catheter insertion

   C. Location of suitable veins

   D. Assessment of needle phobia

2. In which of the following ways are Steps 1 and 2 related?

   A. They describe the steps for inserting a needle.

   B. They explain why patients have needle phobias.

   C. They provide alternative choices in the directions.

   D. They include procedural signal words to show the order of steps.

3. Which of the following are key terms in the passage that signify order?

   A. First, when, before

   B. Follow, insert, look

   C. Carefully use, secure it

   D. Advance the needle slowly

4. Which of the following steps contradicts Step 4?

   A. Step 2

   B. Step 5

   C. Step 7

   D. Step 8

5. Which of the following steps is missing from the procedure?

   A. Then, ask the patient if they have ever had a reaction to needle insertion.

   B. Next, advance the needle slowly and carefully until you feel resistance.

   C. Explain to the patient that you are inserting the needle.

   D. Review with the patient the steps that you performed to ensure understanding.

R.1.4 — Locate specific information in a text

Often, when you read a text, you are reading for the purpose of finding specific pieces of information. You might need to learn about a new procedure or the steps to take to fix an appliance. You might also want to find out what is going on across the world.

Texts contain all sorts of information, but you will not always have time to read everything that is available about a subject. Often, you will need to make a decision or solve a problem quickly. In these situations, it is important to know how to find the specific information you need in a text. Fortunately, there are a lot of tools at your disposal to help you accomplish this. Additionally, you can develop the skills you need to find *relevant* information. You can learn how to approach a text with the right questions in mind to locate the most helpful answers, and you can use text features and navigational tools to skip directly to the information you need.

The TEAS will test how well you can locate specific information in a text. To do well on questions in this TEAS task, you should be able to locate **headings** and **subheadings**, identify various text features, and use navigational tools to find information in digital texts.

> ## Objectives
>
> This objective includes, but is not limited to, the following examples of knowledge, skills, and abilities.
>
> - Select relevant information (e.g., to solve a problem, to inform a decision).
>
> - Ask questions to determine information missing in a text needed for a given purpose.
>
> - Use textual features to locate information (e.g., headings and subheadings, keys, legends, boldface, italics, footnotes, glossary, index, table of contents).
>
> - Use navigational tools in media to find information such as search query or engine.

FINDING RELEVANT INFORMATION

Not all information in a text will be relevant to your specific needs. Relevance is determined by your purpose for reading a text. A car owner's manual can contain all sorts of interesting and useful information about the function of your car, but if you have a broken alternator, the section on alternators and how to fix them is the relevant information in that **context**. To determine what is relevant information, you first need to ask yourself a question, such as "What problem am I trying to solve?" or "What decision am I trying to make?"

One other way to find relevant information in a text is to use textual features or navigational tools. You will look at those in more detail shortly, but first, it is important to determine what information is not contained in a text.

---

relevant. Connected to the idea being discussed.

heading. A title within a text, commonly used by authors to organize information.

subheading. A title of a subdivision of information within a larger division of a text.

context. Surrounding words or ideas within a sentence or passage that affect the meaning of a word and influence how it is understood.

ASKING QUESTIONS TO DETERMINE MISSING INFORMATION

Texts do not always have all the answers you need or want. Often, you will need to read to discern what information a text does not contain, so you can try and find it elsewhere.

Just like discerning relevant information, to find out what is missing from a text, you first should have an idea of what information you need. What is the specific purpose you have for reading a text? To help you clarify your purpose, write it down, and then make a list of what you think you need to know. For instance, you might be reading to discover the steps you must follow to assess damage to an air conditioning unit. You can make a list of the things you need to know, such as how to access the components, how to check the function of the components, and how to perform these steps safely. Using your list, you can then compare and contrast the relevant information you have found in the text with your ideas about the information you need.

To determine missing information, you can also ask a series of who, what, when, where, and how questions as you read. To return to the example of the malfunctioning air conditioning unit, you can read a passage that mentions that you need to check the electrical circuits by using a method called hopscotching. By asking questions, you can then determine if the text tells you what hopscotching is, why it is useful, and how to do it. If you find that the text does not answer these questions, then you know that you need to find this information elsewhere.

Sometimes, texts will tell you that there is missing information in the text and how or where to find it. It can be difficult to find everything you need in a complex or technical text. However, texts like these usually have text features such as section headings, subheadings, *footnotes*, and endnotes. These features will help you sort through categories of information faster than reading every word in the text.

USING TEXTUAL FEATURES TO LOCATE INFORMATION

Textual features are parts of a text that are designed to stand out from a larger text for a specific *reason*. Some additional examples of textual features include bold print, italics, glossaries, *indexes*, and tables of contents. Textual features in many texts can be used to help you quickly locate relevant information.

Glossaries, Indexes, and Tables of Contents

In a longer text, like a book or journal, the first place you can look for textual features to identify relevant information are the *table of contents*, index, and *glossary*. Tables of contents and indexes contain the titles of chapters and provide a page reference so you can quickly find the topics you are looking for. Indexes are alphabetized lists of key details and concepts, such as names, and provide page number references. The index tends to be at the back of a book. The glossary is an alphabetized list of key terms, sometimes with definitions provided. This resource also tends to be at the back of a book.

It is a beneficial practice to consult these features to identify if key terms, concepts, and other pieces of information are covered in your text, and where to find them if so.

---

footnote. Comment at the bottom of a page that provides additional information about something within the text.

reason. A basis or fact to support an idea.

index. A text feature usually found in the back of a book that includes an alphabetized list of key details and concepts and the page numbers where that information can be found.

table of contents. Text feature usually found in the front matter of a book that lists chapter titles and page numbers.

glossary. A text feature usually found in the back of a book that includes an alphabetized list of key terms and their definitions.

Headings and Subheadings

Headings and subheadings are some of the most common text features authors use to help readers understand how a text is organized. Read this example, which contains headings and subheadings.

SUMMER STAFF BARBECUE

The hospital event planner is looking forward to organizing a wonderful staff barbecue this Summer. This year's picnic will include both indoor and outdoor games and activities, as well as a catered meal of delicious barbecue favorites.

Eligibility

All medical staff and their families are invited to attend the barbecue. There will be games and activities suitable for all ages. The barbecue menu will have something for everyone, including those with food allergies.

Location and Time

The barbecue will be at the city park's south end. The time will be from 1 pm to 5 pm in an effort to accommodate the greatest number of staff.

In this example, "Summer Staff Barbecue" is the heading. "Eligibility" and "Location and Time" are subheadings. Notice that the heading appears in bold type and is larger than the subheadings and the explanatory text. The subheadings also appear in bold type, but they are set in a smaller font size. Sometimes, subheadings are italicized as well. These features break up the text and organize it by main idea and topic. The heading and subheadings indicate the main idea or topic each section covers. If you need to find relevant information in a text quickly, you can skim the headings and subheadings, looking for the topic you want to find, and go directly to that section for the information you need. Indentation is another text feature that a writer might use to help organize and clarify a text for readers.

Identifying Features

Some text features are easily identified by where they appear on a page. **Sidebars**, footnotes, and **legends** are some examples of these types of text features. Sidebars are often used in history textbooks. The main text in the book might focus on a world leader's work and major accomplishments associated with a particular social or political movement. A sidebar can include a photograph or image of the leader, along with an additional detail or two about their personal life.

> **For example**
>
> Sidebars like this one can offer readers additional information about a text that might not be provided in the main text.

---

sidebar. Text feature that is set apart from the main body of a text; often includes additional information, charts, graphs, and/or images.

legend. Map feature that explains symbols and other elements that represent information on the map, such as routes, populations, and capital cities.

UNDERLINED, BOLDFACED, AND ITALICIZED PRINT

Some other common text features include underlined, boldfaced, and italicized print. These text features can sometimes be more confusing to interpret because there are many reasons why text might be italicized, boldfaced, or underlined. Likewise, formal style guides used by writers, reporters, and scholars use different sets of rules for italicized, boldfaced, and underlined print. For example, some style guides advise to boldface print for emphasis, while others prefer to italicize words to convey emphasis.

It is sometimes up to a reader to infer why a portion of text appears different from the text around it. There are, however, some standard uses for text features. Italics, for example, are used for titles of longer works (e.g., books), for foreign words or phrases, and, as previously mentioned, for emphasis.

A broadly accepted rule is that writers use text features to draw attention to specific portions of text for specific reasons. Here are some simple questions you can ask yourself if you notice that part of a text has a different appearance than the text around it.

- Is the text a title?
- Is the text a quotation that the author is using to help prove a point, introduce an idea, or make a statement?
- Is the text introducing a different section that will cover a new topic or idea?
- Is the text feature being used for aesthetic reasons only?
- Does the text feature help to organize information?
- Does the text feature have something to do with the type of text? (A script, for example, might include boldface type to indicate characters' names and italics to indicate actions of characters.)

FOOTNOTES

Footnotes are often used in informational texts to offer readers more in-depth information about a topic. Texts that use footnotes usually use numbers in **superscript**. Here is an example.

> *Dr. Benjamin F. Wells will be the special speaker at the graduation ceremony.[4]*

The example indicates that at the bottom of this page, readers can find additional information about this statement next to the number 4.

---

superscript. Small characters, usually numbers, set slightly above a line of text; used to refer readers to a footnote or endnote that provides additional information about a topic.

LEGENDS

Legends are a text feature invaluable to readers wanting to understand information included on a map. Legends often translate symbols included on a map to reduce clutter and make the map easier to read. For example, many maps indicate the population of towns and cities by assigning different styles of dots depending on the population range of a location.

The legend, usually placed somewhere on the edge of the map, indicates which style of dot is assigned to each population range. Large urban centers with populations greater than one million people might be marked with a large black star with a circle around it, whereas small towns might be marked with a very small black dot. Rather than having to guess what each symbol means, readers can look to the legend for help interpreting the map.

USING NAVIGATIONAL TOOLS IN MEDIA

A useful feature in online or computerized media are **search engines** or **query functions**. These tools allow you to enter a **term** or phrase and will provide you a list of instances in which that term or phrase occurs in the text. Often, these features also allow you to jump directly to where that term or phrase is located within the text.

---

search engine. A software tool used to locate information online or within a digital text.

query. query function. (1) A question. (2) A feature in digital texts that allows readers to search for key words and topics within a text.

search term. A word or words used to find information via a search engine.

Practice Problems

Read the passage and answer the following questions.

While reviewing the upcoming semester's course list, you see a course that grabs your attention, so you review it in the course catalog.

COURSE 623 — Historiography of Early England. (3 cr)

This course introduces how the history of England from 410–1066 CE has been theorized, discussed, and framed.

This course is offered in the History Faculty library. See the attached map for its location.

Prerequisites

Enrollment in the Medieval History, Medieval Studies, or Medieval Languages course

Preferred: Knowledge of Old English and/or Latin

Student Comments

"This course gave me a new perspective on the discipline of history and helped me to hone my own ideas and find my own voice as a historian."[1]

1. If you didn't know the meaning of the term "Historiography," which of the following text features could help you?

   A. Sidebar

   B. Glossary

   C. Table of contents

   D. Italics

2. Which of the following information is included in a sidebar?

   A. Campus map

   B. Prerequisites

   C. Course description

   D. Footnote

3. Which of the following pieces of relevant information for the course are not included in the text?

   A. The course prerequisites

   B. Where lessons are held

   C. The name of the course instructor

   D. How many credits are available for the course

4. Which of the following terms from the text would produce the best results when using a search engine on the online course catalog to discover this specific information?

   A. 1066 CE

   B. Course 623

   C. History

   D. Latin

5. Which of the following text features would help you navigate your way to the History Faculty library on the map?

   A. Italics

   B. Headings

   C. Index

   D. Legend

R.1.5 — Analyze, interpret, and apply information from charts, graphs, and other visuals

Informational texts such as textbooks, newspapers, and manuals often contain **graphic** features. Graphic and pictorial images allow readers to comprehend important verbal and written ideas quickly and easily. Most graphic **representations** include titles and subheadings that summarize complex information. Graphics can also assist readers in portraying the key parts that make up a whole. Graphics can also be used to solve problems and differentiate relevant from irrelevant information. Graphic representations include bar, pie, and flow **charts**; **graphs**; maps; pictographs; and illustrations. When you take the TEAS, you will likely be tested on your knowledge of these tools and your ability to analyze, interpret, and apply the information they provide.

LOCATING IMPORTANT AND RELEVANT INFORMATION IN A GRAPHIC TO SOLVE A PROBLEM

Graphic representations illustrate diverse topics and designs, but common features include titles (for example, "Nursing Positions" and "Degrees Required," as in the example below); subheadings ("Registered nurse (RN)," "ICU nurse," and so on); keys/legends, such as a box noting that a heart symbol indicates a nursing degree; and **scales** such as you might find on a map, indicating, for example, that 1 inch equals 100 miles. As you learn how to identify important and relevant graphic information, you will sharpen the skills needed to interpret the information.

> ### Objectives
>
> This objective includes, but is not limited to, the following examples of knowledge, skills, and abilities.
>
> - Locate important and/or relevant information from a graphic.
>
> - Interpret graphic representation of ideas (e.g., in maps, pictographs, bar graphs).
>
> - Identify evidence that is misleading or biased.
>
> - Use important and/or relevant information needed to solve a problem.
>
> - Distinguish between relevant and irrelevant ideas or arguments presented in a text.
>
> - Determine additional evidence needed to strengthen an argument or better meet the author's purpose.

graphic. A diagram, graph, illustration, or other piece of artwork.

representation. A portrayal, depiction, expression, presentation, substitution, sign, or symbol of something; an artistic image or likeness.

chart. A type of diagram that graphically represents data.

graph. A type of diagram that displays data mathematically.

scale. Ratio of distance expressed to actual measurement.

Look at the following table to identify the relevant degrees needed for each type of nursing position. As you can see, there are multiple pathways that lead to becoming a licensed nurse. However, suppose that you want to maximize your options. Which degree would provide you with the greatest number of nursing position options? If you answered a BSN, you are correct. This degree qualifies you for at least four different nursing positions.

Nursing Position	Degrees Required
Registered nurse (RN)	ADN or BSN
ICU nurse	BSN, preferred; CCRN certification
Home health nurse	Nursing diploma, ADN, or BSN
Nurse case manager	BSN or MSN
Clinical nurse specialist	MSN or PhD

INTERPRETING GRAPHIC REPRESENTATIONS OF IDEAS AND SOLVING PROBLEMS

Readers need to be adept at identifying the features and information in graphic representations, just as they need to be able to use that information to solve problems.

Look at the map of a college campus. Then, refer back to it for the remainder of the lesson.

When you read a map, you interpret graphic information. The map to the right includes the common elements of a map: title, legend, and scale. The title, "Nursing College Campus Map," communicates the subject of the map. The legend clarifies what each symbol, color, or shape represents. Lastly, the scale represents distance. In this example, every half inch of space equals 0.1 mile. The legend combined with the title tells the reader that the map illustrates the location of buildings on the nursing college campus. The features on the legend—buildings, walking paths—demonstrate the accessibility of each building via the walking paths.

Use the map to solve the problem of calculating the distance from the main office and faculty building to the women's dorm using the walking paths. (It is a little more than 0.2 mile.) Which information is not relevant in helping you solve this problem: the distance from the main office and faculty building to the biology lab or the distance from the biology lab to the cafeteria? (The distance from the biology lab to the cafeteria—walkers do not need to visit the cafeteria to get to the women's dorm from the main office and faculty building.)

College campus map

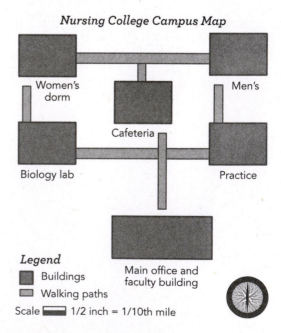

Practice

You are standing near a building on campus and want to solve the problem of orienting yourself. Based on the map compass, which of the following statements is accurate?

    A. The practice clinic is northeast of the main office and faculty building.

    B. The men's dorm is southwest of the cafeteria.

    C. The women's dorm is northeast of the cafeteria.

    D. The biology lab is northwest of the men's dorm.

Rationales

- Option A is correct because the main office and faculty building are at the south end of the map and the practice clinic is accessible by traveling in a northeastern direction.

- Option B is incorrect because the men's dorm is northeast of the cafeteria.

- Option C is incorrect because the women's dorm is northwest of the cafeteria.

- Option D is incorrect because the biology lab is southwest of the men's dorm.

Diagrams vary in their design depending on their purpose and content. Interpreting diagrams requires many of the same skills used in reading informational writing. For example, a diagram usually includes a combination of titles, subheads, summaries, descriptions, images representing ideas, content vocabulary, steps in a process, and other data. Sometimes, the information has already been analyzed for readers. More often, though, readers are required to interpret and analyze the diagram.

The illustration on the following page exhibits some features typically used in diagrams.

Practice

Based on your interpretation of the diagram of the right shoulder, which of the following views are included?

    A. The coracoclavicular ligament is seen in the anterior view of the shoulder.

    B. The thoracoacromial artery and vein are seen in the posterior view of the shoulder.

    C. The suprascapular nerve is seen in the anterior view of the shoulder.

    D. The coracohumeral ligament is seen in the disarticulated view of the shoulder.

Rationales

- Option C is correct because the illustration shows that the suprascapular nerve is labeled number 24 in the anterior view of the shoulder.

- Option A is incorrect because the illustration shows the coracoclavicular ligament is labeled numbers 3 and 9 in the posterior view of the shoulder.

- Option B is incorrect because the illustration shows the thoracoacromial artery and vein are labeled number 16 in the anterior view of the shoulder.

- Option D is incorrect because the illustration shows the coracohumeral ligament is labeled number 25 in the posterior view of the shoulder.

---

diagram. A symbolic representation used to convey information, especially a drawing that shows an arrangement or relationship among the parts of something.

Diagram Example: Right Shoulder

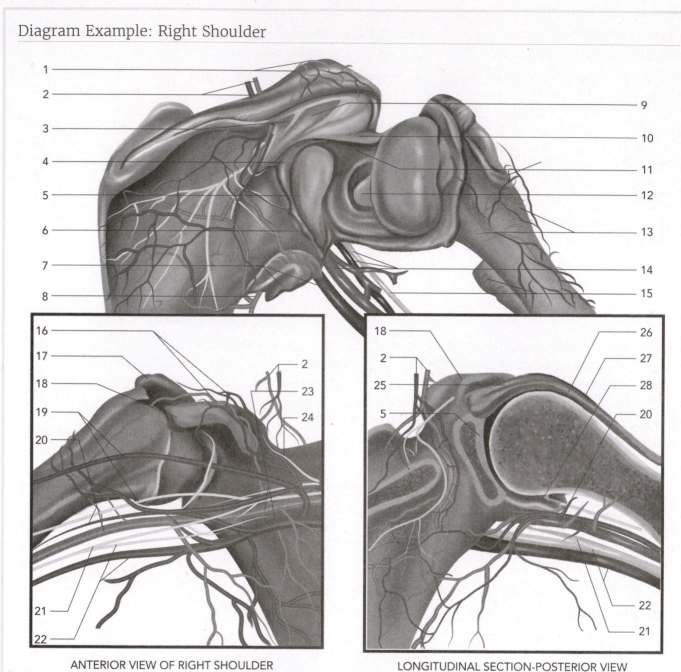

ANTERIOR VIEW OF RIGHT SHOULDER

LONGITUDINAL SECTION-POSTERIOR VIEW

1 Acromial branches of thoracoacromial artery and vein
2 Transverse scapular artery and vein
3 Coracoelavicular ligament (conoid portion)
4 Glenoidal lip: branch of supraseapular nerve
5 Glenoid cavity
6 Cut edge of articular capsule
7 Long head of triceps brachii: basilic vein
8 Scapular circumflex artery and vein

9 Coracoclavicular ligament (trapezoid portion)
10 Cut edge of coracohumeral ligament
11 Tendon of long head of biceps brachii: anterior humeral circumflex artery and vein
12 Tendon of subscapularis
13 Posteror humeral circumflex artery and vein: teres minor muscle
14 Acillary nerve: brachial artery and vein
15 Radial nerve: teres major muscle
16 Thoracoacromial artery and vein
17 Acromion

18 Coracoid process
19 Cephalic vein: musculocutaneous nerve
20 Brachial artery and vein
21 Median nerve
22 Ulnar nerve: basilic vein
23 Axillary artery and vein
24 Suprascapular nerve
25 Coracohumeral ligament
26 Tendon of long head of biceps brachii
27 Intertubercular mucous sheath
28 Articular capsule

IDENTIFYING BIASED OR MISLEADING INFORMATION IN GRAPHICS

Information provided in charts, graphs, and other graphics can be valuable in helping you understand, analyze, and evaluate new ideas. However, do not accept everything you read in a graphic as fact. Like text, graphics can contain **biased** or misleading information. For example, imagine that the "Occupational Outlook for Registered Nurses" infographic was instead titled "Occupational Outlook for Registered Nurses Average over the Next Nine Years." The word "average" implies a bias on the part of the composer. If a job is expected to grow 10% over a 10-year period, economists generally consider that growth good or healthy. The projected growth rate for registered nurses is 12%, which is slightly better than good. By introducing a word such as "average," the composer shows their bias against the profession. A composer can also introduce misleading information. Note that the infographic says that the 12% growth is "much faster than average." If 10% is the average expected growth, is 12% "much faster"? Probably not. To spot biased or misleading information, pay attention to word choice and design, and then question the composer's purpose in using certain words, designing a visual in a particular way, or including or excluding specific information.

USING GRAPHICS TO STRENGTHEN ARGUMENTS

Visual features such as bar graphs, pie charts, and line graphs can have a **persuasive** effect on an **audience**. Statistics, which appeal to the audience's sense of logic, sometimes can be more easily understood if presented graphically or spatially. Pictorial images and photos often evoke emotion or a sense of morality in an audience. All three appeals—logic, emotion, and morality—can be persuasive for an audience.

---

bias. Tendency toward or against a preconceived idea.
persuasive argument/persuasive writing. Argument in favor of a position intended to make the reader agree with an idea, thesis, or claim.
audience. The intended consumers of information.

Practice Problems

Use information from the infographic to answer the questions.

Occupational Outlook for Registered Nurses

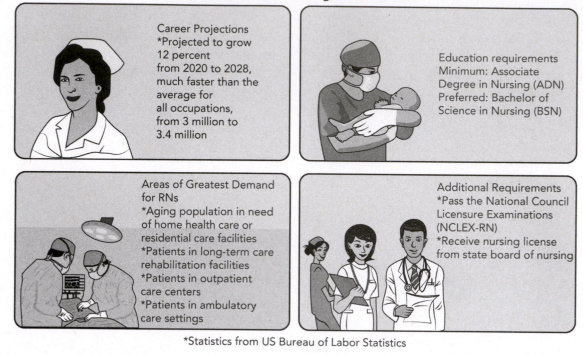

Career Projections
*Projected to grow 12 percent from 2020 to 2028, much faster than the average for all occupations, from 3 million to 3.4 million

Education requirements
Minimum: Associate Degree in Nursing (ADN)
Preferred: Bachelor of Science in Nursing (BSN)

Areas of Greatest Demand for RNs
*Aging population in need of home health care or residential care facilities
*Patients in long-term care rehabilitation facilities
*Patients in outpatient care centers
*Patients in ambulatory care settings

Additional Requirements
*Pass the National Council Licensure Examinations (NCLEX-RN)
*Receive nursing license from state board of nursing

*Statistics from US Bureau of Labor Statistics

1. In which of the following ways does the number range "3 million to 3.4 million" relate to the claim regarding 12% growth?

   A. It contradicts the claim regarding 12% growth.

   B. It states the growth in an alternate way for readers.

   C. It suggests that the growth may be 15%.

   D. It is repetitive and irrelevant information.

2. In the second panel, imagine that the words "Minimum" and "Preferred" were replaced with the words "Worst" and "Best." Which of the following describes this change?

   A. Helpful information

   B. Prejudice

   C. Factual information

   D. Bias

3. Which of the following patients will demand greater nursing care in residential care facilities?

   A. Youth population

   B. Patients requiring rehabilitation

   C. Aging population

   D. Patients requiring ambulatory care

4. Which of the following is the NCLEX?

   A. Nursing Committee Licensing Exam

   B. National Council Licensure Examination

   C. Nursing Coalition for Licensing Expertise

   D. National Corporation Licensure Excellence

5. Look at the images in the infographic. Which of the following information is misleading?

   A. Nurses must be young adults.

   B. Nurses work in a variety of settings.

   C. Nurses help with patient care.

   D. Nurses are required to keep records.

R.1.6 — Interpret events in a sequence

The term "sequence" refers to order and pattern. Recognizing a text's sequence is beneficial because it helps with remembering, understanding, and analyzing information in the text for better comprehension.

The adjective form, "sequential," refers to a fixed order in which there is a consistent, logical pattern. Pages in a book, for example, are sequential, as are steps in a process, because they occur in a set pattern, one after the other. The term "**chronological**" refers to time order, in which events are ordered by when they occur. In some stories, events are not always presented in chronological order, and the reader has to use cues to recognize flashbacks or flash-forwards and determine the overall chronology. For example, a movie might begin in the present day, then go backward in time to hundreds of years ago, and then return to the present day again.

IDENTIFYING AND EVALUATING THE WORDS OR PHRASES THAT INDICATE SEQUENCE OF EVENTS

Sequential order is signaled by words such as the following.

first	third	next	last
then	finally	while	before
second	now	when	after
at the beginning	prior to	afterward	subsequently

The following passage contains sequential order words in bold.

> Marcus, an RN at a children's hospital, offered to work a shift for a fellow nurse, Roberta. **First**, Marcus asked what hours Roberta needed him to cover. Then Marcus received approval from their nursing supervisor to cover the shift for Roberta. **Prior** to working that shift, Marcus learned about Roberta's patients. **Subsequently**, Marcus was able to effectively meet the needs of those patients.

Because of the use of sequence signal words, there is no question about the logical order of Marcus's preparations to cover Roberta's shift.

Objectives

This objective includes, but is not limited to, the following examples of knowledge, skills, and abilities.

- Identify and evaluate the words or phrases that indicate sequence of events (e.g., first, second, third).

- Identify the language in a text that creates cohesion between events in a sequence including transition words (e.g., today, finally) and verb tense (e.g., past or future tense).

- Draw conclusions based on a series of events presented in a text.

- Identify gaps in the sequence conveyed in a text.

- Order events chronologically (e.g., where the text uses flashback or flash-forward).

---

chronological. In order by time.

IDENTIFY LANGUAGE THAT CREATES COHESION IN ORDERING EVENTS

Chronological signal words, or *transition words*, help readers determine a sequence of events or the relationship between steps in a text that may or may not be written sequentially—that is, from first to last or when one step clearly follows right after another. Further, there are a variety of ways to describe time passing in texts or to indicate durations of time. Chronological signal words also describe such things as when an event occurs; when an event begins and ends; and when two events happen simultaneously, or at the same time. Readers must be aware of these terms, which function as adverbs. They refer to when something happens, how often an event occurs, or the length of time an event occurs.

The following is a list of adverbs that signal chronological events.

When	How Often	Length of Time
today	always	all month
tomorrow	frequently	all season
earlier	occasionally	all week
now	never	since
last month	seldom	two hours

Verb tense also gives the reader information about time and sequence. Past tense refers to events that have already happened or concluded, while present tense refers to events happening now. Past perfect tense refers to events that happened before those in the past tense, and future tense refers to those that have not yet happened. Writers sometimes use past tense or past perfect tense to indicate flash-backs, which are jumps backward in time that relate information about events relevant to a current situation or present time. Similarly, future tense or future perfect tense can indicate flash-forwards, which similarly jump forward in time.

The following is a passage with the chronological order words in bold and the verb tenses underlined.

> **Since the beginning** of your studies, you <u>have worked</u> toward the day you <u>will graduate</u>. **Every day,** you studied diligently, and you **frequently** <u>sought</u> help from your teachers when needed. You **always** <u>attended</u> class and **never** <u>missed</u> a test. **Now,** you <u>will be rewarded</u> with a graduation ceremony. **Today,** you can <u>celebrate</u> your achievement!

Chronological signal words are essential for assisting readers in keeping track of when the events they read about in narratives and informational texts occur. In the preceding passage, the chronological signal words and verb tenses help the reader put all the events in sequential order in their mind to create meaning.

---

transition words. Words that link ideas in a text; used to help readers discern steps in a procedure or a chronology of events, such as when things happen and for how long.

DRAWING CONCLUSIONS BASED ON A SERIES OF EVENTS

Texts that include a series of events often lead the reader to a logical conclusion. When reading a sequential text, consider the topic and the purpose of the text. A perceptive reader can draw a conclusion about a text based on the events described.

The example that follows leads the reader to a logical conclusion.

To set up your new tablet, first press the power button, then wait for the device to power on. When prompted, enter a name for your profile. Next, select a theme. Finally, you can follow the tutorial guide, or you can skip this step by closing the window. Enjoy your new tablet!

The reader can conclude that the completion of these steps means the tablet is ready to use and that following the tutorial is not required in order for the tablet to function properly, but the other steps are required.

IDENTIFYING GAPS IN A SEQUENCE

Not all texts are perfect. Occasionally, information can be left out of a sequence of events. You can identify gaps in a sequence relayed within a text if the logical order is interrupted or does not make sense, or if signal words are used but do not follow a logical pattern (e.g., if the words "first" and "third" are used, but "second" is not). When you encounter gaps in a sequence of events in a text, you may be able to infer the missing information. However, if this inference is not possible, you may need to seek help in interpreting the text.

Practice Problems

Read the following passage. Then answer the questions.

Prior to graduating from high school, Tim knew he wanted to become a nurse practitioner. In fact, he often imagined himself working as a nurse practitioner one day like the health care professional who cared for him and his family. Tim then talked to his nurse practitioner to determine the path he needed to take to fulfill his career goal. He learned that he must first choose one of three ways to become a registered nurse: a nursing diploma program, an associate degree in nursing (ADN), or a Bachelor of Science in Nursing (BSN). Tim also learned that nursing students often begin with the diploma or ADN. They can then later participate in an RN-to-BSN program, known as a bridge program, while they gain experience working as nurses. This seemed to be a good plan, because he could start his career sooner. Finally, Tim learned that he would subsequently need to earn his Master of Science in Nursing (MSN) degree in order to become a nurse practitioner.

1. Which of the following words or phrases from the passage indicate sequential order?

   A. One day

   B. Prior to

   C. Later

   D. Often

2. Which of the following words or phrases from the passage are chronological signal words that do not indicate sequence?

   A. One day

   B. Subsequently

   C. Prior to

   D. Then

3. Which of the following phrases appears to be out of sequence?

   A. Tim then talked to his nurse practitioner

   B. he must first choose one of three ways

   C. he could start his career sooner

   D. later participate in an RN-to-BSN program

4. Place the following degrees in the correct sequence needed to become a nurse practitioner.
   MSN, ADN, BSN

5. Which of the following conclusions can the reader draw based on this passage?

   A. Tim will earn a BSN after he graduates from high school.

   B. Tim will pursue a bridge program.

   C. Tim will continue to research paths to becoming a nurse.

   D. Tim will forgo earning an MSN in order to start his career sooner.

Craft and Structure

R.2.1 — Distinguish between fact and opinion to identify misconceptions and biases

One of the challenges readers face is determining what information they can trust in a text. Texts are written by human beings, and all human beings have **opinions** and biases. Similarly, all writers are capable of misleading readers, whether unintentionally, through errors or faulty reasoning, or intentionally, in order to deceive. It is important for readers to equip themselves to understand the **point of view** of a text's author, distinguish fact from opinion, and be aware of a writer's misconceptions and biases. In this TEAS task, you will learn to hone these skills.

RECOGNIZING FACTUAL WRITING SUPPORTED BY EVIDENCE

When information is presented as factual in a text, the reader must check that the author has provided support or citations for those facts. Quality factual evidence, clearly deployed, is essential whenever a writer is making an argument. The evidence must be credible and appropriate to the topic. Evidence can be found in reliable sources and incorporated in a number of ways.

If evidence is presented as factual but no citation is presented to support the evidence, or if the evidence does not adequately or appropriately support the claims, it cannot be accepted as factual.

Review the following table to consider the types of sources that authors can use to support their ideas. This table also provides methods that can be incorporated as evidence in your writing.

Types of Sources	Examples in Texts
Print and electronic sources	Quotations, *paraphrases*, summaries
Observation	Descriptions
Interviews	Quotations, paraphrases, summaries
Surveys	Statistics and data
Experiments	Charts and graphs
Personal experience	Descriptions, photographs, illustrations

Objectives

This objective includes, but is not limited to, the following examples of knowledge, skills, and abilities.

- Identify factual writing supported by evidence.

- Identify an author's point of view in a text.

- Identify an author's tone and explain how it causes a text to be more biased or less.

- Identify biases in a text (e.g., stereotypes, ethnocentric references).

- Distinguish between fact and opinion.

---

opinion. Statement that cannot be proven; an author's beliefs, as opposed to facts or reasoning, presented in a text.

point of view. The narrative voice an author uses to tell a story or relate information; can be first person, second person, or third person.

paraphrase. To explain an idea in one's own words.

When reading a text, the reader should make sure to identify the evidence the author uses to support their argument. The reader should also be prepared to check the evidence for credibility and appropriateness. In most cases, readers can check evidence by confirming the citations or looking up the studies, statistics, and facts that authors present as evidence.

IDENTIFYING AN AUTHOR'S POINT OF VIEW AND VIEWPOINT

The term "point of view" refers to the author's narrative voice—first person, second person, or third person. The term "*viewpoint*" refers to an author's opinions or beliefs about a topic. To identify point of view, determine whether the author is a participant in the text. If so, the author will use first-person pronouns such as "I," "me," or "we." If not, the author will use third-person pronouns such as "he," "she," or "they." An author can also speak directly to readers, as in a procedural text, and use the second-person pronoun "you." Once an author determines their point of view, they approach the task of writing with their own set of life experiences, beliefs, expertise, and ideas that inform their viewpoint. It is impossible to encounter a text that is not in some way influenced by the viewpoint of the author(s). This reality does not mean that you cannot trust any text. An effective reader learns to identify and understand an author's viewpoint based on diction and text details.

There are several ways to identify an author's viewpoint. First, locate the topic of a text. Next, determine what ideas and evidence the writer presents about the topic. Last, consider the ideas and evidence to determine the writer's opinion. As you read, you should ask questions such as: Who is the author? What argument are they presenting? What evidence do they favor? What is their reasoning as they connect evidence to claims to make an argument? Does the author deliberately reveal their own preferences and ideas? What are the *connotations* of the author's word choices? All of these questions and more can be used to identify the author's viewpoint.

TONE AND BIAS

The *tone* of an author's writing is similar to the tone of voice a person can use when speaking. The term "tone" refers to the writer's attitude toward a topic or general feeling about a topic. If viewpoint is an opinion, then tone is the way the writer speaks about that opinion. The tone of a text is usually described by an emotive word, such as "joyful," "ominous," or "detached." To determine tone, take into consideration the context, the event or circumstance, and the audience for the text you are reading. Then, read the text carefully, looking for terms that have to do with emotions. Watch for punctuation, such as exclamation points and question marks, that expresses emotion. Determine how a writer feels about a topic by examining whether their ideas are serious, sarcastic, or show another emotion. These steps will lead you to the tone of a text.

Tone can also help you to identify an author's biases. "Bias" is the term used to explain how an author leans more toward one argument, position, or affiliation than another. Fans of a sports team tend to show bias toward that sports team and its success. This bias can lead them to believe that their team is more worthy of success than their rivals, although such a belief can have no basis in fact.

Tone is an effective guide for detecting bias, because the reader can identify which subjects, concepts, or types of evidence an author takes more seriously than others. An author who routinely makes jokes or sarcastic comments in a text concerning a particular scientist whose work they consider ridiculous

---

viewpoint. An author's beliefs or opinions about a topic.

connotation. An implied meaning of a word or idea created by the emotions and assumptions attached to it.

tone. The author's implied or explicit attitude toward a topic.

reveals their bias against that scientist and their work. On the other hand, a writer who rigorously maintains a serious tone, free of emotive language, when discussing a heated debate between rival scholars signals to the reader that they are trying to present all the arguments fairly.

DETECTING BIAS

Determining the tone of a text is only one way to identify biases and **stereotypes**. Stereotypes reveal themselves through stock characters or general, superficial ideas that stand in for real people and things. Stereotypes drop people, ideas, and events into simplified categories. They are sometimes useful when an author wants to discuss a topic briskly or to illustrate an example. However, in general, stereotypes can be misleading if the reader is not aware they are being used. A bad stereotype disguises a complex reality with a simple categorization. It is important to recognize stereotypes and bias in what you read. Stereotypes and bias can present opinions as facts, as shown in the following table.

	Stereotype	Bias
Definition	A generalized belief that characterizes each person of a group in the same category	An unfair or close-minded opinion for or against an idea, person, group of people, or a belief
Example	All tall people are good at basketball.	Rigorous, sustained cardiovascular exercise is the only way to improve health.
Characteristic	The writer makes general statements about groups of people or uses evidence from unreliable sources about groups.	The writer uses emotionally charged words to describe a topic or purposefully omits facts that contradict ideas about an issue.

How can readers detect stereotypes and bias about the topic of a text? One way is to read multiple texts about a topic. Reading widely about a topic allows the reader to compare how ideas are presented and to evaluate the available evidence for ideas. Another way to avoid stereotypes is to imagine an author's side and the opposing side in a debate. This exercise allows the reader to understand a topic from multiple viewpoints. Yet another important technique for identifying stereotypes and biases and countering their effects is to seek out texts written by people with the identity or experience that is under discussion. Authors can never be truly objective about their own experiences, but the subjective experience of a person or group commonly stereotyped by outsiders is always a useful corrective to negative or oversimplified portrayals of stereotyped people, groups, identities, and ideas.

Review the preceding table again for ways you can recognize stereotypes and bias, and think about how identifying biases and stereotypes can help you read critically.

DISTINGUISHING BETWEEN FACT AND OPINION

Another aspect of reading critically is to determine whether a statement is a fact or opinion. To identify a fact, a reader must first evaluate whether a statement can be proven true. Next, the reader must decide whether the evidence that supports the statement is credible and reliable. If a statement is supported by multiple reliable sources and evidence, it can be considered a fact. If a statement describes an author's beliefs and is an idea that other people might disagree about, it is an opinion. Opinions can be used to mislead or persuade a reader.

---

stereotype. Simplified categorization of an idea or person based on superficial ideas that stand in for real people and things.

Consider the following examples of a fact and an opinion about nursing degrees.

Fact	Opinion
According to Rasmussen University, nurses with associate degrees earn around $67,000 a year, whereas those with master's degrees earn more than $90,000 a year.	The best way to increase your earning potential as a nurse is to earn an advanced degree.

The first statement is a fact that can be checked through **research**. This university's data about average nursing salaries can be studied and validated. In addition, universities are usually considered reliable sources, and whether a university is trustworthy can be verified by looking up the university to check its reliability and consistency. Conversely, the second example is an opinion. The writer's belief is that an advanced degree is the best way to increase earning potential. Although earning an advanced degree can increase earning potential, other people can disagree about whether this is the best way to do so. When a writer claims that an idea is the best or worst of several options, it is likely that the statement is an opinion. To compare and contrast facts and opinions about a topic, read multiple texts about that topic. The more texts you read on a given topic, the easier it will be to identify agreed–upon facts and distinguish them from the opinions of individual authors.

Practice Problems

Read the following passage. Then answer the questions that follow.

There are many reasons to consider making physical education (PE) mandatory in schools. According to the National Institutes of Health, regular physical activity improves cardiovascular health and promotes a healthier lifestyle. It can also help students build strength, can reduce the risk of certain illnesses, and can even improve mental health. Some studies suggest that students who participate in daily PE improve their grades. PE in school can also help students reach the daily recommended 60 min of physical activity. It is likely that many students will not achieve the goal of 60 min of exercise outside of school because they spend so much time on electronic devices. Sedentary students need to participate in team sports. Requiring exercise also rewards students who are naturally athletic, so this is another consideration for mandatory PE.

1. Which of the following are facts that supports the author's claim that PE should be mandatory in schools? (Select all that apply.)

   A. Students spend too much time on electronic devices.

   B. Regular physical activity improves cardiovascular health.

   C. Sedentary students need to participate in team sports.

   D. It rewards athletic students.

   E. Studies suggest that PE can improve student grades.

2. Which of the following statements indicates a stereotype?

   A. Students who spend time on electronic devices are not physically active.

   B. Physical activity helps students develop stronger bodies and reduces illnesses.

   C. Students should learn to participate in team sports.

   D. Physical activity helps promote better mental health among students.

3. The passage illustrates a third-person point of view. Which of the following describes the author's viewpoint regarding PE?

   A. PE rewards students who are naturally athletic.

   B. PE does little for students who spend time on electronic devices.

   C. PE requires participation in team sports.

   D. PE should be mandatory in schools.

4. Which of the following describes the tone of this passage?

   A. Pessimistic

   B. Optimistic

   C. Informative

   D. Irritated

5. In three to five sentences, describe how this passage uses facts and opinions. Then, discuss whether you are persuaded by the argument.

research based. Reliant on ideas backed by study.

R.2.2 — Interpret the meaning of words and phrases using context

Perhaps you have heard the phrase "context is everything." This phrase means that the circumstances surrounding an event often shape it. Context also affects the meaning of words and phrases. The context in which a word is used affects the meaning of the word and how the word is understood. Context can refer to surrounding words, sentences, or ideas within a sentence or passage. Context can also refer to the writer's tone or attitude toward a topic. For this TEAS task, you will be asked to interpret the meanings of words and phrases using the context of sentences and passages, including distinguishing between denotative and connotative meanings of words and between literal and **figurative language**.

USING CONTEXT CLUES

When confronted with unknown terms, use **root** or base words and affixes to determine word meanings. Consider the word "fracture." The root is fract and the suffix is –ure. In this instance, fract means "to break" and the suffix –ure means "the act or process of." So, the meaning of "fracture" is "the act or process of breaking."

> ### Objectives
>
> This objective includes, but is not limited to, the following examples of knowledge, skills, and abilities.
>
> - Infer the correct definition of a word or phrase using context clues.
>
> - Recognize the cumulative effect of word choice on meaning or mood.
>
> - Distinguish between the denotative and connotative meaning of words or phrases based on context clues provided.
>
> - Distinguish between literal and figurative language using context clues.

Another way to determine the meaning of a word or phrase is to evaluate the surrounding text for clues. For example, synonyms, words with identical or similar meanings, can provide clues about the intended meaning. Take the word "reservation," which has different meanings. The sentence below demonstrates how a synonym can provide the meaning of a word.

> *Reece was uncertain about what to do next, but Gloria knew his reservations were unfounded.*

The word "uncertain" provides a clue that this instance of "reservations" refers to feelings of doubt.

Sometimes the context of a sentence provides the definition of a word. Consider this sentence:

> *Becoming a CPA, or a certified public accountant, requires passing a series of exams.*

In this example, the definition of "CPA" is provided following the term.

Another strategy for using context clues is looking at words in a series. The meaning of each word should fit with the meanings of the other words in the group. Consider the meaning of the word "coach" in the series "the coach, athletes, and trainers." Does the word "coach" mean a horse-drawn carriage, or a person working with a team? The words "athletes" and "trainers" make it clear that here, a coach is a person involved in sports. Analyzing the context of a word in a series will help you determine word meaning.

---

figurative language. Language meant to create imagery, comparison, or an association for the reader; usually a metaphor, a simile, or personification.
root word. A word element, or morpheme, from which other words are built.

Another type of context clue is the use of an example or illustration. Consider the following sentence:

> The neonatal intensive care unit (NICU), where medical professionals care for premature or critically ill infants, requires staff with special certifications.

Here, the reader understands that the NICU is an area of a hospital specifically designated for the care of infants.

Signal phrases in a sentence can also help illuminate word meanings. Notice the introductory phrase in the following sentence:

> Unlike many other careers, cartographers are required to understand both geography and design.

In this example, the introductory phrase provides a clue about the meaning of the word "cartographer." A cartographer engages in a career that involves both geography and design.

You can also find context clues to word meanings by using logical inferences about the cause and effect of events in a sentence. The following sentence describes a cause and effect that can help you determine the meaning of the word "solution."

> Miguel studied the mechanical failure and came up with a brilliant solution to work around it.

In this sentence, the cause of events is that "Miguel studied the mechanical failure." What effect did this have? The effect is a "solution." You can infer that in this instance, a "solution" refers to a way of solving a problem.

Finally, the general ideas of a passage can provide clues to the meaning of a word. If you know, for instance, that the setting of a story is a spaceship, then you can determine that a reference to a "hatch" probably refers not to the verb that means "to emerge from an egg" but rather to the noun that means "a small door."

THE EFFECT OF WORD CHOICE

Comprehension of a text can depend on a reader's ability to infer the meaning of a word by reading between the lines. In addition to assisting comprehension, authors can influence the emotional effect of a text on the reader. A word's denotative meaning is the meaning that appears in a dictionary, while its connotative meaning includes the emotions and assumptions attached to it. A reader's experiences will determine the positive and negative connotations of a word. Ultimately, the tone (the author's feelings toward the subject) affects the **mood** (the reader's feelings elicited from the text).

For example, each of the following words is similar, yet experience and use result in diverse meanings.

Word	Definition	Connotation
old	advanced in age	feeble, needing care
mature	fully developed	experienced, competent

Here, the denotative meanings of the words are the same, but the connotative meanings are different.

---

mood. How the elements in a text, such as word choice, affect the reader.

FIGURATIVE LANGUAGE

Many authors employ creative ways to state ideas and make unfamiliar settings and objects more accessible to the reader. They often use figurative language meant to create imagery, a comparison, or an association for the reader. Unlike literal language, which is straightforward and means what it says on the most basic level, figurative language goes beyond the ordinary meanings of words. Figurative language is often metaphorical, allegorical, or symbolic. If a reader becomes aware of common figurative devices, then the text will be more manageable and comprehensible.

Figurative Device	Definition	Example
Metaphor	Comparison between unlike things without using "like" or "as"	Shanaya's phone was a dinosaur.
Simile	Comparison between unlike things using "like" or "as"	The hurdler cleared the barriers as gracefully as a gazelle.
Personification	Giving human attributes to something nonhuman	The gurney groaned under the weight of the injured wrestler.

Practice Problems

Read the passage below then answer the following question.

While the other windows shone with candlelight, the opaque window was completely dark.

1. Which of the following defines the word "opaque" as it is used in the sentence?

   A. Not transparent

   B. Warmly glowing

   C. Partially broken

   D. Mostly visible

Read the passage below then answer the following question.

Uncle Anton placed the sandpaper, saw, plane, and T square in his shop.

2. Which of the following defines the word "plane" as it is used in the sentence?

   A. Model aircraft

   B. Imaginary flat surface

   C. Tool for working wood

   D. Clearly visible

Read the passage below then answer the following question.

The cunning dog hid his stolen treat in the backyard so the other dogs could not find it.

3. Which of the following has a similar connotation to the word "cunning"?

   A. Villainous

   B. Mischievous

   C. Brilliant

   D. Guileless

Read the passage below then answer the following question.

The hazy fog slithered between the gravestones, creating eerie shapes that crept along the grass.

4. Which of the following describes the mood created by the word choices in the sentence?

   A. Happy

   B. Disappointed

   C. Excited

   D. Fearful

Read the passage below then answer the following question

The overland trip required passing through the rugged Brazilian wilderness, which proved to be a formidable opponent.

5. Which of the following figurative devices is used in the sentence?

   A. Personification

   B. Connotation

   C. Denotation

   D. Simile

R.2.3 — Evaluate the author's purpose in a given text

Part of being an astute reader is determining the purpose of a text. Determining an author's purpose, or the reason a particular piece of text was written, can help you focus on the most important details of a text. This skill is especially important if a text is lengthy or complex. As you read, ask yourself whether the author is trying to persuade, inform, or entertain you. It is important to remember that a text can have more than one purpose. In preparing for this TEAS task, practice determining the author's purpose for all texts you encounter.

DETERMINING AND DRAWING INFERENCES ABOUT THE AUTHOR'S PURPOSE

Knowing a writer's purpose (also called "**authorial intent**") is an important component of comprehension. Authors write for one of five main purposes.

- To inform
- To persuade
- To entertain
- To describe
- To explain

When trying to determine authorial intent, it is helpful to ask yourself a series of questions as you read. Some especially helpful questions include the following.

- Where does the text appear?
- What is the structure of the text?
- What is the author's tone?
- Who is the intended audience of the text?
- What does the author want the audience to do in response to the text?

authorial intent. The reason an author creates a text; also called the author's purpose.

In most texts, the author will not state their intent outright. Readers can infer an author's intent based on what is included or not included in the text.

Informative Writing
Includes facts
Utilizes text features
Does not give opinions

Persuasive Writing
Argues in favor of a position
Includes facts and opinions
Can include a call to action
Can use emotional, logical, and ethical language

Entertaining Writing
Includes fiction or *anecdotes*
Can use action, drama, and/or humor
Includes the elements of storytelling: plot, conflict, setting, characterization, and *theme*

Descriptive Writing
Uses sensory details to create vivid mental pictures for readers
Tells about people, places, things, and events of all kinds

Expository Writing
Explains how to do something
Utilizes text features, particularly numbered steps

anecdote. A short story that illustrates a concept or point and creates a connection between the author and reader.
theme. A broad concept or universal concern that an author addresses through a given medium.

DISTINGUISHING BETWEEN FACT AND OPINION

Part of determining an author's purpose is analyzing the text for facts and opinions. What differentiates these types of information?

Facts are information that can be objectively confirmed through a reputable source. Examples of facts include the following.

- The United States was founded in 1776.

- Apples are a type of fruit.

- Some fabrics are made of natural materials, while others are synthetic.

Opinions, on the other hand, are the author's beliefs. For example, the following are opinions.

- The U.S. is the best nation in the world.

- Apples are an essential part of a balanced diet.

- Natural fabrics are the right choice for consumers who care about the earth.

These statements cannot be objectively verified—people other than the author can think differently about these topics.

RECOGNIZING THE AUTHOR'S TONE

Sometimes, determining an author's purpose involves examining the specific words used in a text to identify the author's tone, or attitude toward the subject. Authors who intend to simply inform readers tend to use a straightforward tone with neutral language that lacks emotional correlation (words that can be defined as exclusively positive or exclusively negative). On the other hand, authors who intend to persuade readers might use an emotionally charged tone created by specific word choices and imagery meant to evoke a specific emotional response in readers.

For example, an advertisement for a premium photo-printing service might ask potential customers, "How much are your memories worth?" These words, placed beneath an image of a grandparent smiling over a newborn child, might suggest that readers should not trust a lower-priced service to print their photos but instead should use the advertiser's services. Paying attention to an author's words can help you determine the intended message.

IDENTIFYING EVIDENCE THAT SUPPORTS THE AUTHOR'S PURPOSE

To understand an author's purpose for writing a text, a reader can search the text for the evidence that supports the purpose. An author's tone and opinions are revealing evidence when it comes to figuring out their purpose. It is also important to consider the facts the author chooses to support their ideas. The author's selection of facts implies the underlying idea that they are building. It is vital to question an author's motivation by considering contradictory facts they may have ignored.

For example, a persuasive text can begin with an emotional appeal, then follow with several opinions supported by reasoning and facts. These opinions, reasons, and facts form the evidence that supports the author's purpose. In contrast, the type of evidence that supports the purpose of entertaining readers might be a humorous tone that narrates a series of events in chronological order.

Practice Problems

Read the following passage. Then answer the questions that follow.

A local hospital published the following announcement for mandatory nurse in-service training.

To: All Nursing Staff

From: Dr. Lynette Smith, MSN, Head of Professional Development

Re: Mandatory In-Service Training

Topic: Transitional Care

All staff is required to attend in-service training regarding transitional care. This involves effective procedures for moving patients from inpatient care to a new facility and discharging patients to go home.

In this training, you will learn in greater detail how to fulfill these five standards encompassed within transitions of care:

(1) Identifying at-risk patients who may transition poorly.

(2) Conducting a thorough assessment for transition of those patients identified as at risk.

(3) Compiling a complete and accurate medication list for each patient.

(4) Developing a care management plan that is dynamic and ongoing.

(5) Transferring all transitions of care information to the appropriate new caregivers or care providers.

1. Which of the following is the author's primary purpose for writing this announcement?

   A. To provide a way for nursing staff to sign up for training

   B. To inform nursing staff about an in-service training

   C. To convince nursing staff to memorize the five standards

   D. To inform nursing staff they can miss a shift to attend training

2. Which of the following is the secondary purpose of this announcement?

   A. To persuade readers to become nurses

   B. To entertain readers with patient anecdotes

   C. To describe a hospital setting

   D. To explain the standards of transitional care

3. Which of the following describes the tone of this announcement?

   A. Sincere

   B. Relaxed

   C. Professional

   D. Urgent

4. Which of the following statements express a fact? (Select all that apply.)

   A. Nurses are required to attend mandatory in-service training on how to manage transitions of care.

   B. Nurses who are dedicated will master the five basic standards involved in transitions of care.

   C. The training includes procedures for discharging patients to home.

   D. Nurses who take time off to attend the transitional care training are committed to their profession.

   E. Nurses are most likely to succeed when they create a transitional care management plan.

5. Which of the following evidence in the announcement supports the author's purpose for writing it?

   A. To: All Nursing Staff

   B. Topic: Transitional Care

   C. All staff is required to attend in-service training regarding transitional care.

   D. Developing a care management plan that is dynamic and ongoing.

R.2.4 — Evaluate the author's point of view or perspective in a given text

Authors choose from several points of view to present varying *perspectives* in the texts they write. Differing narrative points of view relay different perspectives, opinions, experiences, and ideas that an author may wish to convey regarding a subject. Developing the ability to identify and distinguish among points of view and perspectives will empower you to evaluate the credibility, relevancy, and accuracy of information in a text.

For this TEAS task, you will need to recognize and evaluate how points of view are used in texts; identify the perspectives that authors offer on their subjects; evaluate the credibility of authors, the *publications* for which they write, and the organizations to which they belong; and evaluate the relevance and accuracy of the information that authors present.

IDENTIFYING POINT OF VIEW

"Point of view" refers to the voice used to narrate a story or relate information.

When a text is written in the first-person point of view, the narrator is involved in events. A hallmark of first-person narration is the use of first-person pronouns such as "I," "me," and "myself." In addition, a first-person narrator cannot report on the thoughts or feelings of other characters. A second-person narrator tells about events and details using the word "you," as if describing things that are happening in the reader's life rather than the author's or characters' lives. The second-person point of view often appears in how-to or procedural texts. A third-person narrator is an outside observer, unconnected to the action or information. Third-person narration uses pronouns such as "he," "she," "they," and "it" to create this effect. An omniscient third-person point of view explores multiple characters' thoughts and feelings within the same text. The third person can be thought of as a camera in the author's control, zooming in and out on particular details and following the action as if the reader is an invisible observer along for the ride. A limited third-person narrator chooses to focus on the thoughts and feelings of one or two characters.

Different points of view are used for varying purposes. Third-person narration is often used when the author wants to relay information in a way that seems objective or unconnected to the author's own feelings. A third-person omniscient (all-knowing) narrator describes events in a story as if the narrator knows all the characters' thoughts and feelings at once. Third person is also a common point of view that readers come across in informational texts and news reporting in which the reporter tries not to insert their own experiences into a story. The first-person point of view is used when the narrator's or author's own thoughts and feelings are crucial to the writing. These might be the author's own beliefs, expressed in an opinion article, or an eyewitness account of a noteworthy event. Texts such as diaries or memoirs are also usually written in the first-person point of view.

The second person is the rarest point of view to encounter because it is unusual for either fictional or nonfictional texts to address the reader directly. Because the second-person point of view addresses the reader as "you," it is sometimes encountered in instructional texts.

Objectives

This objective includes, but is not limited to, the following examples of knowledge, skills, and abilities.

- Identify different perspectives presented in text.
- Evaluate the credibility of the text source (e.g., author, publication, organization).
- Evaluate the relevancy and accuracy of information.
- Determine the author's point of view or perspective.

perspective. The narrator's or author's particular thoughts, feelings, or perceptions about people, ideas, or events in a story or text.
publication. The printing, publishing, and/or distribution of a text; a published work.

IDENTIFYING PERSPECTIVES IN A TEXT

"Perspective" refers to the narrator's particular thoughts, feelings, or perceptions about people, ideas, or events.

When reading a text, there is always at least one perspective. The perspective can be that of the author, or it can be a perspective the author has adopted or assigned to a narrator in a particular text. In some texts, especially fiction, it is common to find multiple perspectives featured in a text. If a story is written from the points of view of several different characters, each of those characters has their own perspective.

Perspective impacts the text in particular ways. Each perspective has its own personality, biases, and interpretations of events. An author might favor certain types of evidence over others, and they might be more familiar with some sources than others. Characters also have their own perspectives. The selfish, wicked king will have a different perspective on the needs of his kingdom from that of the peasant leader who seeks to overthrow him. Different authors, characters, and narrators have different perspectives, even when they are describing the same information.

To identify different perspectives, read carefully to understand what perspective each character or author offers about a given subject or event. Pay attention to the connotations of word choice and to what information is included or excluded.

When reading informational texts, especially for research, a helpful way to identify the perspective of a particular author is to read multiple texts on the same subject and compare and contrast them. Even if the subject matter is the same, the authors' perspectives will differ.

EVALUATING A SOURCE

When reading, it is vital to determine if the source of the information presented is credible. Credible information is reasonable and verifiable. To evaluate a text's reliability, an important first step is to evaluate the source of the text, making sure the information comes from reputable online or print dictionaries, encyclopedias, official government reports, periodicals, or university websites that share their research. Authors who write multiple texts develop a reputation that you can check. The same is true for the publishers or publications for which authors write and the organizations they support.

For example, when researching the benefits of following a particular diet, such as the keto diet, you might stumble onto a **blog** that appears to be a source of useful, factual, and scientific information. However, when you click on the "About" tab at the top of the page and read about the blog's author, you discover that the author is the founder of a company that sells products and memberships related to the keto diet and lifestyle. Therefore, the author's purpose is more likely to grow their business and entice the general public to follow the keto diet and participate in the keto lifestyle community than to provide a truly objective summary of the advantages and disadvantages of the diet. This assessment does not mean that the information included in the blog is necessarily untrue; much of it might be factual. However, you should be aware of the writer's purpose and seek out other sources of information to ensure that you have the most accurate information possible.

It is also worth bearing in mind that even publications with good reputations sometimes publish texts that are unreliable, biased, poorly researched, or otherwise problematic. It is up to the reader to do their own research and read critically.

---

blog. A website that is usually informal and independently run.

EVALUATING RELEVANCY AND ACCURACY

While a text can be full of information, not all of this information will necessarily be accurate or relevant to the issue being discussed. One of the reader's jobs is to evaluate the relevance and accuracy of any information provided in a text. Information is relevant if it deals appropriately with the issue being discussed. It is accurate if it is truthful or, at least, well supported by evidence.

Political speeches illustrate this point well. In a political debate, the participants' aim is not necessarily to answer questions posed to them objectively, but rather to provide answers that reinforce the themes and priorities of their campaigns. It is the job of the audience to evaluate the information that candidates provide in their answers for relevance and accuracy. Relevance can be determined by asking whether the information provided actually addresses the question posed. Accuracy can be determined by comparing and contrasting the information to other sources, conducting independent research, or consulting knowledge that one already has.

Such evaluations are a helpful tool for uncovering the perspective of a particular author. Authors reveal their perspectives through their word choice and their use of evidence, arguments, and reasoning. Likewise, knowing an author's perspective beforehand can help readers determine whether the information they provide is relevant or accurate.

Practice Problems

Read the following passage. Then answer the questions that follow.

A nurse educator at a long-term care facility is preparing a lesson on preventing falls. She wants to include information, examples, and hands-on exercises addressing why falls happen and how to prevent them. She is considering the following three sources of information.

(1) A website features articles and videos from a medical facility. Renowned professionals provide insight on numerous topics. Their credentials and bios are included.

(2) A website sponsored by a nurse-staffing organization provides qualified nurses for travel assignments. The site includes stories from nurses. It also includes lists of services provided, qualifications for nursing staff, and related resources.

(3) A blog by a popular nurse influencer has a substantial following. They share stories about their experiences in the nursing profession. They also write promotional posts for various advertisers of products and services relevant to nursing.

1. Which of the following sources should the nurse educator use to gather reliable research?

    A. Blog by a nurse influencer

    B. Website by a nurse staffing organization

    C. Website from a medical facility

    D. Advertisements for nursing products

2. Which of the following features would support the reliability of a source?

    A. Links to newspaper articles that give information and details

    B. Links to special promotions for regular customers

    C. Links to customer testimonials

    D. Links to a site where an author's books can be purchased

3. Which of the following is a reason the credentials of an author are important to know when evaluating a source?

    A. To understand the author's personal experience

    B. To evaluate the author's expertise

    C. To support an opinion about the author

    D. To understand the author's personal beliefs

4. Which of the following is a reason to evaluate the credibility of sources on fall prevention?

    A. To use only hospital-approved information as a reference

    B. To locate an alternate perspective

    C. To understand a nurse's point of view

    D. To verify the accuracy of the information

5. Read a blog online, and identify the point of view that the blogger uses in their writing and the blogger's perspective on the subject matter. Decide whether the blogger uses credible sources of information to support the topic or argument. Identify at least two reasons why the blog is or is not credible.

Integration of Knowledge and Ideas

R.3.1 — Use evidence from the text to make predictions, inferences, and draw conclusions

Often, writers leave out certain details about a story or topic, and it is up to readers to use evidence from a text to understand the author's intended meaning. Readers draw conclusions and make reasonable interpretations, inferences, and **predictions** based on details they find in a text. Being able to cite specific evidence explaining how you came to a conclusion will help you gain credibility as a reader and can be a benefit to others wanting to better understand a writer's work. For this TEAS task, you will need to be able to successfully identify and cite evidence from a text to support predictions, make inferences or interpretations, and draw conclusions.

> ### Objectives
>
> This objective includes, but is not limited to, the following examples of knowledge, skills, and abilities.
>
> - Cite evidence from the text to support a prediction.
> - Cite evidence from the text to support interpretations.
> - Cite evidence from the text to support a conclusion.

CITING EVIDENCE

Effective readers cite evidence to support their ideas about texts.
Evidence in a text can take many forms. Sometimes, the structure of a text can help readers make predictions about what an author will include as the text progresses. For example, if the text includes a numbered list, a reader might predict that the author will be giving instructions in a sequence or providing a list of items in order of their importance. A title is a text feature that can also help readers make predictions about what might be included in the text.

One thing that readers often must infer in all types of texts is word meanings. When readers come across an unfamiliar word, they might make an educated guess about its meaning before consulting a dictionary. Context is usually a helpful guide to the meanings of words. Often, words that surround an unknown word can provide clues about the meaning of the word.

Whether or not writers intend their readers to predict, infer, interpret, or draw conclusions, it is likely that every text at some point will require a reader to perform these skills. In a sense, all readers are experimenters who are trying out words, exploring meanings, and predicting events and outcomes.

---

prediction. A reader's guess of events to come or what a text will be about.

MAKING PREDICTIONS

A prediction is an informed guess about what will happen later in a text. A reader can make a prediction by paying attention to text details. Suppose an author begins a story with the sentence "If I had known I would end up in the hospital, I never would have gone to the gym that day." This opening line alone captures readers' attention and establishes a situation. It invites the reader to make a prediction about what will happen next. Did this person get into an accident on the way to the gym? Did this person do something at the gym that was too difficult, such as try to lift weights that were too heavy? Readers can make reasonable predictions about what might have happened based on details introduced in this opening line.

INFERENCES AND INTERPRETATIONS

An inference is similar to a prediction. A prediction uses details from a text to speculate about what will happen next. An inference combines text details with a reader's background knowledge to fill in gaps of information in the text. What do you know about a character that is not directly stated in the text, and how do you know it? An inference can support a reader's interpretation regarding the meaning of a text or its significance.

Read the following passage to make inferences about the characters and events presented.

> The young woman stood alone in the corner looking down at the gym floor. She wanted to participate in a deadlift competition but was not sure if she was strong enough to lift weights significantly beyond her normal limits. Little did she know that her decision to go for it would change her life for years to come.

Because the passage ends with the idea that the young woman's decision to compete would "change her life," readers might predict that the woman will be injured or be successful. Readers can also infer ideas about the character. Because the woman "stood alone in the corner looking down," a reader can infer that she was feeling unsure or nervous in this competitive situation. Being alone also suggests that she did not approach others for advice before making her decision. These inferences are based on details provided in the text but also on readers' own experiences with common human behavior in new situations. Readers might interpret the character's gender as having something to do with her nervousness. She might not be sure that she will be accepted in a male-dominated field.

DRAWING CONCLUSIONS

By studying details in a passage, readers can draw logical conclusions that are not directly stated in a text. While the evidence for conclusions is not directly stated, it is present in the text. Readers can discern this evidence by making connections. To draw conclusions, think about the details contained within a text, and combine them with information from within the text or from other sources.

For example, a text might include a scene in which a narrator provides a detailed description of a tree in a forest. The narrator tells the reader what type of tree it is, what conditions are ideal for the tree to grow, what fruit it produces, and what organisms (such as moss and wildlife) live on or near the tree. Although it has not been directly stated, the reader can draw the conclusion that the narrator is an expert on nature and trees. The reader might also then infer, based on specific details and how they are presented, that the narrator came by this expertise either through education or through simply living with and observing this kind of tree for some time.

Drawing conclusions about a text is thus similar to detective work. The evidence for conclusions exists within the text, but it is up to the attentive reader to put it together and interpret its meaning.

Practice Problems

Read the following passage carefully and answer the questions that follow.

Nikita's mother loves to tell anyone who will listen that she had to enroll her daughter in gymnastics to keep her safe. She would often find baby Nikita precariously perched on the highest limb of a tree or attempting double flips from the top of her bureau onto her bed. The gym was Nikita's haven growing up, but now that haven was a sheer rock face in the Sierra Nevada Mountains. Nikita clung to minuscule fissures in the rock as her climbing partner, Ivan, watched from below. His muscles tensed as he watched her, ready to belay her ropes to catch even the tiniest slip or fall. Nikita looked down and made eye contact with Ivan. She detached her ropes and let them fall.

1. Which of the following is a prediction based on the last line of the passage?

   A. Nikita will panic because she lost her ropes accidentally.

   B. Nikita will attempt a freestyle climb without ropes.

   C. Ivan will run for help because Nikita has lost her ropes.

   D. Ivan will climb up and help Nikita reattach her ropes.

2. Which of the following is an inference that could be made about Nikita?

   A. Nikita is afraid of heights.

   B. Nikita is athletic and adventurous.

   C. Nikita is a professional climber.

   D. Nikita has traveled to many mountains.

3. Which of the following is a reasonable conclusion to draw about Nikita's childhood and her present situation?

   A. Nikita is drawn to the outdoors and risk taking.

   B. Nikita's mother discouraged her climbing.

   C. Nikita has a deep love of geology.

   D. Nikita wanted to become an Olympic gymnast.

4. Which of the following definitions can be inferred for the meaning of "belay" in the passage?

   A. To let go of

   B. To fasten on a cleat

   C. To exert tension on

   D. To loosen

5. Read the back cover or online summary of a biography. Make a prediction about the events in the biography based on details from the summary. Cite the evidence you use to make the prediction.

R.3.2 — Compare and contrast the themes expressed in one or more texts

A theme is a broad concept or universal concern that an author addresses through a given medium. The theme of a work is different from its subject. The subject of a story might be living in Alaska, but its theme might be that resilience can help one overcome challenges, such as the challenges of living in the wilderness. This theme, which can be stated as a complete thought, is revealed by the interactions among setting, characters, and plot. At the same time, theme informs a reader's understanding of the story and its characters while offering insight into a truth or message about life. Many stories with different settings, characters, and plots share similar themes.

This TEAS task requires several skills related to comparing and contrasting themes: identifying a common theme that appears in different works; finding differences or variations in themes between two texts; and comparing and contrasting how a theme appears in different media, literary genres, and cultures.

Objectives

This objective includes, but is not limited to, the following examples of knowledge, skills, and abilities.

- Identify a theme appearing in different works on the same topic.

- Distinguish variation in themes between two texts.

- Compare and contrast themes across media, genres, and/or cultures.

IDENTIFYING A THEME

Themes are present in short and long works of fiction and nonfiction. Short stories, novels, poems, and other written materials have themes, as do nonprint materials such as films and radio broadcasts. Sometimes themes are obvious because they are stated directly, as often occurs in fables, for example. However, themes are more often implicit, requiring a reader to make inferences based on the outcome of a plot or changes in a character. When reading a story, watching a film, or looking at a work of art, ask yourself: What message, lesson, or big ideas about life are being communicated through the narration, setting, dialogue, and/or plot? What does the author or creator want the audience to know?

All of the parts of a story work together to build a theme. To identify a theme, pay close attention to each of these story elements.

- **Narration/Exposition.** Big ideas and messages often come through narration and exposition. Look for how characters change as a result of story events.

- **Setting.** Authors choose settings that will enhance the plot and thus the theme. For example, an author might choose to set a story on a space station where the last human beings must live because humanity has taken Earth and its natural environment for granted. The theme can be that people should take care of nature because protecting Earth means protecting humanity.

- **Characters.** The journeys and adventures—emotional or physical—that characters endure and the obstacles they overcome throughout the course of a story give hints about the themes in texts. A character who must overcome many physical and emotional hardships and is rewarded for their efforts might suggest the theme that endurance is a key quality of survival.

- **Dialogue.** Like narration and exposition, the words that characters speak in stories often reveal insights into the ways characters change as a result of plot events.

- **Plot.** Like settings, a story's plot helps readers determine its themes. In a story with a theme such as "Crime doesn't pay," for example, the story's plot must reflect the theme: the criminal character must be caught by the end. As another example, in a story with the theme "Love conquers all," the protagonist (or main character) will triumph over the obstacles they face along the way by expressing or acting out of love.

SIMILARITIES AND DIFFERENCES ACROSS THEMES

A work of literature can have more than one theme. Novels often engage readers by exploring many themes, and sometimes the themes are interconnected. For example, Shakespeare's *Romeo and Juliet* suggests that learned violence sometimes provides a rite of passage within a culture, but that same violence can also lead to the destruction of a culture or family. In addition, different works can explore similar themes in different ways. Suppose you are reading two works of historical fiction about pioneering nurses Clara Barton and Florence Nightingale. One text might suggest that advancements in the medical field are the result of hard work by all. The other text might suggest that the medical field did not advance without the struggle for equal opportunities for women.

SIMILAR THEMES ACROSS MEDIA, GENRES, AND CULTURES

Common themes across classic works of literature often studied in the U.S. relate to power, gender, freedom, and privilege. Much can be learned about politics, economics, and sociology from the themes present within the works of literature of a particular culture, geographic area, or time period. Recurring themes regarding oppression in the literature of a time period or culture, for instance, can be evidence of an oppressive regime or **social structure**. Universal themes appear across literary genres and cultures and signal common struggles addressed by people. Topics of universal themes include love, the quest for power, good vs. evil, and humanity vs. nature.

Different creators can address similar themes differently depending on the medium. One particular medium can be better suited to a creator's viewpoint on a theme than another medium. Many works of fiction and nonfiction deal with the subject of compassion, for instance, but different creators communicate different messages about compassion. One creator might focus on the theme that compassion is healing in times of difficulty. For this theme, the creator might choose the medium of film so that the audience can experience the healing power of compassion along with the characters. Another creator might choose the medium of a photo essay to address the theme that compassion requires sacrifice and often yields sorrow and pain. The still images of this medium could simultaneously capture multiple elements of the theme: compassion, sacrifice, sorrow, and pain.

Visual media such as film and photography explore themes through elements such as light, color, and angle—and, in the case of film, sound. For example, a director might choose to highlight a theme regarding powerlessness by using camera angles that look down on a group rather than head-on or from below. Camera angles showing a subject from below can depict characters as more powerful or important than those around them. Scenes that show a subject as a small part of the screen in comparison with a vast landscape can also depict a theme related to powerlessness.

Literary genre often affects how a theme is addressed. A poem and a play might explore the theme that compassion is healing in very different ways. The poem would feature imagery and meter, for example, and work to capture the feeling of compassion for readers. The play, on the other hand, would reveal the theme through character development and plot.

Once you become adept at inferring themes in all artistic genres, you will more easily be able to evaluate one creator's treatment of a theme in relation to another. Likewise, you can begin to examine themes as **social commentary** and analyze them in relation to cultural or historic movements that might have influenced a creator.

---

social structure. The systems and relationships between groups in a society.

social commentary. Use of rhetoric or themes to make statements about current culture.

Practice Problems

Read the following poem and passage. Then answer the questions that follow.

Our lives, discolored with our present woes,

May still grow white and shine with happier hours.

So the pure limped stream, when foul with stains

Of rushing torrents and descending rains,

Works itself clear, and as it runs refines,

Till by degrees the floating mirror shines;

Reflects each flower that on the border grows,

And a new heaven in its fair bosom shows.

By Joseph Addison, c 1700

The fire crackled in the hearth as Hilda pulled the blanket closer to her for warmth. It had been a long day in the fields, with little to eat afterward. The overseer had been especially harsh that day, with horrifying threats if anyone paused for breath. Hilda looked toward the small opening in the wall and saw the full moon shining through. When the moon waned and waxed just once more, it would be time to run. It would be time to head North.

1. Which of the following is a common theme in the poem and the passage?

    A. Racism poisons people's lives.

    B. Hope sustains people through difficulties.

    C. Hard work brings success.

    D. Nature can be harsh but beautiful.

2. Which of the following describes how the writer develops the theme in the passage?

    A. The character is cold and tired after a long day of work.

    B. The moon reflects the hope of escape.

    C. The story takes place on a Southern plantation.

    D. There is a conflict between the enslaved people and the overseer.

3. Which of the following describes how the writer develops the theme in the poem?

    A. The writer uses a setting, or suitable location.

    B. The writer uses hyperbole, or exaggeration.

    C. The writer narrates a story with characters.

    D. The writer has characters speak for themselves.

4. In which of the following ways does the theme vary between the poem and the passage?

    A. The poem discusses nature, while the passage discusses the city.

    B. The poem discusses daytime, while the passages discusses night.

    C. The poem discusses general human woes, while the passage discusses a historical social situation.

    D. The poem discusses present woes, while the passage discusses poverty on farms.

5. Read the passage again. Describe two themes the writer is exploring in the story. Make sure to state each theme as a complete thought. Provide evidence that supports each theme.

R.3.3 — Evaluate an argument

The word *argument* can be a synonym for the word *conflict*, but in writing, it often means something slightly different. An author's argument is made up of multiple parts: a claim about a debatable issue, background information, reasoning and evidence, appeals, and responses to **counterclaims**. To evaluate the relevancy, sufficiency, credibility, and effectiveness of an argument, you must be able to identify and evaluate how each part of the argument contributes to the whole. To do well with this TEAS task, you need to be able to identify and evaluate the parts of an argument, its **rhetorical devices**, and its sources, as well as identify false or misleading statements by the author.

IDENTIFYING THE CLAIMS AND COUNTERCLAIMS

First, identify the author's topic. One topic could be dairy products. Second, ask yourself about the author's claim or opinion regarding the topic. For example, an author can make a claim that "plant-based milks are better for the environment than cow's milk." Third, check to ensure that the author addresses counterclaims, or conflicting opinions. For example, the author will need to acknowledge and respond to those who would claim the opposite, that "cow's milk is better for the environment than plant-based milks." If the author fails to address counterclaims, this weakens their credibility with audiences.

A claim requires reasoning and evidence from reputable sources for support.

Objectives

This objective includes, but is not limited to, the following examples of knowledge, skills, and abilities.

- Identify the claims and counterclaims made in an argument.

- Evaluate whether evidence made to support an argument is relevant and sufficient.

- Compare texts from different sources and opinions in terms of their credibility in support of an argument.

- Evaluate the effectiveness of cited evidence from primary and secondary sources.

- Identify false or misleading statements or data used to support an argument.

- Analyze how effectively the author uses rhetorical devices (e.g., appeal to crowd mentality, appeal to logic using facts and data) to persuade the audience.

EVALUATING EVIDENCE AND SOURCES

A writer should provide clear reasoning and credible evidence to support why their claim should be accepted by readers as true or valid. For the claim that "plant-based milks are better for the environment than cow's milk," the writer might choose a compare-and-contrast reasoning structure. This structure will allow the author to say how plant-based milks are similar to and different from cow's milk and then why plant-based milk is superior for the environment. For this reasoning structure, the author can choose two or three points of comparison and contrast, such as greenhouse gas emissions, water usage, and ecosystem effects.

For each point of comparison and contrast, the author will introduce reputable evidence in the form of facts, statistics, and quotations that support each point in favor of plant-based milks and against cow's milk.

---

counterclaim. A conflicting opinion that an author acknowledges and responds to when making an argument.

rhetorical devices. Appeals used in arguments to persuade readers emotionally, morally, and intellectually.

However, some evidence is better than other evidence. Evidence drawn from sources that are known to be reputable and based on sound research will likely be more reliable and help support a claim better than evidence drawn from sources that are not. When evaluating sources, ask yourself about the author's credentials, whether the source is *peer-reviewed*, and how current the source is.

If a writer cites a *primary source*, review the evidence to ensure that it is accurate and credible. Review data in context in the original source. If a writer cites a *secondary* or *tertiary source*, look it up and read it for yourself. Decide whether the writer has interpreted the source correctly in their argument.

Some authors use evidence that is somewhat unrelated to the argument. This practice might be accidental; however, sometimes presenting unrelated evidence is a diversion strategy. When you are evaluating the validity of an argument and its evidence, think about how closely the evidence aligns with the claim being presented. If the evidence is inconsequential or out of alignment with the claim, perhaps the author does not have enough support for the presented position.

Some authors may not provide enough evidence to support their claims. Stronger and more daring claims require greater evidence. Ask yourself whether the evidence given is great enough in scope to fully support the claim.

Evidence can even be falsified, or it can be true but presented in a misleading manner. For example, a research study might show that children who eat candy daily have a high rate of tooth decay. An author can present this as evidence in favor of the claim that "candy causes rotten teeth." While the evidence is not false, it is used in a misleading manner because it is true only under a specific set of circumstances.

ANALYZING RHETORICAL DEVICES

Rhetorical devices are not evidence, but a writer can use them to great effect in a persuasive argument. In short, rhetorical devices are strategies for framing information. For example, a writer can use a personal anecdote to illustrate a point and create an emotional connection with the audience. A writer can employ an analogy, or comparison, to show how an unfamiliar situation is similar to a familiar one. Another writer can appeal to a crowd mentality, giving the audience the sense that everyone agrees with a particular position. Take note of these devices and the responses they evoke. Are they logical? Do they elicit a strong emotion or a sense of ethics? Does the author try to convince the reader of their expertise on the subject? Do they provide a simplified view of a complex topic, or vice versa? Lastly, for what purpose is the author employing the device—to strengthen a point or to deceive?

Recognizing the parts of an argument and evaluating corresponding evidence is important. These skills make you a better-informed citizen and less susceptible to manipulation.

---

peer-reviewed journal. Published writings that have been analyzed by experts in the field.

primary source. A firsthand document or source created at the time in question.

secondary source. Secondhand account of events.

tertiary source. A compilation of primary and secondary sources.

Practice Problems

Read the following passage. Then answer the questions that follow.

Milk is a part of diets around the world, and milk from cows, goats, and even camels is used as a beverage and to make dairy products such as yogurt, Skyr, butter, and cheese. People believe that milk is healthy because it is a natural product, but recent research suggests that drinking milk is harmful to human health. Ingesting milk has been linked to heart disease and cancer. Several studies have shown a high positive correlation between milk consumption and mortality rates from heart disease. Most large-scale studies indicate that high dairy consumption increases the risk of prostate cancer. Many people cannot digest the sugars in milk, and it is likely that millions of people suffer from undiagnosed digestive tract illnesses as a result of repeated ingestion of indigestible sugars. Proponents of milk argue that the nutrients provided by milk are important to health. Although milk does contain these components, these macromolecules can also be found in foods that do not promote disease.

1. Which of the following is the primary claim of the passage?

   A. Milk is a part of diets around the world.

   B. Milk is healthy because it is a natural product.

   C. Ingesting milk has been linked to heart disease.

   D. Drinking milk is harmful to human health.

2. Which of the following correctly states whether the evidence fully and sufficiently supports the claim?

   A. The evidence does not fully support the claim because the studies cited are misleading.

   B. The evidence does not sufficiently support the claim because only heart disease and cancer are discussed.

   C. The evidence fully and sufficiently supports the claim because primary and secondary sources are used.

   D. The evidence fully and sufficiently supports the claim because several sources provide multiple reasons the claim is true.

3. Which of the following is a false or misleading claim?

   A. Milk can be used to make yogurt and Skyr.

   B. Millions of people likely suffer from undiagnosed illnesses due to consuming milk.

   C. High dairy consumption increases nutrients in the diet.

   D. Milk contains macromolecules that can also be found in other foods.

4. Which of the following is a counterclaim in the passage?

   A. Milk is a natural product.

   B. Milk can be obtained from cows, goats, and camels.

   C. The nutrients in milk can be found in other foods.

   D. The nutrients provided by milk are important to human health.

5. Many schools require students to wear school uniforms. Write a short argument about whether you agree with this policy. Include a claim, reasoning, and sufficient supporting evidence. You can also provide any needed background information and respond to at least one counterclaim. Use at least one rhetorical device to support your argument.

R.3.4 — Evaluate and integrate data from multiple sources across various formats, including media

Information comes in many forms and from many sources. Sometimes these sources include charts, graphs, and diagrams that help to explain an idea shared in a text. If multiple sources of information are not already included in a particular text, it is often a good idea to locate additional sources that provide more information about a topic.

Doing so will help you develop a more complete understanding of an issue, which will leave you better equipped to speak and write more meaningfully about a topic. Most documents produced in postsecondary coursework and by professionals require the author to integrate knowledge from multiple sources. This TEAS task will test your ability to synthesize, organize, and analyze data from multiple sources.

SELECTING DATA RELEVANT TO A PURPOSE

As with any reading task, you should begin by clarifying the author's purpose. Only when you know the author's purpose can you determine which data is relevant to that purpose. For instance, an author can write to support the claim that studying a foreign language in school leads to better employment outcomes in later life.

Objectives

This objective includes, but is not limited to, the following examples of knowledge, skills, and abilities.

- Organize data from various sources.

- Analyze various data sources.

- Select data relevant to a given purpose (e.g., claim or argument).

- Evaluate whether additional evidence is needed to draw a conclusion or to make an inference.

- Evaluate the utility of ideas that, if added, would make a text argument more logical, relevant, or useful.

- Synthesize data from texts, charts, or graphs.

- Synthesize information from multiple sources to form a prediction, make an inference, and draw a conclusion.

With the purpose clarified, you can proceed to ask yourself what sort of data is relevant to this purpose. Two data sets are recommended immediately by the claim about foreign language study: employment statistics and data on how many students study a foreign language in school. Not all employment statistics, however, are relevant to this purpose. The author should focus on statistics that will show the career trajectories of those who learned languages and those who did not. Additionally, data about earnings across a career will help support the claim. If the author includes other data, it can be misleading or show bias or faulty reasoning.

ANALYZING VARIOUS DATA SOURCES

After you have clarified the author's purpose and assessed the initial data, you will want to ask yourself, "What additional sources of information might the author provide?" Another way to think about is question is, "What information is missing from the argument?" It is a good idea in general for authors to gather data from several different sources. Multiple sources will help authors identify and analyze trends in data and identify outliers or unusual results more easily. Another reason to use several data sources is that doing so helps add texture and depth to an argument. For example, **quantitative data** on the number of people who report having a good experience using a particular service might produce dry reading for the audience. Such data can be enriched by **qualitative data** in the form of interviews with people describing the service and how they benefited from it. If a text relies only on anecdotal evidence in the form of stories or interviews, however, it may not be persuasive. Statistical data is an important appeal to the logic of readers.

ORGANIZING DATA FROM VARIOUS SOURCES

Once you have read related information from several sources, the next step is to organize your notes in a logical manner to clarify your thinking on the subject. Clear organization will help you keep track of evidence and reasoning so that you can evaluate their effectiveness. The method of organization you use should be one that makes the best sense of the evidence. For example, if you have read about how a particular technology developed, an efficient way to organize the data would be to put it in chronological order. Another method is to classify data in order of its importance. The data that most clearly demonstrates a claim or provides the greatest body of evidence could all be grouped together, as could the data of lower priority, validity, or usefulness.

There are many technology tools that can help organize information in meaningful ways. These tools can help people organize articles, data, and notes into electronic files and folders. Using technology to help organize information can save money by eliminating printing costs and time sorting through pages of information to locate what is most relevant.

EVALUATING EVIDENCE AND IDEAS AND DECIDING IF MORE EVIDENCE IS NEEDED

Before using your assembled and organized data to form predictions, make inferences, and draw conclusions about a topic, you should take one more vital step. It is necessary to evaluate whether your assembled data is sufficient for your understanding the issue and, if not, to determine what additional evidence you need to strengthen your understanding.

One way to test whether evidence is sufficient is to summarize your understanding of the issue by answering the reporter's questions: who, what, where, when, why, and how. If you find that there is a gap in your understanding, then you know that you need to read additional information. Moreover, you should have a clearer idea of what sort of evidence you will need to locate in your additional reading.

Another technique is to ask relevant questions about the subject. Are the answers to your questions located in your notes? If so, your notes might be complete. If not, you may need to do additional reading and note-taking to add this missing information.

---

quantitative data. Information that can be counted, measured, or compared on a numerical scale.
qualitative data. Information describing qualities and characteristics that can be observed and recorded, but not objectively measured.

SYNTHESIZING DATA TO FORM PREDICTIONS, MAKE INFERENCES, AND DRAW CONCLUSIONS

After organizing and evaluating the information, ask yourself, "How does all of this data fit together, and what does it mean?" This stage is often called *synthesis* because you have taken information from many sources, pulled it apart, and thought about it, and now you must put it all back together in a meaningful way. By synthesizing data, you bring together different types of information from different sources and combine them to form a clear and concise understanding of the information.

Texts, charts, and graphs are all different sources of data. How can these different sources be synthesized? Your synthesis should be guided by your evolving understanding of the subject. Different data sets can be compared and contrasted to produce a fuller picture than one data set standing alone might provide. You might also discover other relationships among data, such as cause and effect or problem and solution.

Your synthesis of data can be used to form predictions, make inferences, and draw conclusions. These techniques help you extend the act of collecting data into thinking critically about the data.

A prediction is an idea about what will happen at a later point in time. When considering your data, ask what trend seems to emerge or in which direction the data seems to point. You can then predict what other data on the same topic might show and test your prediction against additional, related data. To make an inference, you combine text evidence with your own knowledge and experiences to fill in gaps in information by thinking beyond what the data explicitly shows. Making logic-based assumptions can lead you to other profitable angles of study. A conclusion is a final summary statement about what the data shows. This conclusion is informed by your reading, note-taking, and knowledge and experiences regarding the subject.

Practice Problems

Read the passage and review the graph. Then answer the questions that follow.

Nurse practitioners were concerned about the growing rate of pregnant patients who do not take prenatal supplements. Expectant patients reported that they believed that taking medication when they had no symptoms made no sense. Some believed the supplements could harm the fetus. Pregnant patients also reported that the supplements were difficult to swallow and had an aftertaste. To investigate ways to increase patient knowledge of prenatal supplements, the nurse practitioners designed a controlled study. The control group received normal individual instruction at the hospital. The treatment group received community instruction at local clinics with other pregnant people. Expectant patients in both groups were given a pretest and posttest on their knowledge of supplements. Results are shown in the graph.

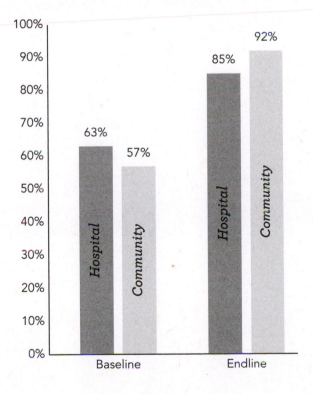

1. Which of the following is a conclusion that can be drawn from the study?

   A. Hospital instruction was more effective than community instruction.

   B. Both types of instruction were equally effective.

   C. Community instruction was more effective than hospital instruction.

   D. Neither type of instruction increased patient knowledge.

2. Which of the following is the treatment in this experiment?

   A. Community instruction

   B. Hospital instruction

   C. Use of prenatal vitamins

   D. Use of a placebo

3. Which of the following describes how the text and graph complement each other?

   A. The graph introduces the experiment, while the data is discussed in the text.

   B. The graph provides evidence that contrasts with the claims made in the text.

   C. The graph introduces a new study that differs from the study described in the text.

   D. The graph presents the findings of the experiment described in the text.

4. Which of the following is an inference that can be made based on the data presented in the text and the graph?

   A. Hospitals are poor tools for staging medical interventions.

   B. People are more willing to accept medical instruction when they feel comfortable and relaxed.

   C. People are less willing to accept medical instruction from doctors than from nurses.

   D. Medical interventions in hospitals have better results than medical interventions at home.

5. Reread the passage and graph. What additional data could be collected to provide more evidence about whether the community intervention helps pregnant people learn more about prenatal supplements?

Reading Key Terms

anecdote. A short story that illustrates a concept or point and creates a connection between the author and reader.

argument. A type of text consisting of a claim on a debatable issue, background information, reasoning and evidence, rhetorical appeals, counterclaims, and responses to counterclaims.

assumption. Supposition of an unstated idea.

audience. The intended consumers of information.

authorial intent. The reason an author creates a text; also called the author's purpose.

bias. Tendency toward or against a preconceived idea.

blog. A website that is usually informal and independently run.

chart. A type of diagram that graphically represents data.

chronological. In order by time.

claim. A statement made in an argument that something about a topic is true.

comprehension. Ability to understand.

conclusion. A deduction made by a reader that takes the details, evidence, and assumptions presented in a text to the next logical step.

connotation. An implied meaning of a word or idea created by the emotions and assumptions attached to it.

context. Surrounding words or ideas within a sentence or passage that affect the meaning of a word and influence how it is understood.

contradiction. A statement, assertion, or instruction in a text that conflicts with information provided elsewhere in the same text.

counterclaim. A conflicting opinion that an author acknowledges and responds to when making an argument.

delineate. Describe precisely or set forth accurately in detail.

denotation. An explicitly stated meaning of a word or idea.

details. Facts, descriptions, and other types of information that support key points.

diagram. A symbolic representation used to convey information, especially a drawing that shows an arrangement or relationship among the parts of something.

evidence. Proof, such as facts, descriptions, and examples, that an author uses to support their ideas and reasoning.

explicit. Describes information that is directly stated in a text.

fact. Statement or data that can be proven or verified through a reputable source.

figurative language. Language meant to create imagery, comparison, or an association for the reader; usually a metaphor, a simile, or personification.

footnote. Comment at the bottom of a page that provides additional information about something within the text.

genre. A group of related writings or other media.

glossary. A text feature usually found in the back of a book that includes an alphabetized list of key terms and their definitions.

graph. A type of diagram that displays data mathematically.

graphic. A diagram, graph, illustration, or other piece of artwork.

heading. A title within a text, commonly used by authors to organize information.

identify. Distinguish a particular idea.

implicit. Describes ideas that are suggested rather than stated directly in a text.

imply. Indicate an idea subtly without specifically stating it.

index. A text feature usually found in the back of a book that includes an alphabetized list of key details and concepts and the page numbers where that information can be found.

inference. A logical assumption, or guess, that can be made about a topic based on evidence, reasoning, and personal experience or knowledge.

irrelevant. Not applicable to the idea.

key points. Ideas that elaborate on and support the main idea about a topic in each paragraph.

legend. Map feature that explains symbols and other elements that represent information on the map, such as routes, populations, and capital cities.

logic. The framework of reasoning used to understand ideas and make sound assumptions, predictions, and conclusions.

main idea. The thesis, claim, or message that an author states or expresses about the topic of a text; the central point in each paragraph.

mood. How the elements in a text, such as word choice, affect the reader.

objective. Describes language that is nonjudgmental, impartial, nonpersonal, and unemotional.

opinion. Statement that cannot be proven; an author's beliefs, as opposed to facts or reasoning, presented in a text.

paraphrase. To explain an idea in one's own words.

peer-reviewed journal. Published writings that have been analyzed by experts in the field.

perspective. The narrator's or author's particular thoughts, feelings, or perceptions about people, ideas, or events in a story or text.

persuasive argument/persuasive writing. Argument in favor of a position intended to make the reader agree with an idea, thesis, or claim.

point of view. The narrative voice an author uses to tell a story or relate information; can be first person, second person, or third person.

prediction. A reader's guess of events to come or what a text will be about.

primary source. A firsthand document or source created at the time in question.

priorities. In written directions, the hierarchy or sequence of which steps must be followed in what order; often indicated by the use of signal words.

procedure. Ordered steps to follow in a set of written directions to complete a task safely, efficiently, and effectively.

publication. The printing, publishing, and/or distribution of a text; a published work.

qualitative data. Information describing qualities and characteristics that can be observed and recorded, but not objectively measured.

quantitative data. Information that can be counted, measured, or compared on a numerical scale.

query. query function. (1) A question. (2) A feature in digital texts that allows readers to search for key words and topics within a text.

reason. A basis or fact to support an idea.

reasoning. A method or structure used to build a valid argument in a persuasive text.

relevant. Connected to the idea being discussed.

rephrase. To explain an idea in different words.

representation. A portrayal, depiction, expression, presentation, substitution, sign, or symbol of something; an artistic image or likeness.

research based. Reliant on ideas backed by study.

rhetorical devices. Appeals used in arguments to persuade readers emotionally, morally, and intellectually.

root word. A word element, or morpheme, from which other words are built.

scale. Ratio of distance expressed to actual measurement.

search engine. A software tool used to locate information online or within a digital text.

search term. A word or words used to find information via a search engine.

secondary source. Secondhand account of events.

sequence. Logical order or pattern of organization in writing or texts.

sequential. Following a set order.

sidebar. Text feature that is set apart from the main body of a text; often includes additional information, charts, graphs, and/or images.

social commentary. Use of rhetoric or themes to make statements about current culture.

social structure. The systems and relationships between groups in a society.

stereotype. Simplified categorization of an idea or person based on superficial ideas that stand in for real people and things.

structures. Ways of logically organizing ideas to enhance comprehension.

subheading. A title of a subdivision of information within a larger division of a text.

superscript. Small characters, usually numbers, set slightly above a line of text; used to refer readers to a footnote or endnote that provides additional information about a topic.

support. Lend credibility to an idea.

table of contents. Text feature usually found in the front matter of a book that lists chapter titles and page numbers.

tertiary source. A compilation of primary and secondary sources.

theme. A broad concept or universal concern that an author addresses through a given medium.

tone. The author's implied or explicit attitude toward a topic.

topic. Subject of a text.

transition words. Words that link ideas in a text; used to help readers discern steps in a procedure or a chronology of events, such as when things happen and for how long.

valid. Proven as true.

viewpoint. An author's beliefs or opinions about a topic.

Practice Problems Answer Key

R.1.1

1. Option C is Correct. This option indicates the common thread among all three paragraphs.
   - Option A is a supporting detail that elaborates on how to take care of the heart.
   - Option B is a supporting detail that justifies why it is necessary to look after the heart.
   - Option D is a supporting detail that elaborates on how to take care of the heart.

2. Option B is correct. The main idea is that diet and exercise can both be used to aid heart health.
   - Option A is a detail about exercise.
   - Option C is a detail about diet.
   - Option D is a supporting detail explaining why exercise helps heart health.

3. Option D is correct. This is the topic sentence of paragraph
   - Options A and B are supporting details.
   - Option C is the main idea of paragraph 3.

4. Option A is correct. It states a detail that supports the main idea of the paragraph.
   - Options B, C, and D are additional details that provide further information on how to achieve the heart-healthy diet detailed in option A.

5. A summary of the passage's main ideas and supporting details could include the following.
   - Nurses can help patients control their weight and lower their risk of heart disease.
   - Exercise is one good way to control weight and reduce health risks.
   - Diet is another good way to control weight and reduce health risks.
   - Food portions should be small and rich in fruits, vegetables, whole grains, and low-fat proteins.
   - Food portions should limit unhealthy fat and salt.

R.1.2

1. Option C is correct. This evidence supports the inference that Danielle has determination, or a willingness to work hard to succeed.
   - Options A and D may support other assumptions that can be made about the character, but they do not support the idea that Danielle is determined.
   - Option B is not enough evidence to support the inference that Danielle is hardworking. Just applying to a program does not necessarily mean that she will work hard once she is accepted.

2. Option D is correct because the author only suggests that Danielle is following in her grandmother's footsteps by including background information about Danielle's grandmother.
   - Options A, B, and C are incorrect because they are clearly stated in the text.

3. Options C and E are correct because the implicit evidence that this program can help Danielle decide if nursing is really right for her supports the idea that the program involves hands-on nursing experiences working at a nearby hospital.
   - The other options are incorrect because the information in the text does not support those conclusions.

4. Option B is correct. This information is explicit evidence in the passage. Nurses in the neonatal intensive care unit (NICU) are responsible for the care of the tiniest patients, the premature newborn infants, as well as critically ill infants.
   - The other options are incorrect because they are not the patient population cared for in the NICU.

5. One possible inference to be made from the passage is that Danielle feels admiration and respect for her grandmother and the life she led. This inference can be made based on the text evidence that Danielle is following in her grandmother's footsteps, as well as many other pieces of evidence in the text, explicit and implicit, such Danielle's determination to succeed.

R.1.3

1. Option B is correct. The passage is about the correct procedure for inserting an IV catheter.
   - Options A, C, and D are parts of the procedure but not the procedure itself.

2. Option D is correct. Steps 1 and 2 use procedural signal words to demonstrate how they are related.
   - Options A and B are false about what is conveyed in the steps.
   - Option C is true in that Step 2 includes an alternative choice about what to do if a patient has a phobia, but it is not an explanation for how Steps 1 and 2 are related.

3. Option A is correct. Order terms signify the relationship among steps.
   - Options B, C, and D are directional terms that explain how to carry out the steps.

4. Option C is correct. Step 4 instructs the user to wear gloves before swabbing the injection site with an alcohol pad, but Step 7 instructs the user to swab the injection site with an alcohol pad before donning gloves.

5. Option B is correct.
   - Option A repeats the same information as Step 2 in the procedure.
   - Option C contradicts Steps 2 and 3.
   - Option D is not necessary and contradicts the use of the signal word finally in Step 8.

R.1.4

1. Option B is correct. A glossary contains the definitions of key terms used in the text.
   - Option C might help you find where it is mentioned but would not define it.
   - Options A and D are both text features that would not help.

2. Option B is correct. Prerequisites for the course are included in the sidebar.
   - Options A, C, and D are included in other parts of the course catalog page.

3. Option C is correct. The name of the instructor of the course is relevant information that the text does not include.
   - Options A, B, and D are all included in the text.

4. Option B is correct. Entering the course number is the most likely term to bring up this page.
   - Option A does not adequately identify this specific page.
   - Options C and D are not specific identifiers for this page.

5. Option D is correct. The map legend would help you understand the map.
   - Options A, B, and C are not features that would help with the navigation of a map.

R.1.5

1. Option B is correct. Stating the same statistic in two different ways may make it understandable to more readers.
   - Options A, C, and D are not correct.

2. Option D is correct. The words "worst" and "best" convey value judgments and demonstrate bias.
   - Options A, B, and C are not correct.

3. Option C is correct. Those patients who are aging and no longer able to care for themselves typically require nursing care in residential care facilities.
   - Options A, B, and D include patients who require care in different types of facilities than residential.

4. Option B is correct. The National Council Licensure Examination (NCLEX)-RN is the exam nurses must pass to qualify for their nursing licenses.
   - Options A, C, and D are fictional variations for the acronym NCLEX.

5. Option A is correct. Nurses may come from a variety of cultural groups and may be of varying ages, genders, ethnicities, religions, and abilities.
   - Options B, C, and D are not correct.

R.1.6

1. Option B is correct. When something occurs prior to something else, that indicates a sequence of steps or events.
   - Options A, C, and D are chronological signal words, indicating a time factor for steps or events to occur.

2. Option A is correct. Chronological signal words can indicate when something will happen that is not specific to sequence, as in the case of "one day" in this passage.
   - Options B, C, and D are words indicating sequential order.

3. Option C is correct. Tim is thinking ahead that if he follows one prescribed plan, it could change his future plans.
   - Options A, B, and D describe events that are sequential.

4. The correct answer is ADN, BSN, MSN. Many nursing students choose to begin with the associate degree in nursing (ADN) and then progress to the Bachelor of Science in Nursing (BSN) followed by the Master of Science in Nursing (MSN) to become a nurse practitioner.

5. Option B is correct. Early in the passage, Tim is described as certain he wants to be a nurse, and the second-to-last sentence states that the option that allows him to begin his career soonest is a good plan. This means he will get either his nursing diploma or an ADN, which also means he will need to apply to a bridge program as the next logical step toward his ultimate goal of getting a master's degree to become a nurse practitioner.
   - Option C is incorrect because nothing in the passage implies that Tim needs further information to make a choice about a career path.
   - Option D is incorrect because an MSN is still necessary even if Tim follows the bridge program that allows him to start his career sooner.

R.2.1

1. Options B and E are Correct. Physical education does promote a healthier lifestyle, and some studies show improved grades for students who participate in daily PE.
   - Options A, C, and D are opinions of the author.

2. Option A is correct. It is a stereotype to believe all students spend too much time on electronic devices.
   - Options B and D are factual statements.
   - Option C is an opinion.

3. Option D is correct. The author believes PE should be mandatory.
   - Option A is an opinion, and options B and C are not conclusions made by the author.

4. Option C is correct. Overall, the author presented information about the benefits of PE. The author does not present this information with optimism about gaining mandatory PE or pessimism that mandatory PE will ever occur. The author uses no words to indicate that there is irritation regarding the topic.

5. Sample answer: The text mostly gives opinions promoting the notion that PE should be made mandatory in schools. A single fact supports this claim, and this fact only provides evidence that regular exercise promotes healthier hearts and lifestyles. This evidence does not support making PE a mandatory school activity, however. The author deploys many opinions about the benefits of PE combined with negative stereotypes about those who do not exercise regularly. I do not find this text persuasive because the author fails to provide solid evidence to support their assertions.

R.2.2

1. Option A is correct. The word "dark" provides a synonym for "opaque."
   - Option B describes the other windows mentioned in the sentence.
   - Options C and D have no basis in context clues.

2. A. This option refers to an airplane, which is not related to the rest of the series.
   B. This is a term from geometry, not woodworking.
   C. Correct. The series of tools listed are all used in woodworking.
   D. This defines a homonym for "plane," "plain."

3. A. This does not imply intelligence.
   B. Correct. The word "cunning" implies intelligence with a craftiness tending toward trickery, similar to that implied by "mischievous."
   C. This does not imply craftiness tending toward trickery.
   D. This does not imply intelligence.

4. Option D is correct. The words "hazy," "slithered," "gravestones," "eerie," and "crept" create a frightful mood. The other options are not implied by the words in the sentence.

5. A. Correct. Personification attributes human qualities to nonhuman entities.
   B. This is a suggestion or implication of a word's meaning.
   C. This is a word's actual meaning.
   D. This is a simile, which uses "like" or "as" to compare unlike things.

R.2.3

1. A. This is part of the task for nurses to complete, but it is not the primary purpose of the announcement.

    B. Correct. The author's primary purpose is to provide information about the in-service training.

    C. This cannot be supported by the evidence in the announcement.

    D. This is not correct because the announcement makes no mention of nurses missing shifts.

2. Option D is correct. The announcement secondarily lists the standards of transitional care.
    - Options A, B, and C are not secondary purposes of the announcement.

3. Option C is correct. The author of the announcement conveys an authoritative, professional tone.
    - Options A, B, and D are not expressed in the tone of the announcement.

4. Options A and C are Correct. Nurses need to know how to manage transitions of care and must attend an in-service training on the subject. Procedures for discharging patients are explicitly included as part of the training.
    - Options B, D, and E are opinions.

5. A. This identifies the audience but does not support the purpose.

    B. This identifies the topic of the announcement, but this does not support the purpose.

    C. Correct. The announcement's purpose is to inform staff of a mandatory training, which is stated in this sentence.

    D. This is a detail about the type of training, which does not support the purpose.

R.2.4

1. Option C is correct. The website by the staff of a medical facility would be the most reliable.

2. Option A is correct. Newspapers verify their sources and information, so links to newspaper articles would be the most reliable.

3. Option B is correct. For an important topic such as preventing patients from falling and sustaining injuries, evaluating authority and expertise would be essential.

4. Option D is correct. Any information pertaining to safety practices should be checked for accuracy.

5. Learner responses will vary. Suitable answers to the question of the blogger's point of view will be first, second, or third person. The perspective will depend on the topic, though it will likely be for or against something. The student should identify the author's priorities and reasons for writing in order to determine the perspective. An influencer is often motivated to build their own presence and brand and sell products for sponsorships; members of a profession or authors writing about serious topics will usually communicate in a way that aligns with professional standards. Other perspectives could be related to the intended audience of the writer. Credible sources will vary; examples include newspapers, encyclopedias, journal articles, authors with academic credentials, and university websites.

R.3.1

1. Option B is correct. Because Nikita detaches the ropes deliberately, the reader can predict she might freestyle climb. Nikita will likely not panic, because she deliberately detaches her ropes. Ivan will not run for help or climb up because there is no evidence to predict that Nikita needs assistance.

2. Option B is correct. Because she has loved to climb all her life, the reader can infer that Nikita is athletic and adventurous. It is unlikely that Nikita is afraid of heights because she loves to climb. There are no details in the passage that suggest that Nikita is a professional climber or has traveled to many mountains.

3. Option A is correct. The reader can use details such as Nikita climbing trees as a baby and her current rock climbing to conclude that Nikita is drawn to the outdoors and risk-taking. Nikita's mother encouraged her climbing by placing her in gymnastics. The passage does not discuss whether Nikita has a deep love of geology or wanted to become an Olympic gymnast.

4. Option C is correct. A climbing partner belays or puts tension on a rope to keep the climber from falling. Letting go of the rope or loosening it would not help the climber. There is no evidence that Ivan has a cleat to fasten the rope to.

5. Answers will vary. One example of a biography is Frida: A Biography of Frida Kahlo by Hayden Herrera. The back of the book states that it is about the life of Frida Kahlo, an important Mexican painter. She was born in Mexico City and was injured in a tram accident. She was involved in international exhibitions and politics. She had many relationships that influenced her and her work. Based on the citation of these details, it can be predicted that the biography will discuss how her injury affected her life and paintings.

R.3.2

1. Option B is correct. Both the poem and passage discuss hope. The poem implies that there is reason for people to hope during a time of woe because such times are like a stream during a rainstorm—eventually, the rain will end, the sun will come out again, and the river will reflect a sunny sky. The same is true for people going through hardship. In the passage, readers learn that the character Hilda can survive harsh conditions by hoping for freedom.

2. Option B is correct. The moon will signal the time to go northward. The other plot elements are not linked to the theme that hope sustains people through difficulties.

3. Option A is correct. The writer develops the theme in the poem by describing a beautiful setting with a stream that becomes clear after the rain has made it muddy. The setting also has flowers growing around the edge of the stream, and after the stream is all clear and the sun comes out, the stream reflects the sky—"a new heaven"—on its surface. Through the setting, which is used as a metaphor, the poem builds the theme of "This too shall pass," meaning that eventually, sad times will come to an end. The writer does not use hyperbole or exaggeration. The poem's writer does not narrate a story or have characters speak for themselves.

4. Option C is correct because the poem discusses a general theme related to human woes and hope, while the passage addresses escape from enslavement. Both texts use nature imagery. Time of day is not stated in the poem. The passage addresses poverty as an aspect of enslavement.

5. Answers will vary. Two possible themes the writer is exploring in the story are resilience in the face of cruelty and the will to survive. Resilience is illustrated by Hilda's ability to keep working despite the overseer's cruelty, and the will to survive is seen in her plans for escape.

R.3.3

1. Option D is correct. The writer is arguing that drinking milk is harmful to human health. The writer provides background by saying that milk is a part of diets around the world and that people believe that milk is healthy because it is a natural product. The fact that ingesting milk has been linked to heart disease is evidence that supports the claim.

2. Option D is correct because the sources mentioned offer enough evidence from primary sources to support the claim. Without reading the studies cited, there is no way to tell if they are misleading, and the argument does not need to cover every aspect of human health in order to be true. Secondary sources are not used in the argument.

3. Option B is correct. This statement is conjecture on the part of the author based on the evidence that some people cannot digest milk sugars. That milk can be used to make yogurt and Skyr and contains macromolecules that can also be found in other foods is background information about milk.

4. Option D is correct. The counterclaim is the opposite of the claim. The opposite of the claim that milk is unhealthy is that the nutrients provided by milk are important to human health. That milk is a natural product and can be obtained from cows, goats, and camels is background information. That nutrients in milk can be found in other foods is a rebuttal to the counterclaim.

5. Answers will vary. Sample answer: Schools should require students to wear school uniforms because it will save families money on clothing. For example, the average teenager needs seven to 10 outfits to wear to school. With a school uniform, this need is cut down to two to three outfits because the student is wearing the same outfit daily. This policy could be the greatest cost savings available to a family of four since the introduction of "kids eat free" Tuesdays at a local restaurant. While some can argue that uniforms cut down on students' ability to show individuality, the schools can still allow students to wear jewelry, hair accessories, and shoes that demonstrate their personalities while also helping with their families' budgets.

R.3.4

1. Option C is correct. Looking at the graph, community instruction was more effective than hospital instruction. This is shown by the larger increase in the percentage points from pretest to posttest. Community instruction increases knowledge by 35 percentage points, whereas hospital instruction increased patient knowledge by 22 percentage points. Both types of instruction increased knowledge, but community instruction increased it by 6 percentage points more.

2. Option A is correct. Community instruction was the treatment in this experiment because it was a new way of presenting knowledge to patients devised by the nurse practitioners to increase patient understanding of supplements. Hospital instruction was the control because it was the normal instruction patients received. This enabled the nurses to discern whether the new method was better than the old method. This study did not test medications or a placebo.

3. Option D is correct. The graph displays the evidence provided by the experiment that is described in the text. The text also provides information on how to read the graph by explaining what each column means.

4. Option B is correct. The evidence supports this inference because the study showed that people were more willing to accept instruction in local clinics in their community. Based on sound reasoning and prior knowledge, it follows that local clinics in a more familiar environment will be less stressful than a hospital environment. The larger increase in acceptance of the intervention when staged in the community suggests that there is something about the community environment in particular that improved outcomes.

5. Answers will vary. One type of additional data that could be collected to provide more evidence would be to interview participants about what they learned. Qualitative studies like this can reveal how patient knowledge differed between groups and what participants felt about the two types of instruction. Patient emotional reactions can enhance or interfere with retention of knowledge.

Reading Unit Quiz

The Apprentice

Luigi, following his friend Matteo, dashed over the cobbled street in the November rain. He'd left his village in the southeast and traveled north to the renowned city of Rome. After several months, the urban environment was becoming more familiar and felt much less chaotic. Above all, Luigi adored art—sculpture, frescos, and mosaics—and Rome contained innumerable artistic treasures. Great masters toiled endlessly: drawing, chiseling, grinding pigments, and mixing paints.

Luigi and Matteo had apprenticed themselves to sculptor and painter Marco de Luca. Luigi's body ached from the intense, grueling work and endless days, but he derived satisfaction from creating works of art out of raw materials and his imagination. However, his greatest desire was to encounter the master of all masters, the young Michelangelo Buonarroti. Luigi and Matteo both deemed Michelangelo's work to be superior to that of all other artists, and the Pietà was their favorite sculpture.

One afternoon, while chiseling a chunk of white marble, Matteo whispered, "After we're done with work today, follow me on an errand for Master Marco. I have a surprise for you." Luigi eyed his companion curiously, then went back to carefully carving a shape in the tough stone.

A little while later, after plodding in the drizzling rain through the muddy streets, lugging a satchel of assorted pigments, Matteo and Luigi entered a large door, navigated a series of hallways, and eventually found themselves in a chapel. Scaffolding blocked considerable sections of the ceiling, but clearly, a great masterwork was in progress. Flowing figures in soft blues, glowing golds, and rowdy reds could be seen through the scaffolding's wooden planks.

"I've brought your requested pigments, sir," squeaked Matteo.

A pale, elongated face framed by brown hair and a scruffy beard appeared over the scaffolding, contrasting with the luminous figures above it.

"Thanks to you and Master Marco, this segment will be completed today!" the man exclaimed. "But painting is secondary for me these days—I prefer sculpture. Surely, you've seen my Pietà?"

Speechless, Luigi gazed up at Michelangelo Buonarroti, master artist of all master artists.

1. Which of the following statements uses relevant details to summarize the story?

    A. One rainy day in Rome, Luigi's friend Matteo asks him to help him run an errand.

    B. Luigi works long hours as an artist. His friend Matteo is also an artist, but Matteo knows famous people.

    C. Luigi moves to Rome to work as an artist. One day, his friend Matteo asks Luigi to accompany him on an errand, and Luigi meets his idol, Michelangelo, as a result.

    D. Luigi meets his idol, Michelangelo, and has the opportunity to see the famous mural on the Sistine Chapel ceiling as it is being painted.

2. Which of the following details supports the main idea in the fourth paragraph that the artist is working on "a great masterwork"?

    A. "Flowing figures in soft blues, glowing golds, and rowdy reds could be seen through the scaffolding's wooden planks."

    B. "Scaffolding blocked considerable sections of the ceiling..."

    C. "A little while later, after plodding in the drizzling rain through the muddy streets, lugging a satchel of assorted pigments..."

    D. "A pale, elongated face framed by brown hair and a scruffy beard appeared over the scaffolding, contrasting with the luminous figures above it."

3. Which of the following best describes what happened immediately after Matteo asks Luigi to follow him on an errand?

   A. Luigi leaves his home to go to Rome.

   B. Matteo and Luigi meet Michelangelo.

   C. Luigi and Matteo find their way to the chapel.

   D. Luigi and Matteo carry a satchel of pigments through the rain.

4. The passage states, "Scaffolding blocked sections of the ceiling." Which of the following is the correct meaning of this phrase?

   A. The scaffolding held up damaged sections of the ceiling.

   B. Parts of the paintings were hidden from view behind the scaffolding.

   C. The scaffolding had been built to cover parts of the ceiling.

   D. Sections of the painting were organized into squares.

5. Which of the following excerpts from the passage includes an opinion?

   A. "Luigi and Matteo had apprenticed themselves to sculptor and painter Marco de Luca."

   B. "Matteo and Luigi entered a large door, navigated a series of hallways, and eventually found themselves in a chapel."

   C. "Luigi, following his friend Matteo, dashed over the cobbled street in the November rain."

   D. "Luigi and Matteo both deemed Michelangelo's work to be superior to that of all other artists."

Use the figure below to answer the question.

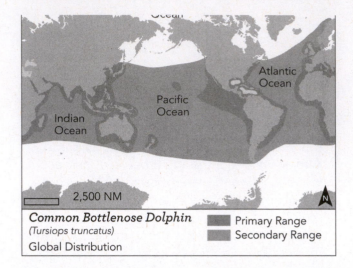

Common Bottlenose Dolphin
(Tursiops truncatus)
Global Distribution

Primary Range
Secondary Range

6. Based on the map, which of the following oceans contains the northernmost secondary range of the common bottlenose dolphin?

   A. Arctic

   B. Atlantic

   C. Pacific

   D. Indian

The Tragedy of the RMS Titanic

Preparation is the key to success, and being prepared for an emergency can mean the difference between life and death. Lack of preparation was one of the key factors in the tragedy of the Titanic, in which more than one thousand people perished in the cold waters of the Atlantic.

The tragedy began when the Titanic hit an iceberg off the coast of Newfoundland in the North Atlantic at approximately 11:40 p.m. on April 14, 1912. The ship eventually sank in the early hours of April 15. However, the profound loss of life of approximately 1,500 people could have been greatly reduced— or even avoided—had there been sufficient planning for the possibility that the ship could sink and was not, in fact, unsinkable. There were only 20 lifeboats available, and they could only hold 1,178 people, but 2,240 were on board. Additionally, during the panic of the tragedy, boats were launched when they were only half-full of passengers. Therefore, too few lifeboats, combined with too few passengers on each lifeboat, resulted in the staggering loss of life.

There was also a difference in the survival of passengers depending on gender, age, and class. The law of the sea dictates that women and children should board the lifeboats first. It wasn't only women and children who were more likely to survive, though; the type of ticket that a passenger had made a difference, too. It is estimated that passengers who were traveling first class were 44% more likely to survive than other passengers. Because of the tragedy of the Titanic, ships today are required to adhere to rigorous safety protocols. These include meeting requirements for the number of lifeboats, having clear directions in cases of emergency, and conducting emergency practice drills before sailing. Because of the Titanic, sailing is much safer today.

Sources: https://www.history.com/topics/early-20th-century-us/titanic#section_6

https://www.britannica.com/topic/Titanic

7. Which of the following supporting details would be included in a summary of the multi-paragraph text?

   A. The Titanic had too few lifeboats and insufficient plans for what to do in an emergency.

   B. The Titanic sank in the icy waters of the Atlantic late at night.

   C. Out at sea, the safety of women and children is prioritized over that of men.

   D. Men, women, and children of all classes lost their lives in the Titanic disaster.

8. Which of the following pieces of information is not contained in the text?

   A. How ships became safer after the disaster

   B. The name of the Titanic's captain

   C. Which groups were most likely to perish

   D. How the accident happened

9. Which of the following events in the passage occurs first?

   A. The Titanic hits an iceberg.

   B. Only a few hours after it hits an iceberg, the Titanic sinks.

   C. Women and children board the lifeboats.

   D. Ships begin to follow rigorous standards, including lifeboat requirements.

10. Which of the following is the purpose of this selection?

   A. To entertain readers with a narrative about events regarding the Titanic

   B. To inform readers about why the loss of life was so high on the Titanic

   C. To persuade readers that the design of the Titanic caused the ship to sink

   D. To describe to readers the design of the lifeboats on the Titanic in detail

Soil Incorporation Composting

To make compost, try soil incorporation, a relatively simple method for composting small amounts of organic waste. Start by digging a hole at least 12 inches deep in your yard. Collect the leftovers you want to compost, such as coffee grounds and vegetables. (Do not include oily or fatty scraps, such as meat, because they can lure hungry animals.) Next, chop up the scraps and mix them into some of the soil you removed; the soil will speed up the decomposition process. Fill the hole about 4 inches deep with the mixture of scraps and soil, and cover it up with at least 8 inches of soil. The buried food wastes will decompose in 1 month to 1 year, depending on the size of the hole, becoming nutrient-rich compost in the process.

Source: https://extension2.missouri.edu/g6957
https://www.baltimorecountymd.gov/Agencies/publicworks/recycling/composting/incorporation.html

11. Which of the following is the conclusion in the process of soil incorporation composting?

   A. Chop up food scraps and mix them with soil for faster decomposition.

   B. Place a mixture of food wastes and soil at the bottom of a hole at least 12 inches deep.

   C. Cover the mixture of food wastes and soil with 8 or more inches of soil.

   D. Wait for the buried food wastes to decompose over time, creating rich compost.

Registering Online for a 5K Run

On the home page of the official website for the 5K race, click on the Register or Sign Up link. Fill in all the fields. You may be asked to provide your birthdate and emergency contact information.

Click on Agree to Terms to read the waiver. Verify that you understand the race legalities by clicking the Agree box. Then, click Continue.

Follow the rest of the steps until you get to the Final Checkout page.

Review all the information entered.

Click on Check Out or Cart and enter your credit card information to pay the entry fee. You may be given the option of buying a race T-shirt. Click Confirm Payment.

Source: https://help.runsignup.com/support/solutions/articles/17000062676-register-for-a-race

12. According to the directions, when should you click the Agree box on the Agree to Terms page?

   A. After you have entered your credit card information on the Final Checkout page and read the waiver

   B. After you have filled out all the fields in the Register section and read the waiver

   C. Before you have filled out all the fields in the Register section or read the waiver

   D. Before you have provided your birthdate and emergency contact in the Register section

Leafy Sea Dragons

Leafy sea dragons are related to seahorses, but they look more like tiny dragons than tiny horses—that is, if dragons could sprout leaves! Found in the ocean off southern Australia, leafy sea dragons can grow to 14 inches. They have a long snout, which is similar to seahorses. The leaflike appendages sprouting all over their bodies do not help them swim, but these protrusions serve an important function. Leafy sea dragons cannot swim fast with their tiny pectoral and dorsal fins, and because their bony bodies are fragile, elaborate camouflage is essential for survival. Leafy sea dragons have been threatened by pollution and climate change and are now a protected species.

Source: https://www.nationalgeographic.com/animals/fish/l/leafy-sea-dragon/

http://www.aquariumofpacific.org/onlinelearningcenter/species/leafy_seadragon

13. According to the passage, which of the following conclusions can be made about the leafy sea dragons' appendages?

A. They enable the leafy sea dragons to swim in deep water.

B. They serve as protective camouflage for the leafy sea dragons.

C. They protect the leafy sea dragons from pollution and climate change.

D. They help the leafy sea dragons quickly swim away from predators.

14. Which of the following is the primary purpose of this text?

A. To entertain readers with a story about leafy sea dragons

B. To persuade readers that leafy sea dragons are worth saving

C. To inform readers about leafy sea dragons

D. To explain that leafy sea dragons are not seahorses

Use the figure below to answer the question.

Cook Time	Power Level	Kitchen Timer
Defrost Time	Defrost Weight	Clock Settings
Pizza	Popcorn	Baked Potato	Hot Dog
	Handy Presets	
Frozen Breakfast	Frozen Dinner	Frozen Vegetable
Fresh Vegetable	Bacon	Boil Water

15. Which of the following buttons on the microwave touchpad should be pressed to cook a 12-oz package of frozen peas efficiently?

A. Defrost Weight

B. Frozen Vegetable

C. Defrost Time

D. Power Level

Memo:

To the residents of the South Washington Condominiums:

During the week of November 3 through 12, hallways on all odd-numbered floors will be painted. This means that we will need access to your apartments to paint the frames of front doors. All residents should make sure the manager has their current contact details for notification approximately half an hour before work begins near their apartment. The schedule for painting even-numbered floors has not yet been determined. Thank you for your cooperation.

16. Which of the following is true according to this passage?

   A. Residents on the third floor should vacate their apartments between November 3 and 12.

   B. Fourth-floor residents should make sure their contact information is up to date.

   C. There are no plans to paint the hallways on the second floor.

   D. Residents on the sixth floor should expect to have their hallway painted between November 3 and 12.

17. Which of the following statements is true based on information in the memo?

   A. The tenth-floor hallways will not be painted after the third-floor hallways.

   B. Residents will not be alerted right before their apartment doors are painted.

   C. Residents do not have to be available at all times for the entire period of the project.

   D. Residents will receive a bill for the cost of the work from the apartment manager.

Desert Garden

She surveyed the wide swath of earth spread out before her as she stepped out of her back door. The ground was cracked, fissures running here and there, but colorful too with lilies, sage, and lavender. She had learned what to plant when water was scarce: what would survive and what wouldn't. She stepped forward and tipped the pail of dishwater, letting it stream onto some tiny green shoots, the dust rising up. She sighed, wondering how long this would last.

18. Which of the following conclusions can be made from the evidence provided in this passage? (Select all that apply.)

   A. The protagonist is an experienced gardener.

   B. Very few plants can survive without a lot of water.

   C. The protagonist lives in an area that is experiencing a drought.

   D. The protagonist is creative about finding ways to save water for the garden.

   E. Some of the plants in the garden are already dying.

19. Which of the following inferences can the reader logically make about the protagonist after reading this passage? (Select all that apply.)

   A. The protagonist lives in a rural area.

   B. The protagonist has a practical outlook.

   C. The protagonist has had a hard life.

   D. The protagonist has endurance.

   E. The protagonist is tired of having to carry water to her garden.

The pond was used to retain excess water and often filled after large rain-storms.

20. Which of the following best captures the meaning of "retain" as used in the sentence?

   A. Remember

   B. Hold

   C. Maintain

   D. Cherish

Alltech Enterprises

Using a product created by Alltech Enterprises will always give users a better experience. For example, the Alltech Desktop Computer is user friendly and less likely to crash and contract viruses than other laptops currently on the market. In addition, when a customer takes the leap of faith and buys multiple Alltech products, such as the Alltech Superphone and Supertablet, there will be a variety of pleasant surprises. The Calendar application on both Alltech's Desktop and Supertablet will sync with the Superphone. Customers can also see texts on all three products simultaneously. Overall, having Alltech products will make a customer's life better and easier.

21. Which of the following pieces of information from the passage is a fact?

   A. Alltech products make a customer's life easier with a variety of features.

   B. The calendar on an Alltech Superphone can sync with the calendar on an Alltech Supertablet.

   C. Using a product created by Alltech always gives users a better experience.

   D. The Alltech Desktop Computer is user friendly.

22. Which of the following statements describes the author's primary claim in the passage?

   A. Having Alltech products will make the user's life better and easier.

   B. Alltech Desktop Computers are less likely to crash.

   C. Alltech products are less likely to contract viruses.

   D. Buying multiple Alltech products results in pleasant surprises.

Annie Oakley: An American Sharpshooter

Annie Oakley (1860–1926) was one of several women of the "Wild West" known for her exceptional talent at wielding shotguns. She traveled with Buffalo Bill's Wild West Show for 16 years, starting in 1885. Because of her talents with a shotgun, the Lakota Sioux leader, Sitting Bull, gave her the nickname "Little Sure Shot." Oakley toured not only the United States but also England and many parts of Europe. She was the first female "international sensation" from the United States. More than that, Oakley was also a strong advocate for women and children. She encouraged and taught women to handle guns for self-protection. When World War I broke out, Oakley offered to create and train an all-female regiment of excellent shooters; however, the government never responded to her offer.

Source: https://www.womenshistory.org/education-resources/biographies/annie-oakley

https://www.pbs.org/wgbh/americanexperience/features/oakley-annie/

23. Which of the following statements expresses the author's perspective on Annie Oakley?

   A. Annie Oakley had an exceptional ability with shotguns and was as adept with a gun as any man.

   B. Annie Oakley was one among many colorful "Wild West" figures whose fame is based on myth.

   C. Annie Oakley accomplished things that no other woman of her time, and few women today, could accomplish.

   D. Annie Oakley was more than just an international star; she also tried to improve the lives of women.

24. Which of the following details from the passage supports the inference that Annie Oakley was not always taken seriously?

   A. Sitting Bull gave her the nickname "Little Sure Shot."

   B. The government ignored her idea of training female sharpshooters.

   C. She traveled in Europe and became the first female international star from the United States.

   D. Sixteen years of her career were spent traveling with Buffalo Bill's Wild West Show.

Morning on Seymour Avenue

All along Seymour Avenue, the blinding white cover that had been yesterday's snowfall had turned to a mass of dingy gray mush. The pollution index had skyrocketed, resulting in overcast skies with a brown, hazy glow. Incandescent lights flicked inside the windows of the cold, repetitive apartment blocks. The smells of fried fish, burning rubber, and gasoline-powered generators mingled with the sounds of factory workers drifting out for the late shift. A lone, wizened woman, her pale hair drawn up in a fierce bun, struck at a stoop with a broom, attempting to eradicate the traces of the stray, mangy dog who had spent the night there.

25. Which of the following statements describes the narrator's perspective?

A. There is little hope for the future here.

B. Pollution is bad for the environment.

C. Factory workers are not to be trusted.

D. Cities are full of interesting people.

26. Which of the following conclusions can be drawn about the woman in the passage?

A. She enjoys living in the neighborhood.

B. She has a partner who works at the factory.

C. She likes to keep her apartment tidy and clean.

D. She is angry at the dog who has slept on her stoop.

27. In what order would a reader perform the following steps to evaluate if the evidence in a passage is fact or opinion? (Use all the steps.)

A. Identify the evidence provided in support of the claim.

B. Read the evidence and determine if it supports the claim.

C. Determine whether the evidence contains feeling words, opinion words, or biased or stereotypical language.

D. Find the source for the evidence and check its reliability.

E. Identify a particular claim.

Do Uniforms Matter?

School uniforms are an invaluable means for educational administrators. They prevent problems within student populations by promoting order and discipline. They help students learn the importance of adhering to regulations and recognizing that deviation from expectations produces consequences. Dressing appropriately for school helps young people learn that life requires different styles of attire, depending on the situation. Uniforms also promote standardization. They limit the promotion of ideas or values that are inappropriate in schools, such as students showing allegiance to a gang or like groups or wearing clothing that others may find offensive. Dr. Karen P. Braun of Southern University, an adolescent behavioral expert, believes that students who wear uniforms are more accepting of their same-age peers.

28. Which of the following evidence would strengthen the claim in the passage?

A. A study that shows students who wear uniforms do better academically

B. A quote from an expert about the need for young people to be individuals

C. A report on the costliness of buying and maintaining school uniforms

D. A series of photographs of students in school uniforms

29. Which of the following is a primary source that could be used to support a counterclaim to the claim made in the passage?

A. The study "Uniforms and Peer Acceptance" by Dr. Karen P. Braun

B. An interview with a school principal who wrote an editorial called "The Harm of Uniforms"

C. A newspaper article that cites several cases about the usefulness of uniforms

D. A catalog that includes different designs and fabrics for school uniforms

Use the figure below to answer the question.

	Price per ounce	Replacement Needed
Soap A	$0.10	3 months
Soap B	$0.11	3 months
Soap C	$0.10	4 months
Soap D	$0.12	4 months

30. A frugal couple is looking to save money and are considering the cost of their hand soap. They are considering four different soap products. Each soap bottle contains 6 oz. The chart shows the cost per ounce and how often the soap would need to be replaced. Which of the following options cost the least over 4 months?

   A. Soap A

   B. Soap B

   C. Soap C

   D. Soap D

31. Which of these sources is most relevant to someone who is seeking information about what it was like to create a particular community garden?

   A. A newspaper interview with local expert gardeners involved in the project

   B. A magazine interview with local business owners who work near the site of the garden

   C. An article in the local newspaper about the effort to create a community garden

   D. A video clip on the local news reporting on a potential community garden

Voting Rights in the United States

Although the majority of those residing in the United States are legally qualified to vote, significant portions of the population are excluded from voting. For example, many people convicted of a crime are not allowed to vote even if they never served time in jail or have completed their prison sentence. In some cases, people who have served their sentences can regain the right to vote, but this is not the case in all states.

People who immigrate to the United States must become a U.S. citizen to vote. Becoming a citizen is a long and sometimes arduous process. In addition, minors—those younger than age 18—cannot vote, although some believe the voting age should be lowered to 16. A person must reach 18 years old before the date of an election, but citizens who are 17 years old can register to vote if they will turn 18 before the date of the election.

Another requirement for voting is a valid U.S. Postal Service street address. This requirement has caused many people to be disenfranchised because their street addresses are not recognized by some electoral boards.

Source: https://www.loc.gov/teachers/classroommaterials/ presentationsandactivities/presentations/elections/who-can- vote-today.html

https://www.scholastic.com/teachers/articles/teach- ing-content/voting-united-states/

32. Based on the opening paragraph of the article, which of the following conclusions can be drawn about the article's purpose?

   A. The article's purpose is to convince readers that fewer people should be allowed to vote.

   B. The article's purpose is to convince readers that the voting age should be 17 years old.

   C. The article's purpose is to convince people that the U.S. government should take steps to enfranchise more voters.

   D. The article's purpose is to convince people that prisoners losing the right to vote is fair.

Women's Suffrage and a Little-Known Warrior

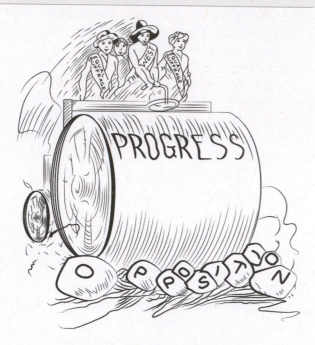

1848 the first women's rights convention, in Seneca Falls, New York, allied strong-minded, resolute women to fight for suffrage—the right to vote. After the Civil War, Congress ratified the Fourteenth and Fifteenth Amendments, which bestowed rights—including suffrage—on males who had been enslaved and continued to exclude women from this significant privilege. In 1872, suffragists intensified their battle, challenging the status quo with lawsuits and by voting illegally. In 1890, women achieved a landmark decision: The state of Wyoming granted women suffrage.

After acquiring support from important politicians, women finally accomplished their objective with the ratification of the Nineteenth Amendment in July 1920. The decisive vote was cast by Harry Burn of Tennessee—who voted "aye" at the urging of his mother, Febb Burn.

33. Which of the following is a common theme in the passage and cartoon?

A. Change will always crush those who are against it.

B. Women are a powerful force for change.

C. Politicians can help people achieve their dreams.

D. Accomplishments come to those who try hard.

34. Which of the following describes how the central ideas in the cartoon and passage are different?

A. The cartoon's central ideas and the passage's central ideas are the same.

B. The passage has a central idea of how men stood in the way of women's suffrage, but the cartoon shows how men helped.

C. The passage displays a central idea that sometimes it is okay to break the law, and the cartoon shows that following the rules leads to progress.

D. The central idea of the passage is that women's suffrage made slow progress, but the cartoon shows opposition to women's progress being crushed quickly.

Choosing a Trailer

A customer who owns an equestrian training business outlines the following criteria when shopping for a preowned automobile. Her vehicle needs to include a preinstalled trailer hitch, and her preference is for a recent model—2017 or later. Another must-have is a powerful eight-cylinder piston engine, and the potential buyer appreciates music, so a high-end eight-speaker sound system is essential. Being ecologically minded, her requirements include achieving at least 17 miles per gallon on long-range highway travel. Finally, the automobile should have fewer than 10,000 miles on the odometer.

		Vehicle A	Vehicle B
Mileage		10,500	8,750
Year		2017	2018
Engine		4 cylinder	8 cylinder
Amenities		Moon roof, trailer hitch	High-performance tires, 8-speaker sound system, heated seats, trailer hitch
Miles per gallon (mpg)	local	14 mpg	15 mpg
	highway	17 mpg	20 mpg

		Vehicle C	Vehicle D
Mileage		7,000	12,200
Year		2019	205
Engine		8 cylinder	8 cylinder
Amenities		Heated seats, back-up camera, 6-speaker sound system	Leather interior, trailer hitch
MPG	local	18 mpg	15 mpg
	highway	21 mpg	18 mpg

35. Which of the following vehicles from the above figure would be appropriate for this customer?

    A. Vehicle A

    B. Vehicle B

    C. Vehicle C

    D. Vehicle D

The First Science Fiction Novel?

Mary Shelley published her novel Frankenstein in 1818. Frankenstein tells the story of a scientist who creates an intelligent but terrifying creature in a laboratory experiment and then is tortured by what he has done. The story is infused with elements of Gothic horror and is representative of the Romantic movement.

Some suggest that Frankenstein should be considered the first true science fiction story. However, while the usage of science and technology is a primary theme of the science fiction genre, a facet of that theme is the explanation of the technology. No scientific explanation for the monster's creation is ever given. Frankenstein focuses heavily on the moral issues and consequences of creating such a beast, themes far more representative of the Gothic novel.

36. Which of the following information from the passage best supports the author's argument that Frankenstein is not a work of science fiction?

    A. The technology behind the monster's creation is not explained.

    B. The scientist uses technology to create a monster in a laboratory.

    C. Frankenstein was published in 1818.

    D. The story contains elements of Gothic horror.

37. Which of the following modern-day news headlines best coincides with the theme of morals and consequences in the novel Frankenstein?

    A. "NASA Spacecraft Lands on Jupiter"

    B. "Radioactive Alligators Threaten Florida Golf Course"

    C. "Advances in DNA Mapping Help to Predict Chances of Heart Disease"

    D. "Engineers Weigh Security Against Privacy in Software Debate"

Brawn GP: A Cinderella Story

The 2009 Formula One season started with what seemed like a disaster for driver Jenson Button and designer Ross Brawn. With the shockwaves of the 2008 financial crisis still spreading throughout the world economy, car manufacturer Honda decided to pull its support from the Formula One team that bore their branding and used their engines.

Brawn, Button, and the rest of the team's employees faced an uncertain future. Even after Brawn bought the team (hastily renamed "Brawn GP" before the start of the season), the chances of getting to the grid for the first race, let alone winning the world championship, seemed like a ridiculous fantasy. They had no sponsors, little money, and even lacked an engine for the car. But an extraordinary sequence of events, fueled by the brilliance of the team and its drivers, led to the latest and perhaps last of Formula One's true fairytale success stories.

38. Which of the following is a prediction about future events supported by details from the text?

   A. The Brawn GP team would be unable to compete in the world championship.

   B. The team would have to be renamed halfway through the season.

   C. The Brawn GP team would win the year's world championship.

   D. Honda would claim credit for the team's success.

39. Which of the following details from the text supports the conclusion that adequate financial resources are usually a deciding factor in Formula One success?

   A. The mention of the brilliance of the car's designer

   B. The mention of the 2008 financial crisis

   C. The mention of the manufacturer of the car, Honda

   D. The mention that the team had no sponsors at first

Quiz Answers

1.   A. This option includes an irrelevant detail about the weather and does not mention that the main characters meet their favorite artist.
    B. This option includes irrelevant details about Matteo and leaves out the relevant detail that the pair meet Michelangelo.
    C. **CORRECT.** This option is correct because it summarizes the passage using the most important relevant details.
    D. This option includes irrelevant details about the mural.

2.   A. **CORRECT.** This option is correct because the detail describes the artist's work using vivid imagery, suggesting that he is a master.
    B. This option does not provide evidence that the artist's work is great.
    C. This option does not provide evidence that the artist's work is great.
    D. This option describes the artist but not the work itself.

3.   A. This event happens before Matteo asks Luigi to follow him on an errand, as shown in a flashback.
    B. This event happens last. However, there are other events that occur after Matteo asks Luigi to follow him on an errand.
    C. This event happens after Matteo asks Luigi to follow him on an errand, but another event happens before this.
    D. **CORRECT.** Just after Matteo asks Luigi to follow him, the two of them walk through the rain with the satchel of pigments.

4.   A. There is no contextual indication that the scaffolding contributes to structural soundness.
    B. **CORRECT.** The word "blocked," in the sense of "created an obstacle," indicates that the scaffolding obstructed the view of parts of the painting.
    C. This explanation misinterprets the meaning of "blocked"; the connotation of the word "blocked" as used in the sentence is not "to cover."
    D. This explanation reflects an incorrect denotation of the word "block" in the sense of a square-shaped chunk of material; the scaffolding did not literally segment the painting in squares.

5.   A. This choice is a factual claim about Luigi and Matteo's activities, rather than an opinion.
    B. This choice describes Matteo and Luigi's actions, rather than giving an opinion about those actions.
    C. This choice describes Luigi's actions rather than giving an opinion about those actions.
    D. **CORRECT.** This choice indicates Luigi's and Matteo's opinion about Michelangelo—that he is a superior artist.

6.   A. The Arctic Ocean does not have any range of the dolphin.
    B. **CORRECT.** The secondary range extends the furthest north in the Atlantic Ocean, off the coast of Europe.
    C. The Pacific Ocean contains substantial portions of the secondary range, but it does not extend as far north as the range in the Atlantic.
    D. The Indian Ocean contains substantial portions of the secondary range, but it does not extend as far north as the range in the Atlantic.

7.   A. **CORRECT.** The Titanic's lack of preparedness is the main idea of the text, and evidence that lives were lost through poor preparation (such as too few lifeboats) is a highly relevant detail to a summary of the text.
    B. This detail is not relevant to a summary of the text, which is about how a lack of preparedness cost lives in the Titanic disaster.
    C. This detail is not relevant to a summary of the text, which is about how a lack of preparedness cost lives in the Titanic disaster.
    D. This detail is not relevant to a summary of the text, which is about how a lack of preparedness cost lives in the Titanic disaster.

8.   A. The text describes the measures taken to make seafaring safer after the accident.
    B. **CORRECT.** This information is not contained within the text. The captain is not mentioned at all.
    C. The text describes how first-class passengers were 44% more likely to survive than others.
    D. The text describes how the Titanic sank after hitting an iceberg.

9. A. **CORRECT.** This event occurs first, at 11:40 p.m. on April 14, 1912.
    B. Several events happen prior to this, including the Titanic hitting the iceberg.
    C. The Titanic hits an iceberg before this happens.
    D. This event happens after all other events in the passage.

10. A. The author's purpose is not to entertain the reader because it does not focus on events or characters.
    B. **CORRECT.** The passage serves to inform readers about the reasons that more than one thousand passengers perished on the Titanic.
    C. The passage does not focus on the design of the Titanic, except for the detail about the lack of lifeboats.
    D. The passage does not describe the design of the lifeboats at all.

11. A. This is the third step, not the final step.
    B. This is a summary of several steps, not the final step.
    C. This is the penultimate step, not the final step.
    D. **CORRECT.** This statement is the conclusion of the process, as it is the final step in this process of creating compost.

12. A. This option is incorrect because a registrant cannot access the Final Checkout page without first clicking the Agree box.
    B. **CORRECT.** The Agree to Terms page appears after the Register section, and the registrant must read the waiver before clicking the Agree box.
    C. The registrant cannot click the Agree box until after clicking Agree to Terms and reading the waiver, so this option is incorrect.
    D. The Agree to Terms link appears after the Register or Sign Up page, which includes the birth date and emergency contact fields, so this option is incorrect.

13. A. The passage clearly states that the leafy appendages are not used for swimming.
    B. **CORRECT.** The passage says that the sea dragon's protrusions "look like strands of kelp or seaweed and can change color," which implies that they serve as camouflage to protect it.
    C. This conclusion is not supported by information in the passage.
    D. The passage clearly states that the leafy appendages are not used for swimming.

14. A. The passage is not a narrative.
    B. Although the endangered status of the leafy sea dragon is mentioned, it is not the main point, and there is no argument about protecting the species.
    C. **CORRECT.** The passage is a brief, informative piece about describing a sea creature that might be unfamiliar to readers.
    D. Even though comparisons are made to the more familiar seahorse, it is done to help readers better visualize and understand the leafy sea dragon; the passage is not a comparison between the species.

15. A. When seeing the word "frozen," one might first think of defrosting, and when seeing "12-oz package" they might think of weight, but the diagram shows that this microwave model has presets that allow for cooking frozen vegetables. Thus, to be efficient, the user should press the Frozen Vegetable button.
    B. **CORRECT.** To be efficient, the user one should press the Frozen Vegetable button.
    C. When seeing the word "frozen," one might first think of defrosting. However, there is no stated time that shows how long the frozen peas must be microwaved. Thus, to be efficient, the user should press the Frozen Vegetable button.
    D. There is no stated power level for cooking frozen peas. Thus, to be efficient, the user should press the Frozen Vegetable button.

16. A. The text does not say that anyone needs to leave during the painting.
    B. **CORRECT.** All residents have been asked to update their contact information; this includes residents on the fourth floor.
    C. The memo does indicate that painting the even-numbered floors is intended, although it is not scheduled yet.
    D. The text says that hallways on odd-numbered floors will be painted at this time. Six is an even number.

17. A. The text indicates that the even-numbered floors will be painted in the future after the odd-numbered floors, even though a specific schedule is pending.
    B. The memo indicates that the manager will contact residents about half an hour before work begins near their apartments.
    C. **CORRECT.** The memo states that residents have to be available half an hour before work begins, but not for the entire duration.
    D. The memo asks for contact information so that access can be given for the painting work. It does not indicate that residents will be billed for the work.

18. A. **CORRECT.** The protagonist is an experienced gardener is correct. The protagonist knows how to care for her garden when water is scarce.

B. Very few plants can survive without a lot of water is incorrect. The passage does not include evidence to support this conclusion.

C. **CORRECT.** The protagonist lives in an area that is experiencing a drought is correct. The cracks and fissures in the earth indicate that the ground is extremely dry, and the protagonist wonders how long "this" will last, indicating that the lack of water is an event or weather pattern.

D. **CORRECT.** The protagonist is creative about finding ways to save water for the garden is correct. The fact that the protagonist has saved dishwater for her plants shows her creativity in finding water sources.

E. Some of the plants in the garden are already dying is incorrect. There is no mention in the passage of plants not thriving.

19. A. The protagonist lives in a rural area is incorrect. The passage mentions a "wide swath of earth" outside of the protagonist's back door, but that doesn't necessarily mean a rural area.

B. **CORRECT.** The protagonist has a practical outlook is correct. The passage notes that the protagonist has learned to adapt her gardening to the available resources and seems to understand that further adaptation may be necessary soon.

C. The protagonist has had a hard life is incorrect. There is no evidence in the passage to support this inference.

D. **CORRECT.** The protagonist has endurance is correct. The protagonist has had time to figure out which plants survive without much water, which suggests she has been doing this for a long time with no end in sight.

E. The protagonist is tired of having to carry water to her garden is incorrect. The passage mentions that the protagonist sighs after watering a few plants, but it does not indicate that she's tired.

20. A. The pond was not used to "remember" the water.

B. **CORRECT.** In this context, "retain" means "to hold," as in holding excess water.

C. The pond was not used to "maintain" the water.

D. The pond was not used to "cherish" the water.

21. A. This statement is an opinion that the company has about its own products, and customers might disagree that their lives were made easier.

B. **CORRECT.** This statement makes a factual claim about the capabilities of the phone and the tablet. This statement could be proven true.

C. This statement is an opinion the company has about its own products, and users might disagree.

D. Because people can disagree about what is "user friendly" for their own needs, this statement is an opinion rather than a factual claim.

22. A. **CORRECT.** The author is trying to convince the reader that having Alltech products will make life better and easier.

B. This statement is evidence to support the claim, not the claim itself.

C. This statement is evidence to support the claim, not the claim itself.

D. This statement describes a rhetorical device used to support the claim, not the claim itself.

23. A. While her ability to handle shotguns is a detail included in the text, the author's perspective is not that she was mostly notable for her shooting ability.

B. The author's perspective is that Oakley's fame as a sharpshooter is deserved, and that she should also be known for her humanitarian goals.

C. The author's perspective is that Oakley was an exceptional woman, but the text does not indicate that the author believes that no other woman, then or now, was capable of such exploits.

D. **CORRECT.** The author's perspective is that Oakley's skills were remarkable, but so was her advocacy and other work on behalf of women and children. The author wants to tell people that Oakley was more than just a good shot and to popularize these other parts of her legacy.

24. A. The text makes it clear that "Little Sure Shot" was a respectful nickname.
    B. **CORRECT.** The government's failure to respond to Oakley's idea to train women to be sharpshooters in the war is evidence that she was not always taken seriously.
    C. That Oakley was invited to perform internationally and became a "star" indicates that her skills were taken seriously.
    D. This detail is evidence that her skills were highly valued and widely respected as part of a famous show.

25. A. **CORRECT.** The narrator's perspective is negative. This hopelessness is shown by the consistently negative and hopeless language used to describe the scene.
    B. This statement describes a belief that the narrator reveals, but it does not describe the overall perspective of the passage.
    C. There is nothing in the passage that suggests this perspective.
    D. The perspective of the passage is not focused on people or how interesting they are.

26. A. There is nothing to suggest that the neighborhood is nice to live in or that she enjoys living there.
    B. The passage does not imply that the woman has a partner.
    C. Although she uses a broom on her stoop, there is no indication that she keeps a clean apartment.
    D. **CORRECT.** This conclusion is supported by the words "fierce" and "struck," words that indicate anger, and her anger seems to be directed at the dog.

27. E. Identify a particular claim is the first step. The logical process is to identify the claim first.
    A. Identify the evidence provided in support of the claim is the second step. Check whether evidence has been provided to support the claim.
    D. Find the source for the evidence and check its reliability is the third step. If evidence has been provided, the reader should find the source for the evidence and check its reliability.
    B. Read the evidence and determine if it supports the claim is the fourth step. The reader should determine the relationship between the claim and the evidence.
    C. Determine whether the evidence contains feeling words, opinion words, or biased or stereotypical language is the fifth step. The reader can evaluate the evidence for feeling words, opinion words, or biased or stereotypical language. With this process complete, the reader can determine if the evidence is factual or not.

28. A. **CORRECT.** This evidence supports the idea that uniforms promote order and discipline.
    B. This evidence provides support against the idea that standardization is important.
    C. This is evidence against uniforms because of the financial burdens they might place on some families.
    D. Although this evidence might illustrate what the uniforms look like, it would not contribute to the overall argument.

29. A. This is a primary source, but it supports the claim.
    B. **CORRECT.** A principal, who has direct experience with school uniforms and is writing about the harm they cause is a primary source, and one that would effectively refute the claim of the passage that uniforms are beneficial.
    C. A newspaper article is a secondary source because it interprets primary sources, which in this example are the cases.
    D. A catalog is a secondary source, and it does not support a claim about uniforms.

30. A. Soaps A and C are the same price per ounce, but Soap C lasts longer. Because Soap A would need to be replaced before 4 months, it would cost $1.20 over 4 months whereas Soap C would cost $0.60.
    B. Soap B is more expensive than Soaps A or C and does not last as long as Soap C.
    C. **CORRECT.** Soap C costs the least over 4 months because, although it is the same price as Soap A, it will last longer and need replacing less.
    D. Soap D is the most expensive; even though it lasts as long as Soap C, it costs more.

31. A. **CORRECT.** An interview with local expert gardeners who were involved in the project would provide a firsthand account of what it was like to work on the garden.
    B. The local business owners do not have firsthand knowledge of what it was like to work on the garden unless they also participated in the project, so this source is not the most relevant.
    C. This information does not provide a firsthand account of what it was like to work on the garden, so it is not the most relevant source.
    D. If the clip is about a "potential" garden, it is not the most relevant source for what it was like to work on the existing community garden.

32. A. The evidence in the paragraph suggests the opposite of this choice; it suggest that voting restrictions are a negative in society.
    B. The statement that 17-year-olds sometimes can register to vote is a supporting detail about the issues with voting, but is not itself the main purpose of the article.
    C. **CORRECT.** The opening paragraph of the article gives multiple and diverse examples of how the government keeps people from voting, so the article is most likely about overcoming these hurdles and enabling more people to vote.
    D. The opening paragraph of the article outlines many of the ways in which voting is restricted, but it gives no indication that the article is arguing in favor of these restrictions.

33. A. This option applies to the cartoon only and states an absolute.
    B. **CORRECT.** This option is correct because both the passage and cartoon portray women as leading progress in society.
    C. This option is illustrated in the passage, but it is not in the cartoon.
    D. This option is best illustrated by the passage only.

34. A. This option is incorrect because, although there are some themes that are similar, there are still key differences.
    B. This option is incorrect because the cartoon does not show men helping.
    C. This option is incorrect because the cartoon does not show a theme of following the rules leading to change.
    D. **CORRECT.** This option is correct because the passage tells the story of how it took decades for women's suffrage to finally be law, while the cartoon implies progress was able to quickly overrun the opposition.

35. A. Vehicle A has too many miles, the wrong engine, and no sound system is mentioned.
    B. **CORRECT.** Vehicle B is correct because it is the only option that meets all of the customer's criteria. The correct answer is revealed through a process of elimination.
    C. Vehicle C does not have a trailer hitch or an eight-speaker sound system.
    D. Vehicle D has too many miles, is too old of a model, and does not mention a sound system.

36. A. **CORRECT.** The author argues that Frankenstein is not a work of science fiction because the technology used to create the monster is not explained in the novel.
    B. This information does not support the author's argument.
    C. This information does not support the author's argument.
    D. This information does not support the author's argument.

37. A. This headline does not coincide with the theme of morals and consequences in the novel.
    B. This headline does not coincide with the theme of morals and consequences in the novel.
    C. This headline does not coincide with the theme of morals and consequences in the novel.
    D. **CORRECT.** Security vs. privacy is an ethical or moral discussion, which coincides with the theme of morals and consequences in the novel.

38. A. This is not supported by the details in the text, which support the prediction of a positive outcome for the team.
    B. There is no evidence in the text to support this prediction.
    C. **CORRECT.** The text refers to the team's brilliance and calls what happens next a "fairytale success" story.
    D. There is no evidence in the text to support this prediction.

39. A. This detail indicates that intelligence can compensate for lack of financial resources.
    B. This historical detail is related to money, but does not have a direct tie to trends in success in Formula One as used in the passage.
    C. There is no direct connection between the detail of the car manufacturer and likely paths to success in Formula One racing.
    D. **CORRECT.** This detail provides context for why the team had a "fairytale success" story, and implies that, without sponsorship or other means of revenue, success is unlikely.

Unit 2: Mathematics

The 15 lessons in this unit cover the tasks from the ATI TEAS test plan for the Math section. These are focused on assessment of basic mathematical skills and are organized into two chapters:

- Number and algebra
- Measurement and data

Each lesson introduces knowledge, skills, and abilities relevant to the corresponding Math test plan task and provides an overview of some essential topics, along with specific examples to highlight important concepts. Practice questions at the end of each lesson will allow you to test your knowledge of select concepts. In addition, there are key terms included at the end of the chapter, followed by a Math quiz. This quiz includes the same number of questions as the Math section on the ATI TEAS and matches the test plan task allocations (shown below). The quiz will give you a good idea of the number and types of questions you will encounter. Keep in mind that these lessons are a great starting point and guide to your studies, but they are not an exhaustive review of all concepts that might be tested in the Math section of the ATI TEAS. You should use other sources (textbooks, online resources, etc.) for additional study and practice in areas that you haven't mastered.

There are 34 scored Mathematics items on the TEAS. These are divided as shown below. In addition, there will be four unscored pretest items that can be in any of these categories.

Section	Number of scored questions
Number and algebra	18
Measurement and data	16

Numbers and Algebra

M.1.1 — Convert among non-negative fractions, decimals, and percentages

Numbers can be written in many ways, including **fractions**, **decimals**, and percentages. For this task on the TEAS, you will need to understand each of these forms and the process of **converting** from one form to another. You should practice converting from one number quantity to another until you have mastered the processes. There are plenty of exercises available on the internet for more practice converting between fractions, decimals, and percentages. The following overview will provide the base of knowledge you will need to succeed at this task.

> ### Objectives
>
> This objective includes, but is not limited to, the following examples of knowledge, skills, and abilities.
>
> - Identify the relationship between the numerator and denominator (part/whole) in a fraction.
>
> - Calculate a percentage.
>
> - Identify place value within decimals.
>
> - Convert between fractions, decimals, and percentages.

RELATIONSHIP BETWEEN THE NUMERATOR AND DENOMINATOR IN A FRACTION

A fraction is a numerical quantity that represents a part of a whole. Fractions can be written in the form a/b or $\frac{a}{b}$, where a and b are **integers**. Integers are **whole numbers** and their opposites. The bottom integer is called the **denominator**. It represents the whole quantity. The top integer is called the **numerator**. It represents the part of the whole number that the fraction represents. So, if you have 1/3 of a cup of flour, you have divided the 1 cup into 3 parts, and you only have one out of the three parts filled with flour.

CALCULATE A PERCENTAGE

Percentage, or percent, means "per 100." A percentage can be used to show a portion or share in relation to the whole. It shows the value of a number in terms of 100. If a product is 100% whole wheat, it means that all of the item is made of whole wheat. If it is 50% whole wheat, only half of the item contains whole–wheat grains. One percent can be interpreted as one one–hundredth, or 1/100, of something.

To calculate a percentage, take the share or portion and divide it by the whole. Then multiply this result by 100. For example, if there are 12 females in a group of 50 people, the percentage of females can be calculated as 12 divided by 50 times 100, which is 0.24 times 100, which is then written as 24%.

---

fraction. A number expressed as a numerator and denominator.

decimal. A number expressed based on place value

unit conversion. Calculating equivalent values between systems of measurement.

integers. Whole numbers and their opposites: ..., −3, −2, −1, 0, 1, 2, 3, ...

whole numbers. The numbers used in counting and zero: 0, 1, 2, 3, 4, 5, 6, 7, ...

denominator. The bottom integer in a fraction.

numerator. The top integer in a fraction.

IDENTIFY PLACE VALUE WITHIN DECIMALS

Another form of number quantity is decimal form. Numbers in decimal form have **place values**, as illustrated by the following **chart**.

This chart shows two examples of decimal numbers and how they are read.

Number	In Words
2134.14	Two thousand one hundred thirty-four and fourteen hundredths
0.00036	Thirty-six hundred-thousandths

The decimal part of any number can be read using the place value of the last nonzero decimal digit. In the case of 0.00036, the 6 is the last nonzero decimal digit. Because the 6 is in the hundred–thousandths place, this is how it is expressed.

CONVERTING FRACTIONS TO DECIMALS AND PERCENTAGES

To convert a fraction to decimal format, take the numerator and divide it by the denominator. For example, the fraction 3/8 can be converted to a decimal by finding 3 divided by 8, which is 0.375.

To convert a fraction to percentage format, first convert the fraction to a decimal. Then convert the decimal to a percentage by multiplying by 100. In connection with the example above, the fraction 3/8 is the decimal 0.375. If you multiply this by 100, you get 37.5%.

CONVERTING DECIMALS TO FRACTIONS

To convert from decimal to fraction form, put the number over the place value of the decimal part and remove the decimal point from the numerator. For the decimal 0.48, simply use 48 as the numerator and the place value of the last decimal digit as the denominator. In this case, the denominator would be hundredths. The decimal 0.48 would be written as 48/100 and read "forty-eight hundredths." If the decimal was 0.048, it would be written as 48/1000 and read "forty–eight thousandths."

When a decimal value is greater than 1, the same process applies. Convert the decimal 3.24 to a fraction. Because the last digit is in the hundredths place, the denominator of the fraction is 100. Removing the decimal point from the number and using it as the numerator gives us the fraction 324/100. The decimal 4.064 converts to 4064/1000 by, again, removing the decimal point from the numerator and using the last digit's place value, thousandths, as the denominator.

---

place value. Numerical value defined by position.

decimal place value. Powers of ten by position away from the decimal point. Going left: units, tens, hundreds, etc. Going right: tenths, hundredths, thousandths, etc.

chart. Information in the form of a table or graph.

CONVERTING PERCENTAGES TO FRACTIONS AND DECIMALS

Fractions are simplified when the numerator and denominator are integers that no longer share common factors. When converting 0.6% to a fraction, start by placing the percentage over 100 and removing the percent symbol. Then, create an equivalent fraction to remove the decimal. In this case, we multiply the numerator and denominator by 10 because the decimal is in the tenths place. Finally, **simplify** the fraction.

0.6% = 0.6/100

0.6/100 × 10/10 = 6/1000

6/1000 ÷ 2/2 = 3/500

To convert a percentage to a decimal, divide the percentage by 100, or move the decimal point two places to the left and drop the percent symbol. For example, the percentage 76.8% can be converted to the decimal equivalent 0.768.

The following chart shows some examples of conversions among percentages, fractions, and decimals.

Percentage	Fraction	Decimal
35%	35/100 = 7/20	0.35
28.4%	28.4/100 = 284/1000 = 71/250	0.284
55%	55/100 = 11/20	0.55
100%	100/100 = 1/1	1
0.09%	0.09/100 = 9/10,000	0.0009

Practice Problems

1. Convert each decimal to a percentage.

    A. 3.25

    B. 0.215

    Convert each percentage to a decimal.

    C. 62.9%

    D. 145%

    Convert each decimal to a fraction.

    E. 0.265

    F. 1.39

    Convert each fraction to a decimal.

    G. 26/10

    H. 16/25

2. What percentage is equivalent to 17/10?

3. Which of the following fractions is equivalent to 56.4%?

    A. 564/1000

    B. 564/100

    C. 564/10

    D. 564

4. What decimal number is equivalent to 3.75%?

5. Which of the following decimals is equivalent to 16/50?

    A. 0.32

    B. 0.68

    C. 1.47

    D. 3.125

simplify. Reduce a fraction or an expression to a simpler form by actions such as cancellation of common factors and regrouping of terms with the same variable.

M.1.2 — Perform arithmetic operations with rational numbers (including positive and negative numbers)

Performing basic computations by hand can, at times, be quicker than using a calculator. Additionally, calculators do not always complete the mathematical order of **operations** in ways you assume they will. For this TEAS task, you need to be competent at performing arithmetic calculations by hand. You will apply the **order of operations**—**addition**, **subtraction**, **multiplication**, **division**, exponents, and roots—and be expected to do so using integers, decimals, fractions, and **mixed numbers**. Practice makes perfect, so it might be helpful to search the internet for additional practice problems.

ORDER OF OPERATIONS

Knowing the order of operations is crucial to success on this task. One mnemonic device for the mathematical order of operations is PEMDAS, which stands for parentheses, exponents (which includes roots), multiplication and division, addition and subtraction. You will need to use parentheses, exponents, multiplication and division, and addition and subtraction in the correct order. To successfully execute these operations, you must follow these rules in order.

- First, perform any calculations inside parentheses.

- Next, perform any calculations involving exponents or roots.

- Next, perform all multiplication and division, completing the operations as they occur from left to right.

- Finally, perform all addition and subtraction, completing the operations as they occur from left to right.

> ### Objectives
>
> This objective includes, but is not limited to, the following examples of knowledge, skills, and abilities.
>
> - Perform computations with integers using the six basic operations (addition, subtraction, multiplication, division, exponents, roots).
>
> - Perform computations with decimals using the six basic operations $(+, -, \times, \div, \wedge, \sqrt{})$.
>
> - Perform computations with fractions, including improper fractions and mixed numbers, using the six basic operations $(+, -, \times, \div, \wedge, \sqrt{})$.
>
> - Perform computations involving the order of operations, excluding complex fractions.

---

order of operations. The sequence of operations that must be followed to simplify an expression.

addition. Calculation of a total of two or more numbers.

subtraction. Removing one number from another; the inverse of addition.

multiplication. Addition of a number to itself a specified number of times.

division. Separation of numbers into parts; the inverse of multiplication.

mixed number. A number formed by an integer and a fraction.

COMPUTATIONS WITH INTEGERS

The following are three basic computations with rationales.

Example 1

$$3 + 5 \times 9$$

$3 + 5 \times 9$	Multiply first.
$= 3 + 45$	Then add.
$= 48$	

Example 2

$$24 \div 3 - 5$$

$24 \div 3 - 5$	Divide first.
$= 8 - 5$	Then subtract.
$= 3$	

Example 3

$$(4 - 1) \times \sqrt{9}$$

$= (4 - 1) \times \sqrt{9}$	Perform operations in parentheses first.
$= 3 \times \sqrt{9}$	Then take the root.
$= 3 \times 3$	Then multiply.
$= 9$	

MULTIPLE-STEP PROBLEMS

The following are several examples involving multiple steps.

Example 4

$$5 + 7 \times (3 + 9) \div 6 - 3^2$$

Solution:

Step 1:	$5 + 7 \times (3 + 9) \div 6 - 3^2 = 5 + 7 \times 12 \div 6 - 3^2$	Parentheses
Step 2:	$5 + 7 \times 12 \div 6 - 3^2 = 5 + 7 \times 12 \div 6 - 9$	Exponents
Step 3:	$5 + 7 \times 12 \div 6 - 9 = 5 + 84 \div 6 - 9$	Multiplication
Step 4:	$5 + 84 \div 6 - 9 = 5 + 14 - 9$	Division
Step 5:	$5 + 14 - 9 = 19 - 9$	Addition
Step 6:	$19 - 9 = 10$	Subtraction

Example 5

$$8 - 4 \div (5 - 3) \times 3 + 11$$

Solution:

Step 1:	$8 - 4 \div (5 - 3) \times 3 + 11 = 8 - 4 \div 2 \times 3 + 11$	Parentheses
Step 2:	$8 - 4 \div 2 \times 3 + 11 = 8 - 2 \times 3 + 11$	Division
Step 3:	$8 - 2 \times 3 + 11 = 8 - 6 + 11$	Multiplication
Step 4:	$8 - 6 + 11 = 2 + 11$	Subtraction
Step 5:	$2 + 11 = 13$	Addition

In the last two examples, you will notice that multiplication and division were evaluated from left to right according to rule 3. Similarly, addition and subtraction were evaluated from left to right according to rule 4.

OPERATIONS WITHIN PARENTHESES

When two or more operations occur inside a set of parentheses, these operations should be evaluated according to rules 2, 3, and 4. This means exponents and roots are completed first, then multiplication and division from left to right. Finally, addition and subtraction are completed from left to right. This is done in the following example.

Example 6

$$225 \div (3 + 2 \times 11) - 4$$

Solution

Step 1:	$225 \div (3 + 2 \times 11) - 4 = 225 \div (3 + 22) - 4$	Multiplication inside parentheses
Step 2:	$225 \div (3 + 22) - 4 = 225 \div 25 - 4$	Addition inside parentheses
Step 3:	$225 \div 25 - 4 = 9 - 4 = 5$	Order of operations to complete the problem

COMPUTATIONS WITH FRACTIONS

When a problem includes a fraction bar, this means we must divide the numerator by the denominator. However, when more than one number exists in the numerator or denominator, it becomes a group. These groups are like parentheses, so we must perform all calculations above and below the fraction bar before dividing. Considering the following example.

Example 7

$$\frac{47 - 5}{5 + 9}$$

Solution:

Perform all calculations above and below the fraction bar before dividing. Thus:

$$\frac{47 - 5}{5 + 9} = \frac{(47 - 5)}{(5 + 9)}$$

Evaluating this expression, we get:

$$\frac{(47 - 5)}{(5 + 9)} = \frac{42}{14} = 3$$

Extensions of the preceding examples include decimals, fractions, and mixed numbers. With decimals, all processes are identical. With fractions, you might need to find a **common denominator** or convert fractions to decimals. With mixed numbers, you might need to convert to improper fractions first. To help prepare for the TEAS, search the internet for order of operations practice and work on your mastery of these types of problems.

---

common denominator. In a set of two or more fractions, an integer that is divisible by each denominator. That is, a multiple of all of the denominators.

Example 8

$$2.8 - 5.1(3.4 + 0.6)$$

Solution

Step 1:	$2.8 - 5.1(3.4 + 0.6) = 2.8 - 5.1(4)$	Parentheses
Step 2:	$2.8 - 5.1(4) = 2.8 - 20.4$	Multiplication
Step 3:	$2.8 - 20.4 = -17.6$	Subtraction

Example 9

$$2\ 1/4 \div 3/5 + 1\ 1/2$$

Solution

Step 1:	$2\ 1/4 \div 3/5 + 1\ 1/2 = 9/4 \div 3/5 + 3/2$	Change the mixed numbers to improper fractions.
Step 2:	$9/4 \div 3/5 + 3/2 = 9/4 \times 5/3 + 3/2 = 15/4 + 3/2$	Division (change to multiplication and take the *reciprocal* of the second fraction)
Step 3:	$15/4 + 3/2 = 15/4 + 6/4 = 21/4$ or $5\ 1/4$	Addition (find a common denominator)

Practice Problems

1. Solve the following problems.

   A. $6 + 8 \times (12 - 9)$

   B. $(14 - 5) \div (7 - 4)$

   C. $7 \times 4 + 8 \div 4 - 3 \times 6$

   D. $\dfrac{50 - 2 \times 7}{6 + 4 \times 3}$

2. Which of the following is the correct value of $3 + \sqrt{4} \times 6 - 4$?

   A. 32

   B. 10

   C. 11

   D. 26

3. Which of the following is the correct value of the expression?

   $$\dfrac{15 + 2 \times 5}{11 - 24 \div 4}$$

   A. 21

   B. 5

   C. ≈ 9.9

   D. ≈ 5.9

4. Which of the following is the correct value of the expression?

   $$50 - (2^3 \times 3) + \dfrac{9 + 6}{3}$$

   A. 31

   B. 35

   C. 131

   D. 135

5. Which of the following is the correct value of the expression?

   $$17 + \dfrac{18 - 2 \times 3}{6}$$

   A. 14

   B. 19

   C. 25

   D. 34

---

reciprocal. One divided by the original number; or, for a nonzero fraction *a/b*, the reciprocal is *b/a*. The product of a number and its reciprocal is 1.

M.1.3 — Compare and order rational numbers (including positive and negative numbers)

DEFINING RATIONAL NUMBERS

A **rational number** is one that can be written as a fraction a/b where a and b are integers and the denominator is not zero. What makes rational numbers unique is that these fractions can be written as either terminating or **repeating** decimals. For instance, ½ can be written as 0.5. This is a terminating decimal. One-third is a repeating decimal because it is equivalent to 0.3 repeating (0.333…). A whole number such as 4, can be written as 4/1 , 12/3, etc., but we usually see it in its simplified form: 4. Integers, like whole numbers, can be written as fractions by simply writing them as the numerator over a denominator of 1. For example, –27 can be written as –27/1. Conversely, **irrational numbers** cannot be written in fraction form. For example, √2 and pi converted to decimals are not terminating or repeating. Other examples of irrational numbers include the square roots of imperfect squares and the natural number e.

Objectives

This objective includes, but is not limited to, the following examples of knowledge, skills, and abilities.

- Identify symbols for "greater than," "less than," and/or "equal to."

- Identify place value with decimals.

- Convert fractions to a common denominator.

- Compare quantities/rational numbers using appropriate symbols (<, >, =).

- Order three or more quantities (e.g., least to greatest, greatest to least).

ORDERING RATIONAL NUMBERS

It is important to be able to put rational numbers in numeric order as well as visualize and predict situations involving ordered quantities. At times, interpreting ordered number inequality statements is as useful as interpreting **equations** (equality statements), but with **inequality symbols** instead of equal signs. The TEAS test requires you to compare and order rational numbers. Try searching the internet using any of the glossary terms to find additional explanations and practice problems.

It is important to note that negative numbers are smaller than **positive numbers**. If a number is to the left of another number on the number line, it is smaller. All negative numbers are to the left of all positive numbers.

To put rational numbers in numeric order (either increasing or decreasing), it can be useful to write the numbers as decimals (unless they are already integers, like –2, –1, 0, 1, 2). Once in decimal form, you can write the numbers vertically, lining up the decimals.

For example, the numbers 4.356, 4.635, and 0.6534 can be stacked this way:

4.356
4.635
0.6534

---

rational number. A number that can be expressed as a fraction.

repeat. Do again.

irrational number. A real number that cannot be expressed as terminating or repeating decimals.

equation. A mathematical statement that indicates the equality of two expressions.

inequality symbols. Less than (<), greater than (>), less than or equal to (≤), and greater than or equal to (≥).

non-negative. Greater than or equal to zero (positive or zero).

Next, analyze the digit with the highest place value (in this case, the ones place) to determine which is the largest or smallest. If you want to put the numbers in decreasing order, start with the highest value. In this example, two numbers start with 4 in the ones place, so it is necessary to compare digits in the tenths place for these two numbers.

In this case, the larger number of the two is 4.635, because 6 tenths is larger than 3 tenths. The next largest number is determined in the same way: 4.356. This process continues until all numbers in the list are in order. The decreasing order and increasing order lists are summarized below.

> *Decreasing order list: 4.635, 4.356, 0.6534*

> *Increasing order list: 0.6534, 4.356, 4.635*

If the numbers are not in decimal form and it is unclear how to order all of them, the fractions or fraction parts can be divided to convert them into decimal form. For instance, for 3 5/6, divide 5 by 6 to get 0.8333 repeating, so the value becomes (approximately) 3.8333. Then, the converted fractions can be compared to the other numbers in decimal form.

COMPARING RATIONAL NUMBERS

You can use comparison symbols to compare and order rational numbers.

Symbol	Meaning
>	Greater than
<	Less than
≥	Greater than or equal to
≤	Less than or equal to

The decreasing order list–4.635, 4.356, 0.6534–can be written as 4.635 > 4.356 > 0.6534.

The increasing order list–0.6534, 4.356, 4.635–can be written as 0.6534 < 4.356 < 4.635.

Inequalities such as 4.356 ≤ 4.635 are also accurate, because 4.356 is truly less than OR equal to 4.635. Here, the qualifying portion is the "or."

You can compare fractions and mixed numbers with different denominators by rewriting the numbers as equivalent fractions or mixed numbers.

To find the lowest common denominator, do the following.

2. Find the **least common multiple** of the denominators (also called the lowest common denominator).

3. Rewrite each fraction as an equivalent fraction using the least common multiple of the denominators.

---

least common multiple. The smallest number that is a multiple of two or more nonzero whole numbers.

Example: Use the lowest common denominator for $\frac{2}{5}$, $\frac{1}{6}$, and $\frac{4}{15}$ to compare and order the fractions.

List the **multiples** of each denominator:

- Multiples of 5 are 5, 10, 15, 20, 25, 30, 35, 40, ...
- Multiples of 6 are 6, 12, 18, 24, 30, 36, 42, 48, ...
- Multiples of 15 are 15, 30, 45, 60, 75, 90, 105 ...

30 is the least common multiple appearing in each list.

Therefore, the **least common denominator** of $\frac{2}{5}$, $\frac{1}{6}$, and $\frac{4}{15}$ is 30.

The equivalent fractions are $\frac{2}{5} = \frac{12}{30}$, $\frac{1}{6} = \frac{5}{30}$, and $\frac{4}{15} = \frac{8}{30}$

Decreasing order: $\frac{2}{5}, \frac{4}{15}, \frac{1}{6}$ or $\frac{12}{30}, \frac{8}{30}, \frac{5}{30}$

Increasing order: $\frac{1}{6}, \frac{4}{15}, \frac{2}{5}$ or $\frac{5}{30}, \frac{8}{30}, \frac{12}{30}$

This method works well for numbers that are not too big. The TEAS test will stick to more manageable numbers.

Practice Problems

1. Write the following in increasing order.

   8, 8 3/4, 8.43

2. Which of the following is a correct comparison of 9.14 and 9 1/6?

   A. 9.14 > 9 1/6

   B. 9.14 < 9 1/6

   C. 9.14 = 9 1/6

   D. 9.14 ≥ 9 1/6

3. Which of the following lists the numbers in decreasing order?

   -4, 0.4, 4 1/5, -0.04

   A. -4, 0.4, 4 1/5, -0.04

   B. -0.04, -4, 0.4, 4 1/5

   C. 4 1/5, 0.4, -4, -0.04,

   D. 4 1/5, 0.4, -0.04, -4,

4. Which of the following lists the numbers in increasing order?

   3/8, 3/4, 11/16, 1/2

   A. 1/2, 3/8, 3/4, 11/16

   B. 11/16, 3/8, 3/4, 1/2

   C. 3/8, 1/2, 11/16, 3/4

   D. 3/4, 3/8, 1/2, 11/16

5. Which of the following lists the numbers in decreasing order?

   -1 3/5, -1.45, -1.8, -1 3/4

   A. -1.45, -1 3/5, -1 3/4, -1.8

   B. -1.8, -1 3/5, -1 3/4, -1.45

   C. -1 3/4, -1.45, -1 3/5, -1.8

   D. -1 3/5, -1.45, -1.8, -1 3/4

multiples of a number. A number multiplied by various integers.

least common denominator. The least common multiple of the denominators of two or more fractions.

M.1.4 — Solve equations with one variable

IDENTIFY THE TERMS OF AN ALGEBRAIC EQUATION

An equation is a statement that shows that two *expressions* are equal to each other. *Algebraic equations* consist of *terms*. A term is a number, variable, or product of numbers and variables. Terms are separated by addition and subtraction signs. A number by itself is called a constant. A variable is a letter that represents an unknown quantity. A *coefficient* is the number being multiplied by a variable. A variable written without a numerical part has a coefficient of one.

To succeed at this TEAS task, you will need to practice solving a *range* of equations with one variable.

Algebraic equations with one variable can have one or more terms with that same variable.

Objectives

This objective includes, but is not limited to, the following examples of knowledge, skills, and abilities.

- Identify the terms of an algebraic equation.
- Apply inverse arithmetic operations.
- Implement a sequence of steps to solve equations.
- Solve proportional relationships (i.e., equations and inequalities) with one variable.

Equation	Variable Terms	Constants	Coefficients
$x + 6 = 10$	x	6 , 10	1
$4x - 7 = 2x + 11$	$4x, 2x$	-7, 11	4, 2

APPLY INVERSE ARITHMETIC OPERATIONS

Inverse mathematical operations are the opposites of each other and cancel each other out. These include but are not limited to:

- addition and subtraction.
- division and multiplication.

For example, to cancel a subtraction operation, use addition. To cancel a division operation, use multiplication. If you want to cancel multiplication of a fraction, you can cancel the multiplication by division. Recall that to divide by a fraction, you need to multiply by the reciprocal of the fraction.

expression. A finite string of mathematical symbols (numbers, operations, variables) that are grouped to show a value.

algebraic equation. A mathematical sentence that includes one or more variables.

term. A number, variable, or product of numbers and variables.

coefficient. The number being multiplied by a variable.

range. The difference between the highest and lowest values in a set.

inverse arithmetic operations. Mathematical operations that cancel each other out.

IMPLEMENT A SEQUENCE OF STEPS TO SOLVE EQUATIONS

To **solve** an equation means to find the value of the variable that will make the equation true (i.e., both sides of the equation have the same value).

Here are some guidelines to follow:

1. **Combine** all **variable terms** on one side of the equal sign using inverse operations.

2. Combine all constants on the other side of the equal sign using inverse operations.

3. Use inverse operations to isolate the variable.

The following examples illustrate using inverse operations to solve algebraic equations with one variable. Notice when the **solution** is substituted into the equation to check the answer, the left side of the equation is equal to the right side.

Solve: $x + 35 = 74$

$x + 35 = 74$	Original equation.
$x + 35 - 35 = 74 - 35$	Subtract 35 from both sides. Subtraction cancels addition.
$x = 39$	Simplify.
$39 + 35 = 74$	Check your answer.
$74 = 74$	

Solve: $(4/5)x = 20$

$(4/5)x = 20$	Original equation.
$5/4 \times (4/5)x = (20/1) \times (5/4)$	Multiply both sides by the reciprocal of 4/5.
$x = 25$	Simplify.
$(4/5) \times (25/1) = 20$	Check your answer.
$100/5 = 20$	

Solve: $x - 8 = -14$

$x - 8 = -14$	Original equation.
$x - 8 + 8 = -14 + 8$	Add 8 to both sides. Addition cancels subtraction.
$x = -6$	Simplify.
$-6 - 8 = -14$	Check your answer.
$-14 = -14$	

Solve: $5x + 5 = 2x - 10$

$5x + 5 = 2x - 10$	Original equation.
$5x - 2x + 5 = 2x - 2x - 10$	Subtract 2x from both sides.
$3x + 5 = -10$	Simplify by combining variable terms.
$3x + 5 - 5 = -10 - 5$	Subtract 5 from both sides.
$3x = -15$	Simplify by combining constants.
$3x/3 = -15/3$	Divide both sides by 3.
$x = -5$	Simplify.
$5(-5) + 5 = 2(-5) - 10$	Check your answer.
$-25 + 5 = -10 - 10$	
$-20 = -20$	

Solve: $4x = 7$

$4x = 7$	Original equation.
$\dfrac{4x}{4} = \dfrac{7}{4}$	Divide both sides by 4. Division cancels multiplication.
$x = \dfrac{7}{4}$	Simplify.
$\dfrac{28}{4} = 7$	Check your answer.

---

solve. Find the answer.

combine like terms. Simplifying an expression by using the distributive property.

variable term. Any term that includes an unknown quantity.

solution. The answer.

SOLVE PROPORTIONAL RELATIONSHIPS (I.E., EQUATIONS AND INEQUALITIES) WITH ONE VARIABLE

A **proportional** relationship between two quantities occurs when the **ratio** of one quantity to another is constant, or when one fraction is equivalent to the other. The constant rate is called the **constant of proportionality** and is represented by the variable k. To solve a proportional relationship with an unknown quantity, a method called "cross multiplication" can be used. Consider the equation below.

$$5/6 = x/18$$

To cross multiply, multiply the numerator of the left fraction by the denominator of the right fraction, and set this equal to the denominator of the left fraction multiplied by the numerator of the right fraction. Then solve the resulting equation by dividing by the coefficient of the variable.

$$5(18) = 6x$$

$$\frac{90}{6} = \frac{6x}{6}$$

$$15 = x$$

Practice Problems

1. Solve the equation below. Which of the following is correct?

   $x - 17 = 48$

   A. 65

   B. 55

   C. 31

   D. 21

2. Solve: $2x - 6 = -4x$

3. Solve: $6x = 19$

4. Solve: $\frac{7}{5}x = 35$

5. Given the equation $6x - 9 = 3x + 12$, which of the following is an acceptable first step toward solving the equation?

   A. Subtract 9 from both sides of the equation.

   B. Add 12 to both sides of the equation.

   C. Subtract 3x from both sides of the equation.

   D. Add 6x to both sides of the equation.

---

proportion. An equality of two ratios.

ratio. Shows the number of times one number is contained within another number.

constant of proportionality. The constant ratio between two quantities.

M.1.5 — Solve real-world problems using one- or multi-step operations with real numbers

Mathematics is a tool we use to observe the world around us, collect and analyze data about our world, and help answer questions and solve problems. Many simple problems can be solved with one or two steps using simple **real numbers**. Being able to recognize the patterns used in these problems will make the solutions easier. Repeated practice will help this process to become automatic and prepare you for success at this TEAS task.

PROBLEM-SOLVING PLAN

Most problems you encounter will not include specific instructions to guide you to a solution. Following are four major ideas and more specific strategies to keep in mind when solving problems.

Objectives

This objective includes, but is not limited to, the following examples of knowledge, skills, and abilities.

- Identify pertinent and extraneous information in a word problem.

- Determine the necessary operation(s) from contextual clues in a word problem.

- Construct an equation to model a real-world situation.

- Perform arithmetic operations with real numbers to solve equations in a real-world context and label the answer with the correct units of measure (e.g., feet, seconds, kilometer).

- Assess the reasonableness of the solution/answer to a problem.

Understand Problem	Devise Plan	Carry Out Plan	Look Back
<ul><li>Identify given information.</li><li>Determine what you need to find or show.</li><li>Determine what is happening in the problem.</li><li>Determine whether you have enough information to solve the problem.</li><li>Determine whether any information given is not needed (*extraneous* information).</li></ul>	<ul><li>Guess and check.</li><li>Make an orderly list.</li><li>Eliminate possibilities.</li><li>Use direct reasoning.</li><li>Solve an equation.</li><li>Look for a pattern.</li><li>Draw a picture.</li><li>Use a model.</li><li>Work backward.</li><li>Use a formula.</li></ul>	<ul><li>Implement your chosen plan.</li><li>If the plan does not seem to be working, try a different approach.</li></ul>	<ul><li>Check to make sure you answered the question.</li><li>Check to see if your answer is reasonable.</li><li>Make sure all of the parts of the problem are answered.</li></ul>

---

real numbers. The set of rational and irrational numbers.

extraneous. Irrelevant.

When you are first in the phase of understanding the problem, look for situations that are modeled by the four operations: addition, subtraction, multiplication, and division. Some of the ways to think about each operation are listed in the following table.

Addition	Subtraction	Multiplication	Division
• joining • putting together	• separating • removing • distancing • comparing differences	• total number of equal groups • *area* • scaling • comparing—multiplication (e.g., three times as much)	• how many in each group/portion • how many groups/portions

REAL NUMBERS IN THE REAL WORLD

Real numbers are used in these problems. Rational numbers are a subset of real numbers that can be represented by fractions. These include integers and all decimals that either **terminate** or repeat. Irrational numbers, such as the square root of five, will not be discussed here.

Most problems will be in a real-world **context**. In the real world, you will likely not have a boss that says, "Solve these 10 quadratic equations and have them on my desk by 5 o'clock." Instead, you will have to take information from several sources, analyze it, determine what the question is that you need to solve, pick out the pertinent information, choose the correct procedure, solve the problem mathematically, and check the reasonableness of the answer. This takes practice.

Practice Problems

1. Jayden wants to use square pavers that are 4 inches on each side to completely surround their flower garden. The garden is 8 feet long and 2 feet wide. How many pavers should Jayden buy?

2. A cat owner gets a vitamin prescription from his veterinarian that lists the dosage as 2.5 mL twice a day. The bottle contains 200 cc. How many days will the bottle last?

3. On Monday, the nurse determined that her patient's total fluid intake for the day was 1,800 mL. On Tuesday, the same patient's total fluid intake was 2,350 mL. If the patient's total fluid outtake over the two days was 1,775 mL, what was his net result?

4. A recipe for 1 batch of cookies calls for 3/4 cup of flour. How much flour is required to bake 1 1/2 batches of cookies?

5. In a small community, 1,225 students take the bus to school. If there are a total of 1,955 students enrolled in the school system, approximately what percentage of students take the bus to school?

---

terminate. To end.

contextual. Related to surrounding content.

area. The amount of space inside a two-dimensional boundary.

M.1.6 — Solve real-world problems involving percentages

PERCENTAGE REVISITED

Percentage is a form of a number quantity. For this task on the TEAS, you will need to understand what percentage means in real-world situations as well as how to work with percentages within these contexts. You will have to find the percentage of a number quantity as well as **percent increase** or **decrease**. You will need to utilize the problem-solving skills discussed in the previous chapter and, if needed, search the Internet for additional practice problems of these types.

Percentage means "per 100," or a value's proportional equivalent compared to 100. One percent can be interpreted as one one-hundredth of something. Examples of percentage expressions are 25%, 19.2%, 50%, 250%, and 0.08%.

When a percentage is less than or equal to 100%, then you can say "out of" 100. For example, 75% is 75 out of 100. However, if a percentage is more than 100%, you need to rethink the wording. It would not exactly work to say that 175% is 175 out of 100, because 175% is 175 for each 100. For example, 175% of 20 is 35.

Following are 100 small squares, and 50 have been shaded.

One way to describe the shading is to say 50% has been shaded—in other words, 50 out of 100. Likewise, 50 cents is 50% of 100 cents (or 50% of $1.00).

Other real-word percentage contexts include percent off for a sale price, annual percent interest rates at a bank, annual percent gain or loss for a company or business, percent commission for a salesperson, percent depreciation of assets, and percentages of ingredients in a mixture or recipe.

You will need to find the percentage of a number to determine a part or portion.

> ### Objectives
>
> This objective includes, but is not limited to, the following examples of knowledge, skills, and abilities.
>
> - Identify quantities needed to calculate a percentage in a real-world situation.
> - Calculate a percentage of a quantity.
> - Use a percentage to calculate a quantity.
> - Find a percent increase/decrease between two quantities.

Example

> At a major airport, 15% of all flights experienced a delay or cancellation due to weather. If there were 220 flights in all, how many flights experienced a delay or cancellation?

15% = 0.15	Rewrite 15% as a decimal.
$220 \times 0.15 = 33$	Multiply 220 by the decimal equivalent.

There were 33 flights that experienced a delay or cancellation due to weather.

---

percent increase. The positive change between two numbers, divided by the first number, multiplied by 100.

percent decrease. The negative change between two numbers, divided by the first number, multiplied by 100.

PERCENT INCREASE OR DECREASE

You also need to find the percentage of a number to solve problems involving increase or decrease. In the next two examples, two methods are presented, but they will yield the same solution.

Example

> Kathryn purchases $60 worth of groceries and pays 8% state tax. How much is her total bill with tax?

Method 1	
8% = 0.08	Rewrite 8% as a decimal.
0.08 × 60 = 4.80	Multiply the decimal equivalent by $60.
60 + 4.80 = 64.80	Add.

Method 2	
100% + 8% = 108%	Add 8% to 100%.
108% = 1.08	Rewrite 108% as a decimal.
60 × 1.08 = 64.80	Multiply the decimal by $60.

Kathryn's total grocery bill is $64.80.

Example

> Haru purchases a new jacket originally priced at $140.00. The store offers a 30% discount. How much does Haru pay for the jacket with the discount?

Method 1	
30% = 0.30	Rewrite 30% as a decimal.
140 × 0.30 = 42	Multiply the decimal equivalent by $140.
140 − 42 = 98	Subtract.

Method 2	
100% − 30% = 70%	Subtract 30% from 100%.
70% = 0.70	Rewrite 70% as a decimal.
140 × 0.07 = 98	Multiply the decimal by $140.

Haru pays a discounted price of $98.00 for the jacket.

Given that you are solving many problems that can have an increase or decrease, remember to pay attention to the type of situation in the problem. Some situations are summarized below.

Increase
Tax, mark up, increased by, gained

Decrease
Discount, markdown, decreased by, depreciation, loss

Practice Problems

1. Your current salary is $55,000. Next year, you will get a 4.5% increase in your salary. How much more money will you make next year?

2. Which of the following is 35% of 900 pounds?

    A. 315 pounds

    B. 595 pounds

    C. 865 pounds

    D. 1,205 pounds

3. While shopping, you find a shirt that is marked 25% off. If the regular price is $50, what is the reduced price?

4. A computer tablet costs $550.00. If the sales tax is 6.5%, which of the following is the total cost of the tablet with sales tax?

    A. $35.75

    B. $514.25

    C. $556.50

    D. $585.75

5. A car salesperson earns $900 each month plus 6% commission on her monthly car sales. If she sells $58,000 worth of cars on a given month, which of the following is her total monthly salary?

    A. $4,380.00

    B. $3,534.00

    C. $3,480.00

    D. $3,426.00

M.1.7 — Apply Estimation Strategies and Rounding Rules to Real-World Problems

METRIC MEASUREMENTS

While the United States still uses standard measurements, you will work primarily with the **metric system** in medical studies. Additionally, for the purposes of the **estimation** strategies and **rounding** rules described by this TEAS task, you will be using metric measurements. It can be helpful to practice thinking metrically in your daily life as well, such as when you shop and drive. You will also want to practice using rounding rules and estimation strategies when solving word problems.

First, you must have knowledge of some simple approximations for common metric units. Study the following table.

Metric Unit	Household Approximation
Millimeter (mm)	The diameter of a pinhead
Centimeter (cm)	Average size of a fingernail
Meter (m)	A doorway is just over 2 m tall
Kilometer (km)	1 km equals about 2/3 of a mile
Gram (g)	The weight of a small paper clip
Kilogram (kg)	The weight of a pineapple
Degrees Celsius (°C)	Zero is freezing, 10 is not; 20 is warm, and 30 is hot!

Objectives

This objective includes, but is not limited to, the following examples of knowledge, skills, and abilities.

- Estimate measurements (e.g., area, length, weight, volume).

- Determine the appropriateness of estimation procedures, including rounding.

- Apply estimation strategies (e.g., using a simpler problem).

- Apply rounding rules (e.g., rounding to ones, tenths, and hundredths; rounding fractions and mixed numbers).

Note that abbreviations for metric units do not have a period after them. Area is measured in **square units**, such as square meters (m^2). **Volume** is measured in **cubic units**, such as cubic centimeters (cm^3). The exponent "3" is used for metric volume, and the abbreviation "cu." is usually used for standard system units. Liquid volume is measured in liters (L) or milliliters (mL). Because carbonated beverages are sold in 2–liter bottles, this is one conversion you are probably already familiar with. One liter contains 1,000 milliliters, or 1,000 cubic centimeters (1 L = 1,000 mL = 1,000 cc). Helpful tip: 1 cc is the same as 1 mL.

---

metric system. International System of Units (French: Système international d'unités, SI) based on powers of ten.

estimation. A rough calculation of numbers.

rounding. Simplifying a number by removing decimal places or changing those places to zero.

square units. Units used to measure area. One square unit is the area of a square with sides that measure 1 unit.

volume. The amount of space taken up by a three-dimensional shape.

cubic units. Units used to measure volume. One cubic unit is the volume of a cube with sides that measure 1 unit.

ESTIMATION AND ROUNDING

Estimating and rounding are two skills that make many problems quicker and easier to solve. Good judgment should be used when deciding if estimating and rounding are appropriate. Sometimes a "ballpark" figure is reasonable. Even in a laboratory setting, where precision and accuracy are extremely important, a quick estimate can tell you whether you have the decimal point in the right place and can help determine if your mathematical procedure was correct.

Estimation strategies that you should be familiar with include *front-end* estimation, in which you focus on the first digits of numbers when adding or subtracting and solving a simpler problem. For example, if you are trying to decide whether to upgrade your kitchen, you can use front-end estimation to get a ballpark idea of how much it would cost. Perhaps you find out that granite countertops will cost $3,250, having cabinets refaced will cost $7,600, and putting in a new stove will cost $985. Using front-end estimation, you learn that it will cost around $11,700 to upgrade your kitchen because 3,000 + 7,000 + 200 + 600 + 900 = 11,700. The actual cost is $11,835 so this is a reasonable estimate to use to determine whether to upgrade your kitchen. There are plenty of other examples of solving a simpler problem and other estimation strategies available on the Internet, so be sure to search these key words and familiarize yourself with these strategies.

The decimal place to which you need to round depends on the problem. When rounding to a decimal place, such as the tenths or the hundredths place, look only at the digit immediately to the right of the place to which you are rounding. For 5 or larger, round up. Less than 5, just remove the digits that follow. Study the following table.

Round to	This place	And the answer is
73.281	Ones	73
73.281	Tens	70
73.281	Hundredths	73.28
0.6467	Thousandths	0.647
0.6467	Hundredths	0.65

When rounding fractions to the ones place, if the numerator is greater than or equal to half of the denominator, round up to the next whole number. If the numerator is less than half of the denominator, round down to the existing whole number. Study the following table.

Round to the ones place	And the answer is
1/12	0
7/12	1
7 2/8	7
7 5/8	8
19 8/20	19
3 4/5	4

Rounding decimals and fractions to whole numbers—which are easier to calculate in your head or quickly with scratch paper—will enable you to estimate whether your detailed calculations are reasonable. One frequent error is when the digits are correct but the decimal point is placed incorrectly.

front-end. An estimation method that focuses on the first digits of numbers when adding or subtracting and solving a simpler problem.

Practice Problems

1. Which of the following gives the best estimate for the equation?

$$\frac{346.8 \times 5.231}{49.6}$$

   A. $(347 \times 5)/50$

   B. $(340 \times 5)/49$

   C. $(300 \times 5)/50$

   D. $(346 \times 6)/49$

2. Round the numbers in the table to the place indicated.

Number	Round to	Your Answer
34.19	Tenths	
6/7	Ones	
7.219	Hundredths	
933.74	Thousands	
2.739	Hundredths	
32.834	Tenths	
37.494	Tens	
23/50	Ones	
7 2/3	Ones	
64.736	Tenths	
547	Tens	
878	Hundreds	

87.357	Hundredths	
32.95	Tenths	
483.34	Hundreds	

3. Which of the following metric units best represents the length of a paper clip?

   A. Meter

   B. Centimeter

   C. Liter

   D. Milliliter

4. Which of the following is best approximated by kilograms?

   A. A pet rabbit

   B. Water spilled from a cup

   C. A piece of paper

   D. A tablet of ibuprofen

5. The value of the equation is closest to which of the following?

$$\frac{873.5 \times 4.72}{59.6}$$

   A. 75,000

   B. 7,500

   C. 750

   D. 75

M.1.8 — Solve Real-World Problems Involving Proportions

Proportional thinking is a valuable real-world problem-solving approach. Proportions come up in scenarios from map reading to money exchange rates. To succeed on this TEAS task, you will need to understand not only what ratios and proportions are, but also how to set up a proportion using ratios, solve it, and identify the **rate of change**, also known as the constant of proportionality. The practice problems in this chapter will provide some examples, but you might want to seek out more practice in other sources as well.

INTRODUCTION TO PROPORTION

A proportion is a ratio in fraction form set equal to another ratio in fraction form. The numerator and denominator of each ratio are "**scaled**" up or down by the same factor. For instance, if one ratio is 3/8, a scaled-up ratio might be 9/24, because 3/8 × 3/3 = 9/24. Similarly, if one ratio is 4/5, the other might be 24/30 because 4/5 × 6/6 = 24/30.

Objectives

This objective includes, but is not limited to, the following examples of knowledge, skills, and abilities.

- Formulate a ratio in a given context.

- Construct a proportion using ratios.

- Solve a proportion with the correct units of measure (e.g., ft/sec, gal/hr).

- Identify a constant of proportionality (e.g., 8:2 as 12:3, proportionality constant is 4).

WRITING AND SOLVING A PROPORTION

One application of proportional relationships is using a map (a type of scale drawing). If the **legend** on a map reads 1 cm = 20 miles and you measure 6.4 cm between destinations, a proportion can be used to calculate how many miles (x) are represented by 6.4 cm. The proportion can be solved using cross multiplication, in which the numerator on one side of the equation is paired/multiplied with the denominator on the other side of the equation. This new equation can then solve to determine the value of x.

$$\frac{1 \text{ cm}}{20 \text{ miles}} = \frac{6.4 \text{ cm}}{x \text{ miles}}$$

1 cm × x miles = 6.4 cm × 20 miles

1x = 128 miles

x = 128 miles

---

rate of change. A rate that describes how one quantity changes in relation to another.

scale. Ratio of graphical representation to actual size.

legend. An explanation of figures used in a chart.

DIRECT PROPORTION AND CONSTANT OF PROPORTIONALITY

Two variables are directly proportional when they increase or decrease at the same rate. This rate is called the constant of proportionality. An equation can be written as $y = kx$, where k is the constant of proportionality.

You might also recall from studying linear equations that equations of lines can be written in the form of $y = mx + b$ (*slope*-intercept form). When $b = 0$ (y-intercept = 0), the equation becomes $y = mx$ (i.e., $y = kx$) and is directly proportional. Because m is the slope, in the case where $b = 0$, m is the constant of proportionality k.

Study the table to see what examples of directly proportional equations look like.

Directly Proportional Equations	Not Directly Proportional
$y = 4x,\ y = 8x,\ y = \dfrac{x}{5},\ y = \dfrac{2}{3}x$	$y = 2x + 9,\ y = x - 3,\ y = \dfrac{4}{x},\ y = 6$

Practice Problems

1. Micah spends 27 hours in a 3-week period practicing piano. At this rate, how many hours will he practice in 7 weeks?

2. The success rate for a salesperson is 2 out of 11 calls. At this rate, which of the following number of sales would the salesperson expect to get out of 55 calls?

   A. 5

   B. 6

   C. 10

   D. 16

3. A company found an average of 4 defective televisions for every 1,000 checked. If the company produced 95,000 televisions in 1 year, which of the following numbers of televisions would be expected to be defective?

   A. 11

   B. 380

   C. 905

   D. 1095

4. On a map, 1 cm = 75 miles. If the distance between two cities measures 8.6 cm, which of the following is the actual distance between the two cities?

   A. 8.7 miles

   B. 66.4 miles

   C. 82.6 miles

   D. 645 miles

5. Which of the following equations is a direct proportion?

   A. $y = x - 5$

   B. $y = 3x - 5$

   C. $y = 3x$

   D. $y = 5$

---

slope. The rate of change, or the steepness and direction, of a line on a coordinate plane.

M.1.9 — Solve Real-World Problems Involving Ratios and Rates of Change

A popular question in every math class is, "When are we ever going to use this?" Ratios and rates are one part of math that is used on a daily basis. How often do you ask the following?

Question	Answer
"How much does a cashier earn working?"	dollars/hour
"How fast is the train going?"	miles/hour
"Do I drink enough water?"	cups/day
"Does my smartphone data plan meet my usage needs?"	gigabytes/month
"Can I afford the mortgage payment for that house?"	(principal + interest + escrow)/month

It is the nature of our world today to think in terms of ratios and rates. Fortunately, the mathematical procedures for working with ratios and rates are quite simple. On the TEAS, you will encounter a range of real–world problems that involve ratios and rates of change, so you will want to understand these concepts and how to put them into practice.

Objectives

This objective includes, but is not limited to, the following examples of knowledge, skills, and abilities.

- Formulate a rate of change (generally expressed as some unit over time) in a given context.

- Use a ratio/rate of change to solve a problem.

- Convert a ratio to a unit rate (e.g., 15 beds for 3 nurses = 5:1).

- Compute a ratio for a real-world situation.

RATIO

A ratio shows how many times one number is contained within another number and is often represented as a fraction, which may or may not be written in the lowest terms. Examples of ratios include 2:3 or 2/3, 7:10 or 7/10, and 7:2 or 7/2.

RATE, UNIT RATE, AND RATE OF CHANGE

Ratios with units are called rates. Examples of rates include (2 cats)/(3 dogs), (7 absent)/(10 present), and (7 miles)/(2 hours).

A **unit rate** is a rate that is expressed per 1 unit. For example, for the rate (7 miles)/(2 hours), the unit rate would be (3.5 miles)/(1 hour), or 3.5 miles per hour. To find a unit rate, simply divide the numerator by the denominator. The unit rate is also called the rate of change.

---

unit rate. A rate that shows how many units of one quantity (in the numerator) correspond to one unit of the second quantity (in the denominator), such as miles/hour.

USING RATIO AND RATE OF CHANGE TO SOLVE PROBLEMS

Elijah manages a small crew of employees at the local utility company that clears trees that fall on electric lines. They use chainsaws that require an oil-and-gasoline fuel mixture with a ratio of oil to gas of 1:50. Normally, Elijah uses 12.8 fluid ounces of oil and 5 gallons of gasoline. Today is a small job, and he plans to use 1 gallon of gasoline. The normal rate is (12.8 fl oz)/(5 gal).

In order to have a 1 in the denominator, divide both numerator and denominator by 5. This is the same procedure we use to reduce fractions. After dividing by 5, the rate has been reduced to approximately (2.6 fl oz)/(1 gal). This is Elijah's unit rate. All rates must also be labeled with the units in the numerator and denominator.

Because rates relate two numbers with units or variables, they can be represented on a **graph**.

Riley keeps a chart on the money she saves each week from her weekly paycheck. By the end of the third week, she has saved $75.00, and by the end of the eighth week, she has saved a total of $200.00.

The graph of this situation is shown to the right.

First, find the rate of change, or slope of the line, containing these two points. To find the rate of change, m, find the change in the y–coordinates $(y_2 - y_1)$ divided by the change in the x–coordinates $(x_2 - x_1)$. The rate of change for Riley's weekly savings (3 weeks, $75) and (8 weeks, $200) is found this way:

m = ($200 – $75)/(8 weeks – 3 weeks)

   = $125/(5 weeks)

   = $25/(1 week)

You do not need to draw a graph to find the rate of change between two rates. To find the rate of change, use the slope formula below, where $(y_2 - y_1)$ is the difference between the y–coordinates and $(x_2 - x_1)$ is the difference between the x–coordinates.

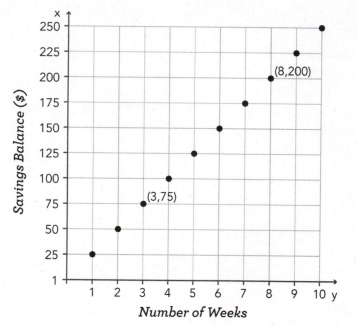

$$m = \frac{y_2 - y_1}{x_2 - x_1}$$

Jorge, who is an artist, has created 256 paintings over the course of four years. He has created paintings that are either portrait (taller than wide) or landscape (wider than tall). He has 145 landscape paintings and 111 portrait paintings.

We can write several ratios from this information.

- Portrait to landscape: 111/145
- Landscape to portrait: 145/111
- Portrait to total: 111/256
- Landscape to total: 145/256

graph. A drawing that represents relationships between numbers or data.

Min-seo works at a bakery. She pulls out a recipe and discovers that the number of cups is unreadable for a cake recipe. Her boss tells her that yesterday, the bakers used a total of 22 cups of cake flour to bake 6 cakes. The ratio of cups of cake flour to cakes is 22 cups per 6 cakes.

Min-seo needs to know the number of cups of cake flour to make one cake, so she writes down the ratio 22 cups per 6 cakes. She calculates the unit rate, or number of cups of flour needed to make one cake, by dividing the numerator and denominator by 6.

$$\frac{22 \text{ cups}}{6 \text{ cakes}} \div \frac{6}{6} = \frac{(22/6)}{1} = \frac{(11/3)}{1} = \frac{3 \ 2/3 \text{ cups}}{1 \text{ cake}}$$

This is the same procedure we use to reduce fractions. After dividing by 6, the rate has been reduced to 3 2/3 cups/1 cake. This is Min-seo's unit rate. All unit rates must also be labeled in the numerator and denominator.

Practice Problems

1. Use unit rates to determine which is the better vacation deal: $900 for 4 nights or $1,443 for 7 nights.

Read the passage and answer the following question.

Jada enters a fitness challenge with her friends at work. They all go walking during lunch to stay fit. Jada decides to track her total steps over 1 month. At the end of the month, she looks back at her records and finds them incomplete. Here is what she sees.

Day	Total Steps Taken This Month at Lunch
3	1,950
7	4,550
20	13,000
22	14,300

3. Which of the following expresses the unit rate in steps per day?

   A. 3 days/1,950 steps = 0.002 days/step.

   B. The unit rate is 1,950 steps/3 days.

   C. The unit rate is 650 steps/day.

   D. The unit rate is 650 steps/1.

4. A box of cereal costs $4.80 for 24 ounces. Which of the following represents the unit rate (price) per ounce?

   A. 5 oz/$1

   B. $4.80/24 oz

   C. 20/1

   D. $0.20/oz

5. Three months into a new Internet/phone/cable plan, Alex has paid a total of $360. Ten months into the plan, they have paid a total of $1,130. Which of the following is the average rate of change for Alex's cable plan between months 3 and 10?

   A. $110/month

   B. $113.33/month

   C. $113.67/month

   D. $114.00/month

6. Joe has a drawer full of 28 different-colored markers. He knows he has 7 red markers and 4 black markers. Which of the following expresses the ratio of red markers to total markers?

   A. 1/7

   B. 1/4

   C. 7/4

   D. 4/7

M.1.10 — Solve Real-World Situations Using Expressions, Equations, and Inequalities

EXPRESSIONS, EQUATIONS, AND INEQUALITIES

Expressions are mathematical phrases that contain numbers, variables, and/or operations. Equations relate expressions that are equal to each other. Inequalities relate expressions that are not equal using comparison symbols, such as greater than or less than.

Some examples are shown.

Expressions	Equations	Inequalities
$9 - 2y$	$9 - 2y = 27$	$9 - 2y < 27x$
$-x$	$x = 8$	$x < 8$
$3(x - 12)$	$-3(x - 12) = 2(3x + 15)$	$-3(x - 12) \geq 2(3x + 15)$

TRANSLATION TO EQUATIONS AND INEQUALITIES

One of the foundational steps of solving problems is translating written text in the problem into algebraic notation. This involves turning words and phrases into variables, numbers, and operations. You will need to understand how those elements combine to create expressions, equations, and inequalities. To be successful at this TEAS task, you will need to practice shifting between the concrete and the abstract.

Objectives

This objective includes, but is not limited to, the following examples of knowledge, skills, and abilities.

- Define/identify the variables (unknown quantities) based on real-world situations.

- Identify the key words which describe specific mathematical operations (e.g., and, difference between, by, is).

- Draw a sketch of the situation, if appropriate, to help clearly identify variables.

- Determine the necessary operation(s) from contextual clues.

- Formulate an expression, equation, or inequality using the identified variables and necessary operations.

- Solve the equation or the inequality to address the real-world situation, and provide a response using the correct units of measure.

- Assess the reasonableness of the solution/answer to the problem.

Translating written language into algebra reduces the information to its most basic level. Phrases become expressions, and sentences become equations or inequalities.

You will be the author of these translations. Think of this as naming characters in your story, using variables as names to represent unknown quantities.

Suppose Xavier attends a local fair. He spends a total of $25.00, which includes $5.00 admission to the fair and 8 rides. When he returns home, his dad wants to know how much it costs for a single ride.

This is a word problem. Identify the extraneous or **erroneous** information. Pick a variable and tell what it represents. This is called defining the variable. Traditionally, x and y are used for variables, but it can be helpful to use a letter that better represents the quantity in the context of the problem.

r = the cost of one ride

Decide what the context of the story tells you about the relationship. "... He spends a total of $25.00, which includes $5.00 admission to the fair and 8 rides." Therefore, the cost of one ride relates to the number of rides. The cost of all rides is the cost of one ride, r, multiplied by the number of rides, 8. The cost of rides and admission combine to create the total cost.

$8r + 5 = 25$

$8r + 5 - 5 = 25 - 5$

$8r = 20$

$r = 2.5$, so each ride costs $2.50. This answer is reasonable because it is a small fraction (in the neighborhood of 1/8) of the total amount of $25.

Vivian is at the supermarket and wants to spend no more than $70 on groceries. She knows that she will spend $45.00 on necessities, but wants to buy pepperoni, which costs $5 per pound. How much pepperoni can she buy while staying within her spending limit?

p = pounds of pepperoni	Define the variable.
$5p$	Total cost of pepperoni.
$5p + 45$	She will spend $45.00 on necessities.
$5p + 45 \leq 70$	Finally, the total is "no more than," or less than or equal to, $70.
$5p \leq 25$	
$p \leq 5$ lb	

She can buy no more than 5 pounds of pepperoni.

---

erroneous. Incorrect.

Practice Problems

1. Naomi decides to collect postcards. She starts her collection with nine cards. Every week, she buys two more cards to add to her collection. Write an inequality that would allow her to find how many weeks until she has more than 35 cards.

2. James is saving money to go to a concert. From his part-time job, he is able to save $20 per week. His older brother gave him $15 to start. If W = number of weeks, which of the following represents the number of weeks until James has saved at least $255?

   A. $20W + 15 = 255$

   B. $(15 + 20)W \geq 255$

   C. $20W + 15 \geq 255$

   D. $20W + 15 < 255$

3. Arya wants to take a taxi to a restaurant. She has only $25 for a taxi ride plus some change in her purse for the driver's tip. The taxi company charges $2.00 to get in the taxi plus $1.75 per mile. If M = miles to a restaurant, which of the following expressions represents the maximum distance to a restaurant that Arya can afford?

   A. $1.75M < 25$

   B. $2.00 + 1.75M > 25$

   C. $(2.00 + 1.75)M \leq 25$

   D. $2.00 + 1.75M \leq 25$

4. Hector spent the morning driving 100 miles. He drives at an average speed of 60 miles per hour. Which of the following inequalities can be used to determine the time, T, it will take to drive at least 350 miles?

   A. $60T < 350$

   B. $100 + 60T > 350$

   C. $100 + 60T \leq 350$

   D. $100 + 60T \geq 350$

Read the passage and answer the following question.

Three more than five times a number x is greater than three times the same number, decreased by nine.

5. Which of the inequalities models the sentence?

   A. $5x + 3 \geq 3x - 9$

   B. $5x + 3 > 3x - 9$

   C. $(5 + 3)x > (5 - 9)x$

   D. $5x + 3 > 9x - 3$

Measurement and Data

M.2.1 — Interpret relevant information from tables, charts, and graphs

You have probably heard the saying, "a picture is worth a thousand words." Now, imagine how much information is packed into a data **table** or graph. You can extrapolate all types of useful details from such data. The amount of information available in our society is multiplying at an incredible rate. Using charts, graphs, and tables helps to relay such relevant information. Charts, graphs, and tables make the presentation of data much clearer. They help readers understand the relationship between quantities, how fast they are changing, and the importance of the data.

For the TEAS, you will need to understand the various parts of these graphical displays and how to interpret information from tables, charts, and graphs. A variety of graphical displays can be used to express data, such as **Cartesian coordinate** graphs, **line graphs**, **scatterplots**, **pie charts**, and **bar graphs**. It is important to choose the right type of display for a set of data. For example, a line graph can be used to track changes over time, whereas a pie chart is used to show parts of a whole.

Objectives

This objective includes, but is not limited to, the following examples of knowledge, skills, and abilities.

- Identify different types of graphical displays, tables, and charts and their components.
- Identify the elements of a graph, chart, or table.
- Identify and interpret the structure of a data table.
- Identify and interpret the labels of a graph or chart.
- Identify and interpret the information in the legend of a graph or chart.
- Identify and interpret the scale of the axes of a graph.
- Identify and verify findings, trends, and relationships.
- Analyze information to summarize and/or form conclusions.
- Predict outcomes based on existing data.
- Select the most appropriate graphical display to use for the data set.
- Formulate graphs, charts, and tables based on a data set (e.g., plot data in a coordinate plane, create a table or chart, label elements).

table. A set of data displayed in rows and columns.

Cartesian coordinates. An ordered pair or ordered triple used to specify a point on a plane or space, respectively.

line graph. A graph that uses lines or line segments to represent data or trends.

scatterplot. A graph that uses dots to represent data points to show relationships between two numeric variables.

pie chart. A circular graph with "slices" suggestive of a pie; the larger the slice, the greater the quantity being represented.

bar graph. A graph that uses vertical or horizontal bars to represent quantities.

GRAPHS AND TABLES

Most graphs you study will represent the relationship between two sets of data or parameters. These types of graphs are **bivariate**. Traditionally, this is shown as a Cartesian coordinate graph. When plotting a **point** or reading the coordinates of a point, remember to move from the origin in the horizontal direction first and then in the vertical direction. This ensures a unique point that corresponds to one pair of coordinates.

Compare the points on the graph with the table of coordinates.

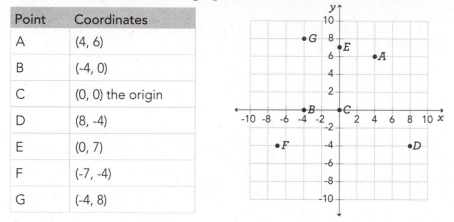

Point	Coordinates
A	(4, 6)
B	(-4, 0)
C	(0, 0) the origin
D	(8, -4)
E	(0, 7)
F	(-7, -4)
G	(-4, 8)

Notice points D and G. Reversing the coordinates results in two completely different points, and in this case, they are even in different **quadrants**.

Graphs tell a story and show the relationship between variables. The graphs you study will not be random collections of points. Consider the graph, Monique's Water Intake on Saturday.

The title conveys what the graph shows: the ounces of water Monique drank on a Saturday. The x-axis displays the time of day, from 8:00 a.m. until 6:00 p.m. The y-axis shows the total number of ounces drank. The scale says 10s of fluid ounces, so 2 on the y-axis represents 20 ounces of water. Using a scale such as this often saves space and makes the graph easier to read. A scale can be shown within a label or in a legend. Any point on the graph can be read as a pair of coordinates.

Can you find the point for 4 p.m. when Monique had drunk 100 ounces of water? What did Monique do between 4 and 6 p.m.? Monique drank another 20 ounces of water. Do you see that by 6 p.m., Monique drank 120 ounces of water? Using the data in the graph as your guide, what would you predict Monique's water intake to be by 8 p.m.? A simple graph can contain a large amount of information.

Monique's Water Intake on Saturday

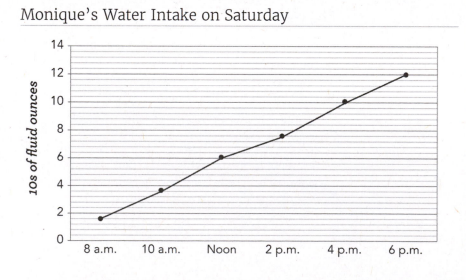

bivariate. Containing two variables.

point on a graph. The location of a value expressed as (x, y).

quadrants. In a Cartesian graph of a plane, the four quarters into which the plane is divided by the two axes. Labeled with Roman numerals, starting with Quadrant I for the upper-right quarter and proceeding counterclockwise.

Practice Problems

1. Which of the following observations based on this graph is correct?

   A. The cost of maintaining a car is constantly increasing each year.

   B. For the first 3 years, it costs $400 to maintain the car.

   C. The average rate of change between year 1 and year 4 is
   $$\frac{\$800 - \$200}{4 \text{ years}} = \$600/4 \text{ years} = \$150/\text{year.}$$

   D. The average rate of change between year 1 and year 4 is
   $$\frac{\$800 - \$200}{4 \text{ years} - 1 \text{ year}} = \frac{\$600}{3 \text{ years}} = \$200 \text{ per year.}$$

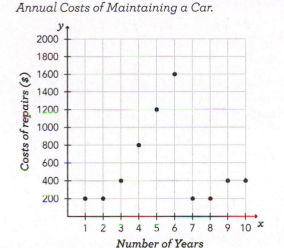

Annual Costs of Maintaining a Car.

2. Which of the following observations based on this graph is true?

   A. Day 3 yielded the most zucchini sold.

   B. The number of pounds of corn sold from days 1 to 3 increased each day.

   C. About 10 pounds of squash was sold over the 3 days.

   D. The most carrots were sold on day 3.

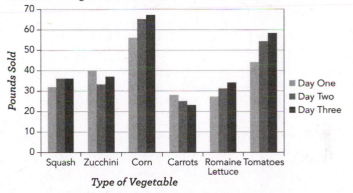

Amount of Vegetables Sold at Frank's Farm Stand

Use this graph to fill in the table and answer the question.

Nights	Dani's Tips	Frank's Tips
Monday		
Tuesday		
Wednesday		
Thursday		
Friday		

3. On what night did Dani's daily tips decrease from the previous night? On what night(s) did Frank earn more in tips than Dani? What is the average rate of change for Frank from Monday to Friday?

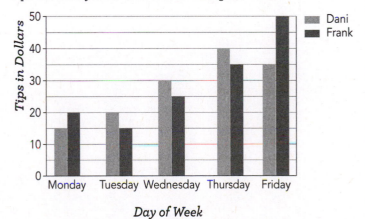

Tips Earned by Dani and Frank During the Week

Practice Problems (cont.)

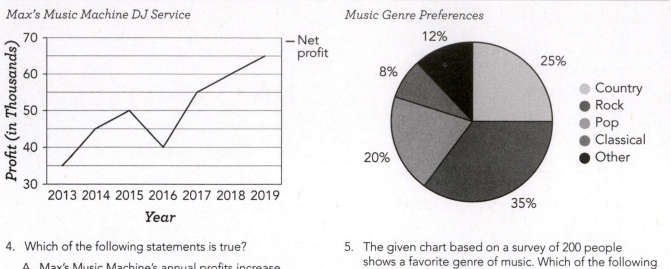

Max's Music Machine DJ Service

Music Genre Preferences

4. Which of the following statements is true?

   A. Max's Music Machine's annual profits increase annually.

   B. The greatest increase in profits was between 2016 and 2017.

   C. Max earned $0 in 2013.

   D. There were two yearly increases of $5,000 between 2013 and 2019.

5. The given chart based on a survey of 200 people shows a favorite genre of music. Which of the following statements is true?

   A. Country music is the favorite of 25 people.

   B. Country music is preferred by 5 more people than pop music.

   C. The most popular music is rock.

   D. There were 40 people who chose neither rock nor country.

M.2.2 — Evaluate the information in data sets, tables, charts, and graphs using statistics

Statistics and data analysis are important parts of what many professionals do quantitatively. These two disciplines help us understand the world of numbers. They help us clear up areas in which there can be uncertainties. The TEAS test requires that you understand some basic concepts and carry out basic statistical calculations. The Internet is a good resource for glossary term definitions, additional explanations, and practice problems.

MEAN, MEDIAN, AND MODE

The mean, median, and mode are three **measures of central tendency**. They are used to summarize a set of data.

Mean. The average. Add all the numbers in a set or list and divide by how many numbers there are in the set

- A number set includes: 3, 3, 3, 7, 8, 9, 9, 14. First, add $3 + 3 + 3 + 7 + 8 + 9 + 9 + 14$, which equals a **sum** of 56. Next, divide the sum by how many numbers are in the set. There are eight numbers, so divide 56 by 8 for a mean of 7.

Median. Median is the middle number of an ordered list. If there are an odd number of terms, there is one middle number. If there is an even number of terms, there are two middle numbers, so the mean of those two middle numbers is the median.

- For the same set of numbers as given for the mean (i.e., 3, 3, 3, 7, 8, 9, 9, 14), there are eight numbers. Because this is an even number, there are two middle numbers: 7 and 8. Next, find the mean of those two numbers to find the median for the number set. The median of this set is 7.5.

Mode. Mode is the number(s) in a list that occurs most often. If a list includes two modes, it is **bimodal**.

- For the same set of numbers as given for the mean (i.e., 3, 3, 3, 7, 8, 9, 9, 14), 3 is the mode because it occurs most often.

---

measures of central tendency. Mean is commonly known as the average; median is the middle value; and mode is the number repeated most often.

sum. The result of addition.

bimodal. Describes a distribution of data with two clear peaks.

RANGE

Range is one measure of **spread** for a data set. To find the range, subtract the minimum value from the maximum value. This is sometimes referred to as the **absolute difference**, meaning the absolute value of the difference of two numbers. For the example given in the table for the mean, median, and mode, 14 − 3 = 11, so 11 is the range. Spread can be determined from a graph as well. The highest y-value is the maximum value, and the lowest y-value is the minimum value. Once these are determined, the same process to find the range is used. The spread reflects the variability of the data. Observations that cover a wide range have a large spread. Observations that are clustered near a single value have a small spread.

Standard deviation describes how data varies from the mean. A standard deviation that is high indicates data that is spread out, whereas a low standard deviation describes a data set where the majority of values are close to the mean.

The **shape** of a data distribution can reveal valuable information. There are several common distribution patterns.

Symmetry

A symmetric distribution can be divided at the center with each half mirroring the other. Dividing the below distribution at 51, both halves mirror each other.

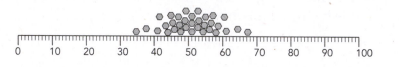

Number of Peaks

Distributions of data can have few or many peaks. A distribution with a single clear peak is called "**unimodal**," and a distribution with two clear peaks is called "bimodal."

Bimodal

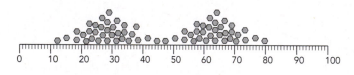

Bell-Shaped, Unimodal

When a symmetric distribution has a single peak at the center, it is referred to as "bell-shaped." A bell-shaped, unimodal peak is also referred to as a "normal distribution."

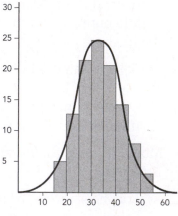

---

spread. The range of values in data distribution.

absolute difference. The absolute value of the difference of two numbers.

standard deviation. A quantity that indicates the extent to which data varies from the mean.

shape. Symmetry, number of peaks, skewness, and uniformity of data distribution.

unimodal. Describes a distribution of data with a single clear peak.

Skewness

Some graphic distributions have more observations that fall on one side of the graph compared to the other. Distributions with fewer observations on the right (toward higher values) are skewed right.

Skewed right

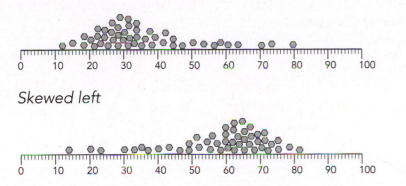

Skewed left

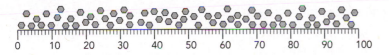

Distributions with fewer observations on the left (toward lower values) are skewed left.

Uniform

When the observations in a data set are spread equally across the range of the distribution, this is a called a "uniform distribution." A uniform distribution has no clear peaks.

TRENDS IN GRAPHS AND TABLES

Data sets in a graph or a table also reveal trends, or patterns, in the data. **Data trends** are usually easy to see in simple data tables, like the one shown below. As the value of x gets closer to 6.0 from either direction, the value of y increases. Trends can be more difficult to find in complicated data tables. This is where graphs can be used. Graphs are valuable because they make trends easier to see. The graph clearly shows that as the value of x increases, the value of y increases, until the value is 6.0. After that, the value of y has a decreasing trend in relation to the value of x.

Does the value of x affect y?	
Value of x	Value of y
1.0	50
3.5	70
6.0	100
8.5	80
11.0	60
13.5	30

Data set models can reveal what are known as **expected values** and **outliers**. An "outlier" is an unexpected value that does not fit any trend or pattern in the data. The graph above illustrates an example of an outlier.

All points on the graph follow along the trend line except the one that is way above the rest of the data. Visually, we can qualify this point as an outlier, or unexpected value. All of the other data points follow the same trend and, thus, are expected values.

PROBABILITY

Data sets often contain information regarding events that can be measured numerically. When trends are identified, the information within the data can also be used to determine the likelihood of an event occurring if another data piece were to be collected.

Simple **probability** can be found by dividing desired outcomes by the total number of outcomes in the data set.

P (event) = (number of desired outcomes)/(total number of outcomes)

For example, a student has taken 12 math tests in a course and has 8 grades in the 90s, 3 grades in the 80s, and 1 grade in the 70s. This data can be used to determine the likelihood that, with equal preparation and level of understanding, her next test score is in the 90s by calculating the probability, P.

Currently, 8 (the desired outcome) of her 12 test scores (the total outcomes) are in the 90s, so $P = 8/12 \approx 0.667$. So it is 66.7% likely that she will score in the 90s on her next test.

data trend. General tendency of numbers in a set.

expected value. The most likely value of a random variable.

outlier. A data point that is distinctly separate from other data; an unexpected value.

probability. The likelihood that an event will occur.

Practice Problems

1. Find the mean, median, and mode of the following data set: 0, 1, 2, 2, 3, 5, 6, 7, 8, 16

Use the graph to answer the following question.

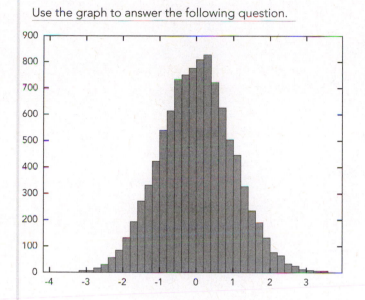

2. Which of the following best describes the distribution portrayed in the graph?

   A. Bell-shaped

   B. Bimodal

   C. Skewed left

   D. Skewed right

Use the graph to answer the following question.

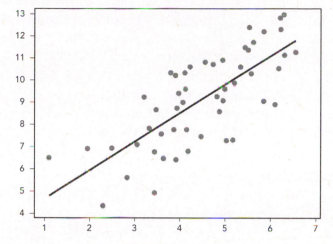

3. Which of the following describes the trend of the data portrayed in the graph?

   A. Decreasing

   B. Increasing

   C. Stable

   D. No trend

4. Which of the following statements best describes a distribution that is skewed left?

   A. The data peaks closer to lower values.

   B. The data peaks closer to higher values.

   C. The data peaks closer to middle values.

   D. There are no clear peaks.

5. Which of the following describes a decreasing trend?

   A. As one set of values decreases, the other set of values also decreases.

   B. As one set of values increases, the other set of values decreases.

   C. As one set of values increases, the other set of values remains constant.

   D. Both sets of values neither increase nor decrease.

M.2.3 — Explain the relationship between two variables

The concept of a variable is one of the most powerful and important ideas in mathematics. Variables allow us to work with both known and unknown quantities. A variable represents a quantity that can truly vary. Much of your work will involve the relationship of two variables and how the change in one causes a change in the other. Being able to mathematically describe or interpret this dynamic relationship between two variables is essential for your success on this TEAS task.

Nothing happens in isolation. When you sit down to study, you increase your knowledge and decrease your free time. When you buy a new video game, your use of technology goes up and the money in your pocket goes down. When you exercise, you increase the calories you burn and decrease your weight.

DEPENDENT AND INDEPENDENT VARIABLES

In all of these examples, one variable depends on another variable. When the first quantity changes, the second quantity changes in response. The first quantity is called the "***independent variable***," and the second quantity is called the "***dependent variable***." Let's look at an example.

As the temperature of a glass of water decreases, the speed at which water molecules move also decreases. The temperature is the independent variable, and the molecule speed is the dependent variable.

You can transfer variables to a graph. The independent variable goes on the x-axis (horizontal **axis**), and the dependent variable goes on the y-axis (vertical axis). This helps you visualize the relationship between the variables. In the following example, you are traveling 100 miles in total. You can see that as your speed (independent variable) increases, your travel time (dependent variable) decreases. These two variables are inversely related.

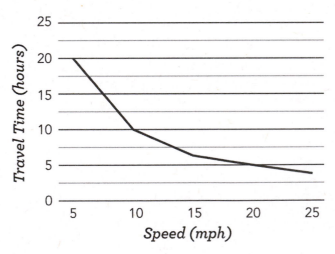

---

independent variable. A variable that determines the value of another variable.

dependent variable. A variable that depends on at least one other variable.

axis. A reference line for measurement of coordinates.

CORRELATION

If you get paid an hourly wage, then the time you spend working at a job is a constantly changing number. For every hour you work, the money you earn increases for that pay period. The time is a quantity that varies. We can represent it with a variable. Let t = the number of hours worked. In between pay periods, the money you earn varies, and it can be represented with a different variable. Let m = money earned from working. As t increases, m increases. The variables t and m are positively (or directly) related.

The monthly bills I owe decrease when I pay them off. I can pay them off when I work and earn money. When I work, I always pay my monthly bills. As the money I earn increases, my monthly bills decrease.

Again, let m = money earned from working. Let b = balance of monthly bills. As m increases, b decreases. The variables m and b are negatively (or inversely) related.

We describe this relationship between variables as **correlations**, or covariance. If both variables increase, a positive correlation exists, and the variables are directly related. If one increases and the other decreases, there is a negative correlation, and the variables are inversely related.

COMPARE AND CONTRAST DIRECT AND INVERSE RELATIONSHIPS

When two quantities have a direct relationship, or **direct variation**, we can relate two variables x and y using the direct variation equation: y = kx, where k is the constant of proportionality, as discussed in previous lessons. To determine the value of k, use known values of x and y and solve for k.

When two quantities have an inverse relationship, or **inverse variation**, we can relate two variables x and y using the inverse variation equation: y = k/x. In order to determine the value of k, use known values of x and y and solve for k.

---

correlation. The way two variables change together, also known as covariation.

direct variation. When two variables increase or decrease at the same rate.

inverse variation. When an increase or decrease in one variable produces a decrease or increase, respectively, in another variable.

Practice Problems

Read the passage and answer the following question.

From 2006 to 2012, it was found that MLB players with higher batting averages tended to score more runs. This relationship makes sense because higher batting averages suggest that the players get more hits onto the field, which in turn, allows teammates already on base to reach home plate and score a run.

1. Which of the following sentences best describes this relationship?

    A. The two variables show a positive correlation.

    B. The two variables are constants and represent fixed points in time.

    C. The batting average is the dependent variable.

    D. The two variables are inversely related.

Read the passage and answer the following question.

The table represents the side of a square compared to its area.

Side	Area
1 inch	1 square inches
2 inches	4 square inches
3 inches	9 square inches
4 inches	16 square inches

2. For this relationship, the side of the square and the area of the square are directly related and show a positive correlation. Based on this relationship, which of the following statements is true?

    A. If these two variables were graphed, the slope of the line between any two points would be negative.

    B. If these two variables were graphed, the side of the square would be the dependent variable.

    C. The points on the graph should be connected with a straight line to show that they represent variables.

    D. If these two variables were graphed, the slope of the line between any two points would be positive.

3. Determine whether each statement is true or false.

    A. Every scatterplot shows an example of covariance.

    B. The more I practice the piano, the better my performance at the recital is. This is an example of positive covariance.

    C. "No pain, no gain" is an example of direct variation, positive covariance.

    D. "The more I cough, the less likely I can run at a fast pace," is an example of direct variation, negative covariance.

4. Which of the following represents a negative correlation?

    A. The more snow we get, the less likely school is open.

    B. The less you drive, the less money you spend on gasoline.

    C. The more snow we get, the more likely school will be closed.

    D. The more you drive, the more money you spend on gasoline.

Read the passage and answer the following question.

The table represents the average daily temperature in degrees Fahrenheit compared to daily sales for a small ice cream stand.

Temp.	Sales
95	$7800
85	$7350
65	$5900
55	$5100
45	$3850

5. Which of the following statements is true?

    A. There is an inverse relationship between temperature and ice cream sales.

    B. There is a negative correlation.

    C. There is a positive correlation.

    D. The rate of change for any two points is always negative.

M.2.4 — Calculate geometric quantities

Geometric quantities, such as **length**, area, and volume, are part of our daily lives. It may never cross your mind, but calculating a geometric quantity is a skill you experience quite often. How long is the route to the grocery store? How big is the living room that needs to be carpeted? What volume of liquid can fit into a container? On the TEAS, you need to be able to calculate length, area, and volume of shapes (regular and **irregular**) using various units.

Length is measured with a tool such as a ruler or tape measure. The table summarizes some **units of length**, some of which are US customary and some of which are metric.

US Customary	Metric
inches (in), feet (ft), yards (yd), miles (mi)	millimeters (mm), centimeters (cm), meters (m), kilometers (km)

PERIMETER AND CIRCUMFERENCE

Both straight and curved figures possess length, or the distance of a side or around a curve. "**Perimeter**" is the distance around an entire shape. Perimeter is the sum of the individual lengths of the parts of the shape going around the shape once. Some shapes have all straight sides (e.g., rectangle, square, trapezoid, triangle).

Objectives

This objective includes, but is not limited to, the following examples of knowledge, skills, and abilities.

- Identify the measure of length as a linear measure.

- Identify the measure of area as a square unit measure.

- Identify the measure of volume as a cubic unit measure.

- Determine the perimeter of a shape.

- Determine the circumference of a circle.

- Calculate linear measures by finding the sum of the lengths of sections with correct units of measure.

- Calculate the area of an irregular shape by finding the sum of the areas of sections.

- Determine the volume of a solid.

---

length. The measure from end to end.

irregular shape. A shape in which not all sides and angles are equal.

linear units. Units used to measure length.

perimeter. The distance around a two-dimensional shape.

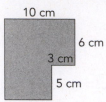

To find the perimeter of a complex shape with straight sides, simply add the lengths of all the sides together. To get the missing long side, add 6 cm and 5 cm. To get the missing short side, subtract 3 cm from 10 cm. The perimeter is then calculated as 10 + 6 + 3 + 5 + 7 + 11 = 42 cm.

Curved figures include circles or **arcs**, which are incomplete circles. The "**circumference**," or distance around a circle, can be found by using the formula $C = 2\pi r$ (π is approximately 3.14, and r is the radius of the circle). A variation of this formula is $C = \pi D$ where D is the diameter, or twice the radius. The length of an arc (part of a circle) can be found by using the formula $C = 2\pi r$ and then multiplying by the following fraction (the fraction of the circle that the arc covers).

$$\frac{\text{central angle measure}}{360}$$

Some shapes are curved, and some have a combination of straight and curved. To find the perimeter of this shape, add 3 + 3 + 6 + the length of the semicircular top.

The length of the semicircle can be calculated by finding half of $C = 2\pi r$, or just πr. The radius is half of 6 in, or 3 in; therefore, the semicircle distance is $\pi \times 3$, or approximately 9.42 in.

Thus, the entire perimeter is approximately 3 + 3 + 6 + 9.42 = 21.42 in.

arc. Part of the circumference of a circle.

circumference. The distance around a circle.

AREA

Area is how much surface space something takes up. It is measured in square units. Area units include square inches (in²), square feet (ft²), square yards (yd²), square miles (mi²), and square meters (m²). Areas can cover a flat surface (such as a shipping crate) or curved surface (such as an orange). Area and **surface area** have one simple, yet important, difference: area is for two-dimensional space (flat), and surface area is for three-dimensional space.

The following table provides basic area formulas with examples.

Shape		Formula	Example
Square		$A = l \times l = l^2$	Length = 4 ft $A = 4 \times 4 = 16$ ft²
Rectangle		$A = l \times w$	Length = 8 cm, width = 6 cm $A = 8 \times 6 = 48$ cm²
Triangle		$A = 1/2 \times b \times h$	Base = 3 m, height = 8 m $A = 1/2 \times 3 \times 8 = 12$ m²
Parallelogram		$A = h \times b$	Height = 6 cm, base = 9 cm $A = 9 \times 6 = 54$ cm²
Trapezoid		$A = 1/2 \times h \times (b_1 + b_2)$	Height = 6 ft, base 1 = 8 ft, base 2 = 5 ft $A = 1/2 \times 6 \times (8 + 5) = 39$ ft²
Circle		$A = \pi \times r^2$	Radius = 5 mm $A = \pi \times 25 = 25\pi \approx 78.5$ mm²
Rhombus		$A = 1/2 \times d_1 \times d_2$	Diagonal 1 = 4 yd, diagonal 2 = 9 yd $A = 1/2 \times 4 \times 9 = 18$ yd²

surface area. The total area of a three-dimensional object's surface.

M.2.4 — Calculate geometric quantities

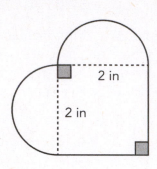

When you have a composite, or irregular, shape, you can use a combination of formulas from the table to find area.

The square area is l × l, or 2 in × 2 in, or 4 in².

For each semicircle, find the area of a circle with a 1 in radius and then divide by 2. This would be π × (1²)/2 ≈ 3.14 × (1/2) or approximately 1.57 in².

Then add the three areas, which comes to approximately 7.14 in² for the combined area.

VOLUME

Volume is how much space a three-dimensional object takes up. It is measured in cubic units. Volume units include cubic inches (in³), cubic centimeters (cm³), milliliters (mL), and fluid ounces (fl. oz). Volume can relate to the amount of matter that is within a three-dimensional solid or to the space within a hollow shape, such as the capacity of a container.

Shape		Formula	Example
Rectangular Prism		$V = l \times w \times h$	Length = 3 cm, width = 2 cm, height = 4 cm $V = 3 \times 2 \times 4 = 24$ cm³
Triangular Prism		$V = \dfrac{b \times h \times l}{2}$	Base = 4 in, height = 3 in, length = 5 in $V = \dfrac{4 \times 3 \times 5}{2} = 30$ in³
Cylinder		$V = \pi r^2 h$	Radius = 2 m, height = 1.5 m $V = \pi \times 2^2 \times 1.5 = 6\pi \approx 18.8$ m³
Cone		$V = \dfrac{\pi r^2 h}{3}$	Radius = 4 cm, height = 6 cm $V = \dfrac{\pi \times 4^2 \times 6}{3} = 30\pi \approx 100.5$ cm³
Rectangular Pyramid		$V = \dfrac{l \times w \times h}{3}$	Length = 6 in, width = 4 in, height = 9 in $V = \dfrac{6 \times 4 \times 9}{3} = 72$ in³
Sphere		$V = \dfrac{4}{3}\pi r^3$	Radius = 2 cm $V = \dfrac{4}{3} \times \pi \times 2^3 = \dfrac{32\pi}{3} \approx 33.5$ cm³

Practice Problems

1. Find the area of the shaded region.

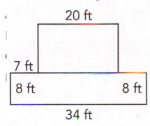

2 m
7 m
10 m
12 m

2. A rectangle and a square align at their bases with the rectangle in front of the square. Which of the following is the perimeter of the front-facing view of these shapes as shown in the diagram?

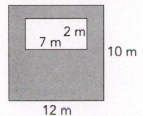

20 ft
7 ft
8 ft   8 ft
34 ft

3. What is the area of the following shape?

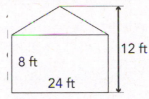

12 ft
8 ft
24 ft

4. What is the area of the following shape?

A
B.
C
D

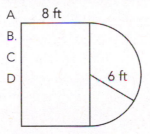

8 ft
6 ft

5. What is the area of the following shape?

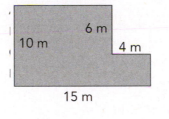

6 m
10 m   4 m
15 m

M.2.5 — Convert within and between standard and metric systems

No matter what career you pursue, you will work with numerical quantities in some form every single day. Equally important to these numbers are the units attached to those numbers. Measuring quantities accurately with the correct units is an extremely important skill to master. The health and safety of clients depend on it. You should be familiar with all of the standard and metric units used in medicine. This primarily involves length, volume, mass, and temperature. The TEAS will test your ability to convert among various values accurately, and you should be familiar with some of the most common conversions.

STANDARD SYSTEM

The following table summarizes some useful conversions within the U.S. customary system.

Original Unit	Equivalent Unit
1 ft	12 in.
1 yd	3 ft
1 mi	5280 ft
I lb	16 oz
1 pt	2 c
1 gal	4 qt
1 t	2000 lb

Objectives

This objective includes, but is not limited to, the following examples of knowledge, skills, and abilities.

- Calculate conversions using dimensional analysis.

- Convert within standard/customary/household systems (e.g., quarts to gallons, teaspoons to tablespoons).

- Convert within metric system (mL to L, mcg to mg, cm to m).

- Given a conversion factor, convert between standard and metric systems (fluid oz to mL, lb to kg, Fahrenheit to Celsius).

You can use **dimensional analysis** to convert from one unit to another. Start the mathematical expression with what you know and end with what you are trying to find.

For example, if an infant weighs 275 oz, you can convert this number to pounds.

$$275 \text{ oz} \times \frac{1 \text{ lb}}{16 \text{ oz}} \approx 17.2 \text{ lb}$$

Multiplying by a **conversion factor** is the same as multiplying by 1. This is because the numerator and denominator name the same quantity. Thus, the value of what we know is not changed; only its representation is changed.

---

dimensional analysis. Applying the technique of multiplication by 1 with rates to convert from one unit to another.
conversion factor. The number used to multiply or divide to convert from one value to another.

METRIC SYSTEM

The metric system was designed to make conversions easier. The units for length, volume, and mass are directly related to each other. The prefixes indicate the degree of quantity of the root, no matter what characteristic is being measured. There are many prefixes for the metric system, but those you will use on a daily basis are limited and shown in the following table.

Prefix	Meaning	Example
kilo	1, 000	1 kg = 1, 000 g; 1 kL = 1,000 L; 1 km = 1,000 m
deca	10	1 dag = 10 g; 1 daL = 10 L; 1 dam = 10 m
deci	1/10	1 dm = 1/10 m, or equivalently, 10 dm = 1 m
centi	1/100	1 cm = 1/100 m, or equivalently, 100 cm = 1 m
milli	1/1000	1 mg = 1/1000 g, or equivalently, 1, 000 mg = 1 g
micro	1/1,000,000	1 mcL = 1/1,000,000 L, or equivalently, 1,000,000 mcL = 1 L

If a provider prescribes 500 mg of medication 3 times a day, how many grams of medication should be given each day?

The number of milligrams per day can be found by: 500 mg × 3 times = 1500 mg/day. Then converting to grams gives:

$$\frac{1500 \text{ mg}}{1 \text{ day}} \times \frac{1 \text{ g}}{1000 \text{ mg}} = 1.5 \text{ g/day}$$

Another way to think about this is moving the decimal in 1500 three places to the left because 1 mg = 1/1000 g. Considering the latter method makes it easier to convert among metric units.

CONVERTING BETWEEN STANDARD AND METRIC SYSTEMS

Here is a table that is useful in converting between U.S. customary system measurements and the metric system.

Original Unit	Equivalent Unit	Original Unit	Equivalent Unit
1 gal	3.8 L	1 mi	1.6 km
I kg	2.2 lb	1 oz	28.35 g
1 in	2.54 cm	1 m	1.09 yd
1 m	3.28 ft		

To convert between units, use dimensional analysis. For example, if you needed to convert 14 pounds to kilograms, the needed conversion factor is 1 kg = 2.2 lb. Multiply what you know by the conversion factor (hint: write it as a fraction).

$$14 \text{ lb} \times \frac{1 \text{ kg}}{2.2 \text{ lb}} \approx 6.4 \text{ kg}$$

As long as you can find the conversion factor, any conversion can be accomplished. One more example: convert 250 g into ounces. The conversion factor is 1 oz = 28.35 g.

$$\frac{250 \text{ g}}{1} \times \frac{1 \text{ oz}}{28.35 \text{ g}} \approx 8.82 \text{ oz}$$

Practice Problems

Read the passage and answer the following question.

Jalen is preparing dinner. He is using a cookbook his aunt sent him from Europe. The recipe calls for 5 mL vanilla extract. Jalen only has a teaspoon for measuring. He finds that 1 tsp equals 4.93 mL.

1. Which of the following calculates the needed amount?

    A. $\dfrac{4.93 \text{ mL}}{\text{tsp}} \times 5 \text{ mL} = 24.65 \text{ mL}$

    B. $\dfrac{4.93 \text{ mL}}{\text{tsp}} \times \dfrac{1}{5} = 0.986 \text{ tsp}$

    C. $\dfrac{4.93 \text{ mL}}{\text{tsp}} \times \dfrac{1 \text{ tbsp}}{14.8 \text{ mL}} = 0.333 \text{ tsp}$

    D. $\dfrac{5 \text{ mL}}{1} \times \dfrac{1 \text{ tsp}}{4.93 \text{ mL}} = 1.014 \text{ tsp}$

Read the passage and answer the following question.

Patricia is in Ireland on vacation. While shopping, she sees a pretty sweater in a shop window. The price is marked €50. Patricia had seen the same scarf in the United States for $45. The conversion rate in the bank window next to the store says €1 = $1.20. Patricia is deciding whether the sweater in the window is a good deal or if she should wait until she returns to the United States to purchase it.

2. Which of the following describes how to solve this dilemma?

    A. Divide €50 by $1.20 per €.

    B. Divide €50 by 12.

    C. Multiply €50 by $1.20 per €.

    D. Divide €50 by $45.

3. In the following table, match the equivalent quantities. Refer to the conversions presented in this lesson. If necessary, you can consult the Internet.

Original Unit	Equivalent Unit
1. 750 mL	A. 12 kg
2. 75 mL	B. 4 cm
3. 26.4 lb	C. 5 in
4. 100° C	D. 75 cc
5. 600 m	E. 212° F
6. 12.7 cm	F. 0.75 L
7. 40 mm	G. 0.72 kg
8. 720 g	H. 0.6 km

4. Approximately how many feet are in 3 m?

    A. 0.9 ft

    B. 1.18 ft

    C. 7.62 ft

    D. 9.84 ft

5. Remi had 5 gal of gas remaining in their tank when they stopped at a gas station in Canada. They added 35 L of gas to the tank to fill the car. How much gas in liters does Remi have?

Mathematics Key Terms

absolute difference. The absolute value of the difference of two numbers.

addition. Calculation of a total of two or more numbers.

algebraic equation. A mathematical sentence that includes one or more variables.

arc. Part of the circumference of a circle.

area. The amount of space inside a two-dimensional boundary.

axis. A reference line for measurement of coordinates.

bar graph. A graph that uses vertical or horizontal bars to represent quantities.

bimodal. Describes a distribution of data with two clear peaks.

bivariate. Containing two variables.

Cartesian coordinates. An ordered pair or ordered triple used to specify a point on a plane or space, respectively.

chart. Information in the form of a table or graph.

circumference. The distance around a circle.

coefficient. The number being multiplied by a variable.

combine like terms. Simplifying an expression by using the distributive property.

common denominator. In a set of two or more fractions, an integer that is divisible by each denominator. That is, a multiple of all of the denominators.

constant of proportionality. The constant ratio between two quantities.

contextual. Related to surrounding content.

conversion factor. The number used to multiply or divide to convert from one value to another.

correlation. The way two variables change together, also known as covariation.

cubic units. Units used to measure volume. One cubic unit is the volume of a cube with sides that measure 1 unit.

data trend. General tendency of numbers in a set.

decimal. A number expressed based on place value

decimal place value. Powers of ten by position away from the decimal point. Going left: units, tens, hundreds, etc. Going right: tenths, hundredths, thousandths, etc.

denominator. The bottom integer in a fraction.

dependent variable. A variable that depends on at least one other variable.

dimensional analysis. Applying the technique of multiplication by 1 with rates to convert from one unit to another.

direct variation. When two variables increase or decrease at the same rate.

division. Separation of numbers into parts; the inverse of multiplication.

equation. A mathematical statement that indicates the equality of two expressions.

erroneous. Incorrect.

estimation. A rough calculation of numbers.

expected value. The most likely value of a random variable.

expression. A finite string of mathematical symbols (numbers, operations, variables) that are grouped to show a value.

extraneous. Irrelevant.

fraction. A number expressed as a numerator and denominator.

front-end. An estimation method that focuses on the first digits of numbers when adding or subtracting and solving a simpler problem.

graph. A drawing that represents relationships between numbers or data.

independent variable. A variable that determines the value of another variable.

inequality symbols. Less than (<), greater than (>), less than or equal to (≤), and greater than or equal to (≥).

integers. Whole numbers and their opposites: …, −3, −2, −1, 0, 1, 2, 3, …

inverse arithmetic operations. Mathematical operations that cancel each other out.

inverse variation. When an increase or decrease in one variable produces a decrease or increase, respectively, in another variable.

irrational number. A real number that cannot be expressed as terminating or repeating decimals.

irregular shape. A shape in which not all sides and angles are equal.

least common denominator. The least common multiple of the denominators of two or more fractions.

least common multiple. The smallest number that is a multiple of two or more nonzero whole numbers.

legend. An explanation of figures used in a chart.

length. The measure from end to end.

line graph. A graph that uses lines or line segments to represent data or trends.

linear units. Units used to measure length.

measures of central tendency. Mean is commonly known as the average; median is the middle value; and mode is the number repeated most often.

metric system. International System of Units (French: Système international d'unités, SI) based on powers of ten.

mixed number. A number formed by an integer and a fraction.

multiples of a number. A number multiplied by various integers.

multiplication. Addition of a number to itself a specified number of times.

non-negative. Greater than or equal to zero (positive or zero).

numerator. The top integer in a fraction.

operation. A mathematical action.

order of operations. The sequence of operations that must be followed to simplify an expression.

outlier. A data point that is distinctly separate from other data; an unexpected value.

percent decrease. The negative change between two numbers, divided by the first number, multiplied by 100.

percent increase. The positive change between two numbers, divided by the first number, multiplied by 100.

perimeter. The distance around a two-dimensional shape.

pie chart. A circular graph with "slices" suggestive of a pie; the larger the slice, the greater the quantity being represented.

place value. Numerical value defined by position.

point on a graph. The location of a value expressed as (x, y).

probability. The likelihood that an event will occur.

proportion. An equality of two ratios.

quadrants. In a Cartesian graph of a plane, the four quarters into which the plane is divided by the two axes. Labeled with Roman numerals, starting with Quadrant I for the upper-right quarter and proceeding counterclockwise.

range. The difference between the highest and lowest values in a set.

rate of change. A rate that describes how one quantity changes in relation to another.

ratio. Shows the number of times one number is contained within another number.

rational number. A number that can be expressed as a fraction.

real numbers. The set of rational and irrational numbers.

reciprocal. One divided by the original number; or, for a nonzero fraction a/b, the reciprocal is b/a. The product of a number and its reciprocal is 1.

repeat. Do again.

rounding. Simplifying a number by removing decimal places or changing those places to zero.

scale. Ratio of graphical representation to actual size.

scatterplot. A graph that uses dots to represent data points to show relationships between two numeric variables.

shape. Symmetry, number of peaks, skewness, and uniformity of data distribution.

simplify. Reduce a fraction or an expression to a simpler form by actions such as cancellation of common factors and regrouping of terms with the same variable.

slope. The rate of change, or the steepness and direction, of a line on a coordinate plane.

solution. The answer.

solve. Find the answer.

spread. The range of values in data distribution.

square units. Units used to measure area. One square unit is the area of a square with sides that measure 1 unit.

standard deviation. A quantity that indicates the extent to which data varies from the mean.

subtend. Form an angle at a particular point on an arc.

subtraction. Removing one number from another; the inverse of addition.

sum. The result of addition.

surface area. The total area of a three-dimensional object's surface.

table. A set of data displayed in rows and columns.

term. A number, variable, or product of numbers and variables.

terminate. To end.

unimodal. Describes a distribution of data with a single clear peak.

unit conversion. Calculating equivalent values between systems of measurement.

unit rate. A rate that shows how many units of one quantity (in the numerator) correspond to one unit of the second quantity (in the denominator), such as miles/hour.

variable term. Any term that includes an unknown quantity.

volume. The amount of space taken up by a three-dimensional shape.

whole numbers. The numbers used in counting and zero: 0, 1, 2, 3, 4, 5, 6, 7, …

Practice Problems Answer Key

M.1.1

1. Solutions worked out:

    A. $3.25 \times 100 = 325\%$; when multiplying by 100, you move the decimal two places to the right.

    B. $0.215 \times 100 = 21.5\%$; when multiplying by 100, you move the decimal two places to the right.

    C. $62.9 \div 100 = 0.629$; when dividing by 100, you move the decimal two places to the left.

    D. $145 \div 100 = 1.45$; when dividing by 100, you move the decimal two places to the left.

    E. $0.265 = 265/1000$, where 265 is the numerator and the last decimal place is the thousandths. This would simplify to 53/200.

    F. $1.39 = 139/100$, where 139 is the numerator and the last decimal place is the hundredths.

    G. $26 \div 10 = 2.6$.

    H. $16 \div 25 = 0.64$.

2. The correct answer is 170%. This is calculated by dividing 17 by 10 and multiplying by 100.

3. Option A is correct. This is calculated by converting to a decimal (0.564) and then writing the 564 over the place value of the last digit in the decimal (1,000).

4. The correct answer is 0.0375. This is calculated by dividing 3.75 by 100 and dropping the percent sign or by moving the decimal two places to the left and dropping the percent sign.

5. Option A is correct. This is calculated by dividing 16 by 50.

M.1.2

1. Solutions worked out:

    A. $6 + 8 \times (12 - 9)$

    First, perform operations in parentheses:
    $12 - 9$
    Then, multiply: 24
    Finally, add: 30

    B. $(14 - 5) \div (7 - 4)$

    First, perform operations in parentheses:
    $9 \div 3$
    Then, divide: 3

    C. $7 \times 4 + 8 \div 4 - 3 \times 6$

    First, multiply and divide from left to right.
    $28 + 8 \div 4 - 3 \times 6$
    $28 + 2 - 3 \times 6$
    $28 + 2 - 18$
    Then, add and subtract from left to right: $30 - 18 = 12$

    D. $\dfrac{50 - 2 \times 7}{6 + 4 \times 3}$

    First, simplify the numerator and denominator.
    Numerator: $50 - 14 = 36$
    Denominator: $6 + 12 = 18$
    Last, divide numerator by denominator: $36 \div 18 = 2$

2. Option C is correct.

    First, determine the root: $3 + 2 \times 6 - 4$.
    Then, multiply: $3 + 12 - 4$.
    Then add: $15 - 4$.
    Then subtract: 11.

3. Option B is correct. Simplify both numerator and denominator first:

    Numerator: $15 + 10 = 25$
    Denominator: $11 - 6 = 5$
    Last, divide numerator by denominator: $25 \div 5 = 5$

4. Option A is correct.

    First, complete the operations in parentheses. Determine the exponent: 8×3.
    Then multiply: 24.
    Then, simplify the fraction: $15/3 = 5$
    Last, add and subtract from left to right: $50 - 24 + 5 = 31$

5. Option B is correct. First, complete the multiplication in the numerator: 6
    Then, complete operations in the numerator: $18 - 6 = 12$
    Next, simplify the fraction: $12/6 = 2$
    Last, complete the addition: $17 + 2 = 19$

M.1.3

1. If $8\frac{3}{4}$ is converted to a decimal, it becomes 8.75. Thus, the increasing order is: 8, 8.43, $8\frac{3}{4}$.

2. Option B is correct. $9\frac{1}{6}=9.1\overline{6}$ is larger than 9.14.

   9.14 is not larger than $9\frac{1}{6}=9.1\overline{6}$.

   9.14 is not equal to $9\frac{1}{6}=9.1\overline{6}$.

   $9\frac{1}{6}=9.1\overline{6}$ is not smaller than, nor is it equal to, 9.14.

3. Option D is correct. If $4\frac{1}{5}$ is written in decimal form, it equals 4.2. The decimals can be stacked to compare.

4. Option C is correct.

   The lowest common denominator for the fractions is 16.

   $$\frac{1}{2}=\frac{8}{16}, \frac{3}{8}=\frac{6}{16}, \frac{3}{4}=\frac{12}{16}$$

   The ordered list is $\frac{3}{8}, \frac{1}{2}, \frac{11}{16}, \frac{3}{4}$

5. Option A is correct.

   If $-1\frac{3}{5}$ is written as a decimal, it is −1.6.

   If $-1\frac{3}{4}$ is written as a decimal, it is −1.75.

   The decimals can be stacked to compare.

M.1.4

1. Option A is correct. To isolate the variable on one side of the equation, add 17 to both sides of the equation.

2. Subtract $2x$ from both sides of the equation as shown.

   $$2x - 2x - 6 = -4x - 2x$$

   Next, divide by −6 on both sides of the equation as shown.

   $$-6 = -6x$$

   $$\frac{-6x}{-6} = \frac{-6}{-6}$$

   $$1 = x$$

3. Divide both sides of the equation by 6 as shown.

   $$6x = 19$$

   $$\frac{6x}{6} = \frac{19}{6}$$

   $$x = \frac{19}{6}$$

4. Multiply both sides of the equation by $\frac{5}{7}$ as shown.

   $$\frac{7}{5}x = 35$$

   $$\frac{5}{7} \times \frac{7}{5} = 35 \times \frac{5}{7}$$

   $$x = 25$$

5. Option C is correct. Subtracting 3x from both sides uses the inverse operation to combine variable terms on the left side of the equation. This is an acceptable first step.

   Subtracting 9 from both sides still leaves constants on each side of the equation.

   Adding 12 to both sides of the equation still leaves constants on each side of the equation.

   Adding 6x to both sides of the equation still leaves variables on both sides of the equation.

M.1.5

1. **Step 1:** Understand the problem.
   - How many pavers should Jayden buy?
   - The square pavers are 4 inches on each side. The garden is 8 feet long and 2 feet wide.

   Step 2: Make a drawing of the garden. Recall that the opposite sides of a rectangle are equal.
   - Because 1 foot equals 12 inches, it takes three 4-inch pavers to equal a length of 1 foot.
   - Add six pavers to both of the 2-foot sides in your drawing.
   - Next, add 24 pavers to both of the 8-foot sides.
   - One extra paver is needed in each corner to surround completely the garden.

   Step 3: Add up the pavers needed.

Length	Number of Pavers Needed
8 feet	24
2 feet	6
8 feet	24
2 feet	6
4 corners	4
TOTAL	**64**

   Step 4: Visualize walking around the drawing, counting three pavers for each foot. Don't forget to step on each corner.
   - 64 pavers is a reasonable solution.

2. **Step 1:** Understand the problem.
   - How many days will the bottle last?
   - The dosage is 2.5 mL twice a day. The bottle contains 200 cc.

   Step 2: Because 1 cc is equivalent to 1 mL, the cat needs to take 5 cc per day (2.5 mL twice daily). Divide the bottle's volume by the dosage.

   Step 3: Perform the division.
   - 200 cc divided by 5 cc/day will equal the number of days.

   Step 4: Evaluate for reasonableness.
   - 40 days is a reasonable time period for a prescription. Each day requires 5 cc, and 200 is much more than 5, so you would expect an answer greater than 1. Two days requires 10 cc, three days 15 cc, and so on. So 40 days requires 200 cc of the vitamin overall.

   $$\frac{200 \text{ cc}}{5 \text{ mL/day}} = 40 \text{ days}$$

3. **Step 1:** Understand the problem.
   - Fluid intake: Monday: 1,800 mL, Tuesday: 2,350 mL
   - Total fluid outtake: 1,775 mL

   Step 2: Add to determine total fluid intake.
   - Total fluid intake = 1,800 + 2,350 = 4,150 mL

   Step 3: Determine net result by subtracting.
   - Net result: Intake minus outtake = 4,150 mL − 1,775 mL = 2,375 mL

   Step 4: Check your answer for reasonableness.
   - 2,375 + 1,775 = 4,150, which was the total fluid intake, so the answer 2,375 mL is a reasonable solution.

4. **Step 1:** Understand the problem.
   - 1 batch of cookies requires 3/4 cups of flour.

   Step 2: Use multiplication to determine the flour needed for 1 1/2 batches.

   Step 3: Multiply a fraction and a mixed number by converting the mixed number to an improper fraction, and then multiply the resulting numerators and denominators.

   $$1\frac{1}{2} \times \frac{3}{4} = \frac{3}{2} \times \frac{3}{4} = \frac{9}{8} = 1\frac{1}{8} \text{ cups}$$

   Step 4: Check for reasonableness.
   - 2 batches would require 3/4 cups two times, or 1 1/2 cups. 1 1/8 cups is between these numbers, making it a reasonable solution.

5. **Step 1:** Understand the problem.
   - 1,225 students take the bus. 1,955 students are enrolled in the school system.

   Step 2: Identify the part and whole.

   1,225 (part), 1,955 (whole)

   Step 3: Divide the part by the whole to determine the decimal equivalent. Then multiply the decimal by 100 to change to a percent.

   $$\frac{1225}{1955} \approx 0.6266 \qquad 0.6266 \times 100\% = 62.66\%$$

   Step 4: Evaluate for reasonableness.
   - Because 1,225 is a little more than half of 1,955, 62.66% is reasonable.

M.1.6

1. Convert 4.5% to decimal form: 0.045.
   Multiply 0.045 × $55,000 = $2,475, which is your salary increase for next year.

2. Option A is correct. Convert 35% to a decimal (0.35), then multiply 0.35 × 900 = 315.

3. The correct answer is $37.50.
   Find 25% of $50 by multiplying 0.25 × $50 = $12.50.
   Subtract $50 − $12.50 = $37.50.
   Alternatively, you can subtract 100% − 25% to get 75%, rename 75% as 0.75, and then multiply 0.75 × $50 = $37.50.

4. Option D is correct.
   Find 6.5% of $550 by multiplying 0.065 × $550 = $35.75.
   Add $550 + $35.75 = $585.75.
   Alternatively, you can add 100% + 6.5% to get 106.5%, rename 106.5% as 1.065, and then multiply 1.065 × $550 = $585.75.

5. Option A is correct.
   Find 6% of $58,000 by multiplying 0.06 × $58,000 = $3,480.00.
   Add $3,480.00 and $900.00 to get $4,380.00.

M.1.7

1. Option A is correct. Rounding each number to the nearest one is an appropriate estimate.
   - Rounding each number to different place values can introduce more error.
   - You cannot ignore decimal place value and round to the first digit only.
   - Rounding every number up to its smallest place value introduces more error than necessary.

2. Solutions worked out.

Number	Round to This Place	Your Answer
34.19	Tenths	34.2
6/7	Ones	1
7.219	Hundredths	7.22
933.74	Thousands	1000
2.739	Hundredths	2.74
32.834	Tenths	32.8
37.494	Tens	40
23/50	Ones	0
7 2/3	Ones	8
64.736	Tenths	64.7
547	Tens	550
878	Hundreds	900
87.357	Hundredths	87.36
32.95	Tenths	33.0
483.34	Hundreds	500

3. Option B is correct. Meters and millimeters both measure length: however, because a meter is close to a yard, that unit would be too large to use. A paper clip is small, so centimeters is the most appropriate unit.

4. Option A is correct. A pet rabbit's weight can be measured in kilograms. Spilled water from a cup, a piece of paper, and a tablet of ibuprofen all have small masses that would be measured in units smaller than kilograms.

5. Option D is correct. In the numerator, round to the nearest hundred and nearest one, and then round to the nearest ten in the denominator. You will have a calculation you can do easily without a calculator.

M.1.8

1. Solution worked out:

$$\frac{27 \text{ hours}}{3 \text{ weeks}} = \frac{x \text{ hours}}{7 \text{ weeks}}$$

Multiplying both sides by 7 weeks yields

$$\frac{27 \times 7}{3} = \frac{x \times 7}{7}$$

Simplifying the left side leads to x = 63 hours

2. Option C is correct.

$$\frac{2 \text{ sales}}{11 \text{ calls}} = \frac{x \text{ sales}}{55 \text{ calls}}$$

Multiplying both sides by 55 calls will give

$$\frac{2 \text{ sales} \times 55 \text{ calls}}{11 \text{ calls}} = x$$

Simplifying the left side leads to x = 10 sales.

3. Option B is correct.

$$\frac{4 \text{ defective}}{1000 \text{ TVs}} = \frac{x \text{ defective}}{95,000 \text{ TVs}}$$

Multiply both sides by 95,000 TVs.

$$\frac{4 \text{ defective} \times 95,000 \text{ TVs}}{1000 \text{ TVs}} = x$$

Simplify the left side: x = 380 defective.

4. Option D is correct.

$$\frac{1 \text{ cm}}{75 \text{ miles}} = \frac{8.6 \text{ cm}}{x \text{ miles}}$$

Multiply 75 by 8.6 cm to get x = 645 miles.

5. Option C is correct. The remaining choices are in the form y = mx + b, where b is nonzero.

M.1.9

1. The 7-night deal is the better deal.

$$\frac{\$900}{4 \text{ nights}} = \frac{\$225}{1 \text{ night}}$$

$$\frac{\$1443}{7 \text{ nights}} = \frac{\$206.14}{1 \text{ night}}$$

2. Option C is correct. The rate has been reduced correctly, and the denominator is one unit.
   - Jada has written the reciprocal of the unit rate.
   - The unit rate should have 1 day in the denominator.
   - A rate must include units.

3. Option D is correct. The rate has been reduced correctly, and the denominator is one unit.
   - Option A is the reciprocal of the unit rate.
   - A unit rate should have 1 ounce in the denominator.
   - A rate must include units.

4. Option A is correct: The rate of change is

$$\frac{\$1130 - \$360}{(10 - 3) \text{ months}} = \frac{\$770}{7 \text{ months}} = \$110/\text{month}$$

5. Option B is correct. The ratio has been reduced correctly.
   - Option A is the reduced ratio of black markers to total.
   - Option C is the ratio of red markers to black markers.
   - Option D is the ratio of black markers to red markers.

M.1.10

1. The question asks how many weeks, so let w = number of weeks.
   - The total number of cards over time would be $2w$.
   - Nine cards to start with can be shown as $+\,9$.
   - More than 35 cards would be shown as > 35.

   The inequality is $2w + 9 > 35$.

2. Option C is correct.
   - "At least" should be greater than or equal to ($\geq$).
   - The $15 is a one-time gift, not every week.
   - Option D gives James less than $255.

3. Option D is correct.
   - The taxi driver charges $2.00 before the taxi starts to move.
   - Option B ensures that the fare will be more than $25.
   - The $2.00 is only paid once, not every mile.

4. Option D is correct.
   - Hector has already driven 100 miles.
   - Option C ensures that Hector drives at most 350 miles.
   - "At least" means greater than or equal to.

5. Option B is correct.
   - 3 is not multiplied by 5, and 9 is not multiplied by 3.
   - Greater than will not be equal to.
   - 9 is not multiplied by x.

M.2.1

1. Option D is correct. The average rate of change on a graph is the same as the slope. Find the slope between year 4 ($800) and year 1 ($200).
   - The cost to maintain the car decreased between years 6 and 7. It is possible that a new car was purchased.
   - The graph shows the expense for each year individually. The total cost for the first 3 years is $800.
   - There are only 3 years between year 1 and year 4.

2. Option B is correct. The number of pounds of corn sold increased each day.
   - The most zucchini was sold on day 1.
   - The scale on the y-axis is 10 pounds, not 1 pound.
   - The most carrots were sold on day 1, not day 3.

3. Dani's and Frank's tips:

Nights	Dani's Tips	Frank's Tips
Monday	$15	$20
Tuesday	$20	$15
Wednesday	$30	$25
Thursday	$40	$35
Friday	$35	$50

   - On Friday night, Dani's tips decreased from $40 to $35.
   - On Monday night, Frank earned $5 more than Dani. On Friday night, Frank earned $15 more than Dani.
   - The average rate of change is

   $$\frac{\$50 - \$20}{4 \text{ nights}} = \frac{\$30}{4 \text{ nights}} = \$7.50 \text{ per night}$$

4. Option B is correct. The greatest increase in profits was $15,000 from 2016 to 2017.
   - There was a decrease in profits from 2015 to 2016.
   - Max earned $35,000, not zero, in 2013.
   - There were three yearly increases of $5000: from 2014 to 2015, from 2017 to 2018, and from 2018 to 2019.

5. Option C is correct. Most people chose rock as their favorite genre of music.
   - Country music was a favorite of 25% of people, not 25 people.
   - There was a difference of 5% of people, not 5 people, preferring country music to pop music.
   - Neither rock nor country was chosen by 40% of people, not 40 people.

M.2.2

1. Solutions:

   Mean

   $$\frac{0+1+2+2+3+5+6+7+8+16}{10} = \frac{50}{10} = 5$$

   Median

   $$\frac{3+5}{2} = \frac{8}{2} = 4$$

   Mode = 2

2. Option A is correct. When most of the data is in the center of a histogram, it is bell–shaped.

3. Option B is correct. As the value of x increases, the value of y increases.

4. Option B is correct. When a data set is skewed left, the data peaks closer to higher values.

5. Option B is correct. When one set of values increases and the other set of values decreases, there is a decreasing trend.

M.2.3

1. Option A is correct. As the batting average goes up, the runs scored also goes up.
   - Variables represent quantities that are changing. They are not constant but instead representative of the time period from 2006 to 2012.
   - When graphing this, the batting average would come first and be the independent variable.
   - Because the values go in the same direction, they are directly related.

2. Option D is correct. For a direct relationship, as one variable increases so does the other. This would have a positive slope.
   - For any direct relationship, as one variable increases so does the other. This would have a positive slope instead of a negative slope.
   - The side of the square determines the area of the square, so it is the independent variable. When collecting data, it will not always be immediately known which variable is independent and which is dependent.
   - The relationship is not linear. Because the area is growing by multiplication, the graph would be curved.

3. Options B and C are correct.
   - A. **False**. If there is no relationship between variables, there is no covariance. If some-times one goes up while the other goes down and vice versa, there is no covariance.
   - B. **True**. The more you practice, the better you perform. This is a belief held by many musicians and music teachers.
   - C. **True**. This statement is usually heard in sports, exercise, and in medical or dental procedures.
   - D. **False**. The two variables are inversely (not directly) related. It is a good example of negative covariance. As your coughing increases, you will likely have difficulty running at a fast pace.

4. Option A is Correct.
   - A. **True**. The more snow on the ground, the less likely schools will be open. As one variable increases, the other decreases.
   - B. **False**. This is a positive correlation because both quantities decrease.
   - C. **False**. The more likely school will be closed is logically equivalent to the less likely school will be open, but the statement as is has a positive correlation.
   - D. **False**. This is a positive correlation.

5. Option C is true because as the temperature increases, ice cream sales also increase.
   - Options A, B, and D are all false because the variables are positively (or directly) related.

M.2.4

1. Find the areas of the outer rectangle and inner rectangle, and imagine "cutting out" the area of the inner rectangle. The area of the shaded region is the area left over after subtracting the inner area from the outer area. Therefore, $(12 \times 10) - (7 \times 2) = 120 - 14 = 106$ m².

2. Option C is correct. The missing horizontal segment is $34 - 20 - 7 = 7$ ft. The missing vertical segments are $20 - 8 = 12$ ft. The combined perimeter is $34 + 8 + 8 + 7 + 7 + 12 + 12 + 20 = 108$ ft.

3. Option B is correct. The height of the triangle is 12 – 8 = 4 ft, and the base of the triangle is 24 ft. To find the total area, add the area of the rectangle to the area of the triangle:

$$(24 \times 8) + \frac{1}{2}(24 \times 4)$$

$$= 192 + \frac{1}{2} \times 96 = 192 + 48 = 240 \text{ ft}^2$$

4. Option C is correct. To find the total area, add the area of the rectangle and the area of the semicircle.

$$(12 \times 8) + \frac{1}{2}(3.14 \times 6^2)$$

$$= 96 + \frac{1}{2} \times 113.04 = 96 + 56.52 = 152.52 \text{ ft}^2$$

5. Option C is correct. To find the total area, imagine the upper right corner is being cut off. Subtract the area of the upper right corner from the rectangular area.

$$(15 \times 10) - (6 \times 4) = 150 - 24 = 126 \text{ m}^2$$

M.2.5

1. Option D is correct. The answer would be rounded to 1 tsp in the kitchen.

   - The mL units do not factor out to leave tsp. This is not set up correctly.
   - Without units on the 5, it is hard to know if this is set up correctly.
   - This is the wrong conversion factor. Teaspoons are smaller than tablespoons.

2. Option C is correct.

$$\frac{€50}{1} \times \frac{\$1.20}{€1} = \$60.00$$

   - Patricia did not use dimensional analysis correctly.
   - (€50)/12 = €4.17. There was no conversion.
   - To compare prices, they both must be in the same monetary unit.

3. Solution:

Original Unit	Equivalent Unit
1. 750 mL	F. 0.75 L
2. 75 mL	D. 75 cc
3. 26.4 lb	A. 12 kg
4. 100° C	E. 212° F
5. 600 m	H. 0.6 km
6. 12.7 cm	C. 5 in
7. 40 mm	B. 4 cm
8. 720 g	G. 0.72 kg

4. Option D is correct.

$$\frac{3 \text{ m}}{1} \times \frac{3.28 \text{ ft}}{1 \text{ m}} = 9.84 \text{ ft}$$

   - The meters units do not factor out to leave feet. This is not set up correctly.
   - The conversion factor is incorrect; 1 m is not equal to 2.54 ft.
   - The conversion factor is incorrect; 1 ft is not equal to 2.54 m.

5. The correct answer is 54 L.

$$\frac{5 \text{ gal}}{1} \times \frac{3.8 \text{ L}}{1 \text{ gal}} = 19 \text{ L}$$

19 L + 35 L = 54 L

Mathematics Unit Quiz

1. Which of the following pairs is equivalent to 6.74%?

   A. 6.74/100, 0.0674

   B. 674/10, 6.74

   C. 6.74/1000, 674

   D. 674/1000, 67.4

$(22 + 14 \div 7) / (17 - 42 \times 3)$

2. Which of the following is the correct value of the given expression?

   A. 5.14/-75

   B. 24/109

   C. 24/-109

   D. 5.14/75

$8x + 3x - 5 = 4x + 16$

3. Which of the following shows the correct steps to finding the solution for the given equation?

   A. 8x + 3x = 11x
   11x − 5 = 4x + 16
   6x = 12x
   x = 2

   B. 3x − 5 = 4x − 8x + 16
   −2x = −4x + 16
   −2x = 16x
   x = −8

   C. 8x − 5 = 4x − 3x + 16
   3x = x + 16
   2x = 16x
   x = 8

   D. 8x+3x = 11x
   11x − 5 = 4x + 16
   11x − 4x = 16 + 5
   7x = 21
   x = 3

4. A doctor prescribes a medication at a dosage of 37.5 mg daily for 45 days. To fill this prescription, the pharmacist cuts a total of 15 pills into smaller 37.5 mg sections. Which of the following is the size of the original pill, and how many sections was each pill divided into?

   A. 112.5 mg, 3 parts

   B. 135 mg, 3 parts

   C. 112.5 mg, 2.5 parts

   D. 150 mg, 4 parts

5. A company is providing performance bonuses to employees at a rate of between 3% to 5% of the employee's salary. Which of the following is the range of possible bonuses for an employee whose salary is $79,200?

   A. $2,400 to $4,000

   B. $2,376 to $3,960

   C. $2,187 to $3,645

   D. $2,370 to $3,950

$9x + 4 = 3x - 8$

6. Which of the following is the solution to the above equation?

   A. x = 2

   B. x = -2

   C. x = 1/2

   D. x = 1

7. A lawn mowing service is scheduled to mow five lawns. The lawns are sized 20 ft by 30 ft, 200 ft by 45 ft, 50 ft by 50 ft, 90 ft by 90 ft, and 150 ft by 95 ft. If the lawns are mowed at a rate of 240 ft²/min, which of the following is how long it will take to mow all five lawns?

   A. 2 hr and 24 min

   B. 2 hr and 20 min

   C. 1 hr and 9 min

   D. 6 hr and 58 min

8. A going-out-of-business sale has marked all items in the store at 55% off the listed price. You found a shirt listed for $17.50 and a pair of pants listed for $37. Which of the following is the reduced total you will pay?

    A. $34.15

    B. $44.87

    C. $24.52

    D. $54.50

9. A recipe for Dijon Chicken that is designed to serve 6 calls for 3/4 of a tablespoon of brown sugar. Which of the following is the amount of brown sugar needed to make the recipe to serve 22 guests?

    A. 2 1/2 tablespoons

    B. 3 tablespoons

    C. 2 3/4 tablespoons

    D. 1 3/4 tablespoons

$7 \times 3 - 8 + 6 \div 2$

10. Which of the following is the correct value if the given expression is simplified?

    A. 3.5

    B. 16

    C. 9.5

    D. 14

11. The interest earned on $1000 is $23. If the interest rate and time period are the same, which of the following is the amount of interest earned on $750?

    A. $17.25

    B. $23

    C. $20.50

    D. $18

12. There are 3,400 students and 200 teachers at a high school. If an additional 250 students are added to the school, then which of the following is many new teachers would be needed to keep the ratio of students to teachers the same?

    A. 15

    B. 25

    C. 35

    D. 50

$5/8, \sqrt{9}, -\sqrt{4}, 3/5$

13. Which of the following lists is in order from least to greatest?

    A. $-\sqrt{4}$, 3/5, 5/8, $\sqrt{9}$

    B. 3/5, 5/8, $-\sqrt{4}$, $\sqrt{9}$

    C. $-\sqrt{4}$, 5/8, 3/5, $\sqrt{9}$

    D. $\sqrt{9}$, $-\sqrt{4}$, 3/5, 5/8

14. A water cooler holds 5 gallons of water, which is enough to serve 40 athletes. There are 17 volleyball players, 25 soccer players, and 67 football players. Which of the following sets represents the correct amount of water to serve each team?

    A. 2 1/2 gallons, 3 3/4 gallons, 8 2/3 gallons

    B. 2 gallons, 3 gallons, 8 gallons

    C. 2 1/8 gallons, 3 1/8 gallons, 8 3/8 gallons

    D. 3 gallons, 4 gallons, 9 gallons

15. An organizer is planning a raffle to raise money for a charity. If the organizer spends $100 on the raffle prize and each raffle ticket (T) costs $2, then which of the following expressions represents the number of tickets that must be sold for the raffle to generate at least $500 in net revenue?

    A. $2T \leq 500$

    B. $2T \geq 500$

    C. $2T < 500 + 100$

    D. $2T \geq 500 + 100$

16. A car wash charges $10 for minivans (x) and $5 for sedans (y). The car wash spends $3 on supplies for each minivan service and $2 on supplies for each sedan service. Which of the following expressions represents the net revenue for the car wash?

    A. $10x + 5x - 3y + 2y$

    B. $10x + 3x + 5y + 2y$

    C. $10x + 3x - 5y + 2y$

    D. $10x - 3x + 5y - 2y$

17. The expenses for a school dance are $3,967 for room rental, $563 for a DJ, $2,311 for decorations, and $500 for security. If the expenses are rounded to the nearest hundred dollars and tickets cost $40 each, then which of the following is the estimated number of tickets that must be sold to repay the expenses?

A. 185 tickets

B. 200 tickets

C. 180 tickets

D. 178 tickets

18. A parking lot has a total of 50 parking spaces. If each space measures 8 ft by 12 ft, which of the following best estimates the area of the parking spaces?

A. 3,750 ft²

B. 5,000 ft²

C. 1,000 ft²

D. 7,500 ft²

Use the figure below to answer the question.

19. Which of the following is the area of the irregular polygon above?

A. 44 square cm

B. 45 square cm

C. 34 square cm

D. 54 square cm

20. Which of the following shows a negative correlation?

A. The more water I drink, the more energy I have.

B. The more I sleep, the more I want to eat.

C. The more I exercise, the less I weigh.

D. The longer I study, the more I remember.

21. A carpet installer is preparing to order carpet for the hallway and waiting room of an office. The hallway is 6 ft wide by 67 ft long and the waiting room is 20 ft wide and 35 ft long, with a semicircular area by the door measuring 10 ft in diameter. Which of the following is the amount of carpet that should be ordered? (Round your answer up to the nearest foot.)

A. 1,102 ft²

B. 1,181 ft²

C. 1,259 ft²

D. 1,142 ft²

Use the figure below to answer the question.

High Schooler Participation in Activities by Year

Activities	Total (%) by year					
	2007	2009	2011	2013	2015	2017
Watch streaming television	6	6.9	7.4	7.7	7.8	6
Use social media	45.5	56	66.9	67.1	77.6	6.7
Participate in sports	14.9	15.5	16.2	14.8	15.5	14.9
Play video games	20	19.9	20.1	19.6	19.2	19
Read comic books	7.5	7.4	7.5	7.3	7.5	7.4
Write poetry	13.4	12.6	11.7	10.3	9.6	8
Volunteer with an organization	11.3	10.8	10.7	10.4	10.6	6.9

22. Based on the data in the table, which of the following statements is correct?

A. The percentage of high school students who play video games has increased consistently from 2009 to 2017.

B. The percentage of high school students who read comic books has remained consistent from 2007 to 2017.

C. The percentage of high school students who use social media has decreased steadily from 2007 to 2017.

D. The percentage of high school students who volunteer with an organization has declined more rapidly than those who write poetry.

Use the figure below to answer the question.

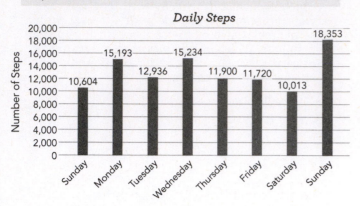

Daily Steps

23. According to the graph, which of the following best represents the median of the data represented?

    A. 12,418

    B. 11,900

    C. 12,936

    D. 13,244

Use the figure below to answer the question.

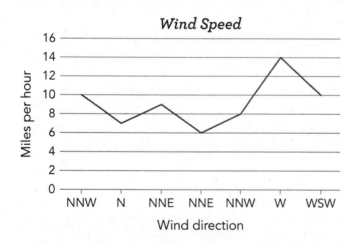

Wind Speed

24. Which of the following conclusions does the graph support?

    A. Winds from the NNE cause wind speeds to increase.

    B. Wind speed is not impacted by wind direction.

    C. The highest wind speed was recorded with winds from the W.

    D. The lowest wind speeds were recorded with winds from the N.

Use the figure below to answer the question.

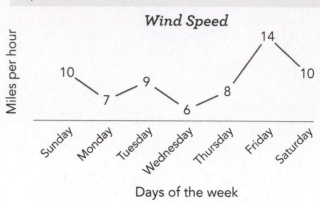

Wind Speed

Days of the week

25. Using the data represented, which of the following is the mean wind speed in miles per hour over the 7 days? (Round to the nearest tenth.)

    A. 9.1

    B. 10.5

    C. 10.7

    D. 9.0

Use the figure below to answer the question.

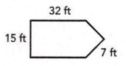

26. If a yard has the above measurements, which of the following is the perimeter? (Assume the angles that make the rectangle shape are right angles, and the triangle has 2 equal sides.)

    A. 84.5 ft

    B. 108 ft

    C. 54 ft

    D. 93 ft

> *4, 11, 38, 15, 22, 17, 42, 41, 19, 38, 22,*
> *29, 42, 11, 8, 6, 27*

27. What is the range of the data set given?

28. Which of the following is an example of a positive correlation?

   A. Decreasing the time spent getting ready in the morning allows more time to sleep.

   B. Increasing a car's fuel efficiency reduces its carbon footprint.

   C. The higher the down payment on a new car, the lower the monthly payment.

   D. The higher the temperature outdoors, the more ice cream is sold.

29. An employee worked 35 hr last week and earned $367.50 in hourly wages. How much will the employee earn in hourly wages this week if they work a total of 27 hr?

30. A shopper is trying to determine if a 1-liter bottle of soda priced at $1.99 is cheaper per liter than a 16-oz bottle of soda priced at $0.99. Which of the following describes how to solve this problem? (1 L ≈ 34 oz)

   A. Multiply the rate of $0.99 per 16 ounces by the conversion factor of 1 L per 34 oz and compare prices per liter.

   B. Multiply the rate of $0.99 per 16 ounces by the conversion factor of 34 oz per 1 L and compare prices per liter.

   C. Multiply the rate of 16 ounces per $0.99 by the conversion factor of 34 oz per 1 L and compare prices per liter.

   D. Multiply the rate of $0.99 per 16 ounces by the conversion factor of $1.99 per 1 L and compare prices per liter.

31. Which of the following would be the best way to display the relationship between time playing video games and college GPA?

   A. Line graph

   B. Pie chart

   C. Bar graph

   D. Scatter plot

32. A student flips a fair, two-sided coin and chooses one card at random from a standard deck of 52 cards. Which of the following is the probability that the coin lands on tails and they choose a 7?

   A. 1/14

   B. 1/26

   C. 9/14

   D. 1/15

33. Michael Phelps' notable wingspan is 6 feet 7 inches long. Which of the following is his wingspan converted to centimeters? (1 in = 2.54 cm)

   A. 200.66 cm

   B. 31.1 cm

   C. 170.18 cm

   D. 189.88 cm

34. A 2 1/2 gallon container of water is half full. Given that there are 16 cups in 1 gallon, which of the following is the number of cups of water that are in the container?

   A. 8 cups

   B. 16 cups

   C. 20 cups

   D. 40 cups

Quiz Answers

1. A. **CORRECT.** This is correct because percent means parts per hundred. Therefore, 6.74% = 6.74/100 = 0.0674.

   B. This is not the correct fraction and not the correct decimal equivalent. Because percent means per 100, 6.74% should be written as 6.74/100, which is the decimal 0.0674.

   C. This is not the correct fraction and not the correct decimal equivalent. Because percent means per 100, 6.74% should be written as 6.74/100, which is the decimal 0.0674.

   D. This is not the correct fraction and not the correct decimal equivalent. Because percent means per 100, 6.74% should be written as 6.74/100, which is the decimal 0.0674.

2. A. Multiplication and division must come before addition and subtraction.

   B. The order of operations was performed correctly, but there is a computation error in the denominator.

   C. **CORRECT.** The order of operations was followed. The problem is solved by first dividing 14 by 7 to get an answer of 2. Then, add the 2 to 22 for a total of 24 in the numerator. In the denominator, multiply 42 × 3 for an answer of 126. Then calculate 17 − 126. This results in −109 in the denominator. The resulting fraction 24/(−109) is already in lowest terms.

   D. The order of operations was not performed correctly, and there is a computation error in the denominator.

3. A. These steps are incorrect because the second step does not combine like terms.

   B. These steps are incorrect because terms were not correctly combined in the first step; 3x and −5 are not like terms and cannot be combined.

   C. These steps are incorrect because terms were not correctly combined in the first step; 8x and −5 are not like terms and cannot be combined.

   D. **CORRECT.** The first step correctly combines 8x and 3x. The second step uses inverse operations to get like terms on the same side of the equation. The third step correctly combines like terms on each side of the equation. The final step divides both sides by 7 to arrive at the correct answer of 3.

4. A. **CORRECT.** The total amount of medication prescribed was 37.5 mg per day × 45 days = 1,687.5 mg. The pharmacy needed 15 pills to fill the prescription, so the milligrams per pill can be calculated by the equation 15x = 1,687.5 mg. Thus, x = 112.5 mg per pill. To determine out how to cut the pill, use the number of milligrams needed per day, which is 37.5 mg. Thus, the equation is 37.5x = 112.5 mg, and x = 3. Each pill must be cut into 3 parts to get the proper daily dose of 37.5 mg.

   B. The milligrams in one pill were incorrectly calculated.

   C. The milligrams in one pill were correctly calculated through multiplication and division. To cut the pill into parts, divide the milligrams per pill by 37.5.

   D. The milligrams in one pill were incorrectly calculated.

5. A. The percent increase is calculated on an incorrectly rounded up salary of $80,000.

   B. **CORRECT.** This is the correct bonus range because these figures represent 3% and 5% of $79,200. The range can be calculated by 79,200 × 0.03 = 2,376 and 79,200 × 0.05 = 3,960.

   C. A mathematical error is made in this option.

   D. The percent increase is calculated on an incorrectly rounded down salary of $79,000, rather than $79,200.

6. A. This is not correct because when subtracting 4 from both sides, there is a negative number on the right leading to a negative number for x in the final division step.

   B. **CORRECT.** This is correct because like terms are first combined by subtracting 3x from both sides of the equation. Then 4 is subtracted from both sides of the equation. Finally, both sides are divided by 6.

   C. This is not correct because both sides are divided by 6 and not by 12.

   D. This is not correct because like terms must first be combined before solving the equation.

7. A. **CORRECT.** The total area of all the lawns must be determined first and then divided by the area mowed in a minute:
$[(20 \text{ ft} \times 30 \text{ ft})^2 + (200 \text{ ft} \times 45 \text{ ft})^2 + (50 \text{ ft} \times 50 \text{ ft})^2 + (90 \text{ ft} \times 90 \text{ ft})^2 + (150 \text{ ft} \times 95 \text{ ft})^2]/240^2 = x.$
This number must then be converted to hours and minutes: x = 143.54 converted is 2 hr and 24 min.

   B. 132 was incorrectly converted to hours and minutes.

   C. The perimeter, and not the area, was used.

   D. The total area was multiplied by 240 and then not divided by 60 min; its decimal form was used as hours and minutes.

8. A. This answer results from taking 55% off the pants but not the shirt.

   B. This answer results from taking 55% off the shirt but not the pants.

   C. **CORRECT.** The total listed cost of the shirt and pants is $54.50. 100% − 55% = 45%, so 0.45(54.50) = $24.52.

   D. This answer results from neglecting to take 55% off the total price.

9. A. When simplifying the proportion, both sides must by multiplied by 22 and then divided by 6, rather than multiplied by 6.

   B. This option is the result of calculating the amount of brown sugar needed for 24 guests, rather than 22 guests.

   C. **CORRECT.** The proportion is 3/4 tablespoons to 6 servings = x tablespoons to 22 servings or 3/4 tablespoons/6 servings = x tablespoons/22 servings.
   Solving for x yields (3/4) × (22/6) = x, where x = 2.75 and then converted back to a fraction is 2 3/4.

   D. Simplifying the proportion involves multiplying both sides by 22, rather than dividing both sides by 22.

10. A. The order of operations was not properly followed.

   B. **CORRECT.** Following the order of operations, the first step is to perform all multiplication and division, completing the operations as they occur from left to right.
   In this equation, 7 × 3 = 21 and 6 ÷ 2 = 3. So, the equation now reads 21 − 8 + 3. The next step is to perform all addition and subtraction, completing the operations as they occur from left to right, which yields 16.

   C. The order of operations was not properly followed.

   D. The order of operations was not properly followed.

11. A. **CORRECT.** The interest rate stayed the same, so the proportion is set up as 23/1000 = x/750. Solving for x yields 23 × (750/1000) = x, where x = $17.25.

   B. Even though the interest rate remained the same, the amount earned is not the same.

   C. The proportion is set up incorrectly.

   D. The proportion is set up incorrectly.

12. A. **CORRECT.** The initial ratio is 200/3400, which is simplified to 1/17. For the additional students, x/250 = 1/17, so x ≈ 14.7. However, because 0.7, or 7/10, of a person is not feasible, the number needs to be rounded up. Therefore, 15 additional teachers are needed to keep the ratio the same.

   B. The ratio would be 1/16.

   C. The ratio would be 1/15.

   D. The ratio would be 1/14.

13. A. **CORRECT.** These are ordered from least to greatest. This is easiest to see by converting all the numbers to decimals:
$-\sqrt{4} = -2, 3/5 = 0.6, 5/8 = 0.625, \sqrt{9} = 3.$

   B. When ordering these numbers, $-\sqrt{4} = -2$ is smaller than 3/5 = 0.6 and 5/8 = 0.625.

   C. When ordering these numbers, 5/8 = 0.625 is greater than 3/5 = 0.6.

   D. When ordering these numbers, $\sqrt{9} = 3$, not −3.

14. A. The ratios were not set up correctly or the calculations were not completed correctly.

   B. The problem did not ask for the answers to be rounded down.

   C. **CORRECT.** The ratio is set up correctly by using the number of gallons of water over the players it serves. For the volleyball team, 5/40 = x/17, then x = 2.125, or 2 1/8. For the soccer team, 5/40 = x/25, then x = 3.125, or 3 1/8. For the football team, 5/40 = x/67, then x = 8.375, or 8 3/8.

   D. The problem did not ask for the answers to be rounded up.

15. A. The amount of the ticket sales has to be greater than or equal to the amount of the total sales, and it does not include the cost of the winning prize.
B. Even though the amount of the ticket sales is more than or equal to the amount of the total sales, it does not include the cost of the winning prize.
C. The income from the sales of the $2 tickets would be less than $500 plus the cost of the winning prize.
D. **CORRECT.** The income from the sales of the $2 tickets must be equal to or greater than $500 plus the amount spent on the winning prize ($100).

16. A. The problem gave the symbol of (x) for minivans washed and (y) for sedans washed, rather than (x) for all cars washed and (y) for all supplies.
B. All numbers are added, and there are no costs subtracted.
C. The cost for supplies has been added to money earned for the car wash, and then the amount of money earned from the two styles of car washed was subtracted.
D. **CORRECT.** This represents $10 per minivan washed (x) minus $3 for the supplies and $5 for each sedan washed (y) minus $2 for the supplies.

17. A. **CORRECT.** This is the result of correctly rounding the prices to the nearest hundred, adding the rounded values together, and then dividing the total by the cost of the ticket.
B. This is the result of rounding expenses to the nearest thousand dollars, rather than the nearest hundred dollars.
C. This is the result of rounding expenses down to the nearest hundred dollars, rather than to the nearest hundred dollars.
D. This is the result of rounding decoration expenses to the nearest thousand dollars, rather than the nearest hundred dollars.

18. A. This results from an error in rounding.
B. **CORRECT.** This is correct because the area of one parking space is estimated to be 10 ft by 10 ft = 100². For 50 spaces, this would become 100 ft² × 50 = 5,000 ft².
C. This is incorrect. When finding area, multiply the length by the width of the space instead of multiplying each dimension by 50.
D. This uses incorrect calculations.

19. A. **CORRECT.** This can be found by breaking the figure down into three rectangles and finding the sum of their areas to get the total area. One rectangle is 4 cm by 5 cm; one is 3 cm by 6 cm; and one is 2 cm by 3 cm. Area is length times width, so 20 cm2 + 18 cm2 + 6 cm2 = 44 cm2.
B. This answer represents the area of a 5 cm by 9 cm rectangle and does not take into account the polygon's irregular shape.
C. This answer represents the sum of the given lengths and the unknown length (2 cm), representing the perimeter of the shape.
D. This answer represents the area of a 6 cm by 9 cm rectangle and does not take into account the polygon's irregular shape.

20. A. This represents a positive correlation because as one variable increases, the other variable increases as well.
B. This is a positive correlation, even though eating more can seem to be a negative.
C. **CORRECT.** As one variable (exercise) increases, the other variable (weight) decreases.
D. This represents a positive correlation because as one variable increases, the other variable increases as well.

21. A. This accurately calculates the area of the hallway and waiting room. However, it does not include the area of the semicircle.
B. This accurately calculates the area of the hallway and waiting room. However, only half of a circle needs to be carpeted.
C. This accurately calculates the area of the hallway and waiting room. However, the diameter of the semicircle is 10 ft, so the radius is 5 ft.
D. **CORRECT.** The area of the hallway (6 ft × 67 ft) is 402 ft². The area of the waiting room (20 ft × 35 ft) is 700 ft². The area of the semicircle is determined by using the formula for the area of a circle (A = πr^2) and then dividing that by 2 because a semicircle is half of a circle. The diameter of the semicircle is 10 ft, so the radius is 5 ft. The equation is thus $\pi(5)^2/2$ ft, which is about 39.27 ft². So, the total area of carpet needed is 402 ft2 + 700 ft2 + 39.27 ft2 = 1,141.27 ft2, which rounded up to the nearest square foot is 1,142 ft².

22. A. This statement is inaccurate because the table shows that the percentage of students playing video games has decreased overall.

    B. **CORRECT.** This statement is correct because the data from 2007 to 2017 in the table showed little change (7.5, 7.4, 7.5, 7.3, 7.5).

    C. This statement is incorrect because the table shows the percentage of students using social media has increased steadily.

    D. This statement is incorrect because the table shows that the decrease in writing poetry (5.4%) is greater than the decrease in volunteering (4.4%).

23. A. **CORRECT.** First, the numbers must be ordered from least to greatest to find the median. Because there are two middle numbers (11,900 and 12, 936), they must be averaged: 11,900 + 12,936/2 = 12,418.

    B. This does not represent the median of the data.

    C. This does not represent the median of the data.

    D. This does not represent the median of the data.

24. A. This is incorrect because the graph shows that winds from the NNE caused wind speeds to both increase and decrease.

    B. This is incorrect because the graph shows the line is not straight, so wind speed must be impacted by wind direction.

    C. **CORRECT.** This is correct because the graph shows the highest recorded wind speed occurred when the winds were from the W.

    D. This is incorrect because the graph shows the lowest wind speeds were recorded with winds from the NNE and not the N.

25. A. **CORRECT.** This answer is correct because it adds all the values together, which totals 64, and then divides it by the number of days, which is 7, to find the mean of 9.1.

    B. This answer is incorrect because it used the total value of 74 instead of 64.

    C. This answer is incorrect because the total value is only divided by 6, and not 7, days instead.

    D. This answer is incorrect because 9.0 is the median and not the mean.

26. A. This answer is incorrect because the area of the triangle was calculated and added to the perimeter of the rectangle.

    B. This answer is incorrect because the base of the triangle was added into the perimeter.

    C. This answer is not correct because all the sides were not added together.

    D. **CORRECT.** The answer is correct because all the sides are added together to determine the perimeter: 15 + 32 + 32 + 7 + 7 = 93.

27. The range is a measure of the spread of a data distribution found by subtracting the lowest data value from the highest data value. The lowest data value here is 4, and the highest is 42, so the range is 42 – 4 = 38.

28. A. This is an example of a negative correlation.

    B. This is an example of a negative correlation.

    C. This is an example of a negative correlation.

    D. **CORRECT.** As the temperature increases, the ice cream sales increase. This is a positive correlation.

29. Let p represent the weekly pay, let h represent the hours worked, and p = kh. 367.50 = k(35)
    k = 10.5
    p = 10.5h
    p = 10.5(27)
    p = $283.50

30. A. This represents an incorrect method for setting up dimensional analysis.

    B. **CORRECT.** This represents a correct way to set up dimensional analysis to convert the unit rate of the item from ounces to liters. Then a comparison can be made between the per liter rates.

    C. This represents an incorrect method for setting up dimensional analysis.

    D. Do not use $1.99/1 L as your conversion factor.

31. A. A line graph is the best choice when you want to display how a variable is affected by a change in time (i.e. how the high temperature in one town changes over the course of a week).

B. A pie chart is used to display how a whole population is broken down into certain parts (i.e. how someone spends the 24 hr in one day).

C. Bar graphs are used to compare things between different groups or responses (i.e. showing the various responses of a population when asked their favorite color).

D. **CORRECT.** Scatter plots are used to represent a correlation (positive, negative, or none) between two variables.

32. A. This answer is the result of multiplying the probability of the coin outcome (1/2) by an incorrect card outcome probability (1/7).

B. **CORRECT.** This answer is the result of correctly multiplying the probability of the coin outcome (1/2) by the probability of the card outcome (1/13, as 4 of the 52 cards are "7" cards).

C. This answer is the result of adding the coin outcome (1/2) by an incorrect card outcome (1/7).

D. This answer is the result of incorrectly adding the denominator for the probability of the coin outcome (1/2) to the denominator of the probability for the card outcome (1/13).

33. A. **CORRECT.** This answer is the result of correctly multiplying the arm span in inches (79) by 2.54.

B. This answer is the result of incorrectly dividing the arm span in inches (79) by 2.54.

C. This answer is the result of incorrectly assuming there are 10 inches in a foot and determining the arm span is 67 inches then multiplying by 2.54.

D. This answer is the result of incorrectly calculating the arm span in inches by converting the feet to inches (72), multiplying by 2.54, then adding the remaining 7 inches as 7 cm.

34. A. This is half of the number of cups in 1 gallon, rather than half the number of cups in 2 1/2 gallons.

B. This is the total number of cups in 1 gallon, rather than half the number of cups in 2 1/2 gallons.

C. **CORRECT.** This is half the number of cups in 2 1/2 gallons. This is calculated by multiplying the size of the container in gallons (2 1/2) by the number of cups in a gallon (16), and then dividing by 2 to determine the number of cups of water if the container is half full.

D. This is the total number of cups in 2 1/2 gallons, rather than half the number of cups in 2 1/2 gallons.

Unit 3: Science

The 27 lessons in this unit cover the tasks from the ATI TEAS test plan for the Science section. These are focused on assessment of knowledge and understanding of scientific information and concepts and are organized into three chapters:

- Human anatomy and physiology
- Life and physical sciences
- Scientific reasoning

Each lesson introduces knowledge, skills, and abilities relevant to the corresponding Science test plan task and provides an overview of some essential topics, along with specific examples to highlight important concepts. Practice questions at the end of each lesson will allow you to test your knowledge of select concepts. In addition, there are key terms included at the end of the chapter, followed by a practice Science quiz. This unit quiz includes the same number of questions as the Science section on the ATI TEAS and matches the test plan task allocations (shown below). The quiz will give you a good idea of the number and types of questions that will encounter. Keep in mind that these lessons are a great starting point and guide to your studies, but they are not an exhaustive review of all concepts that might be tested in the Science section of the ATI TEAS. You should use other sources (textbooks, online resources, etc.) for additional study and practice in areas that you have not mastered.

There are 44 scored Science items on the TEAS. These are divided as shown below. In addition, there will be six unscored pretest items that can be in any of these categories.

Section	Number of scored questions
Human anatomy and physiology	18
Biology	9
Chemistry	8
Scientific reasoning	9

Human Anatomy and Physiology

S.1.1 — Demonstrate knowledge of the general orientation of human anatomy.

This TEAS task requires an understanding of the general anatomy and physiology of the human body. You will be required to locate body structures using **anatomical positions**, planes, directions, and regions. There are many resources available on this subject, including print textbooks, online content and quizzes, and free online textbooks. These are excellent for both learning the concepts and committing them to memory.

Objectives

This objective includes, but is not limited to, the following examples of knowledge, skills, and abilities.

- Identify the standard anatomical position.
- Apply knowledge of anatomical planes.
- Apply knowledge of anatomical directions.
- Apply knowledge of anatomical regions.

ANATOMICAL TERMINOLOGY

For the TEAS assessment, you will need to describe the position and location of features in the human body. You will need to use standard anatomical terminology, as shown in the following diagram.

Cephalic - head
Cranial - skull
Facial - face
Cervial - neck
Axillary - armpit
Brachial - arm
Antecubital - front of elbow
Antebrachial - forearm
Carpal - wrist
Palmar - palm
Pollex - thumb
Digital or phalangeal - fingers
Femoral - thigh
Patella - front of knee
Crural - shin
Pedal - foot
Tarsal - ankle
Digital or phalangeal - toes
Dorsum - top of foot
Hallux - great toe

See below
Sternal - breastbone
Thoracic - chest
Mammary - breast
Abdominal - abdomen
Umbilical - navel
Coxa - hip
Pelvic - pelvis
Inguinal - groin
Pubic - pubis
Dorsum - back of hand
Manual - hand

Frontal - forehead
Temporal - temple
Orbital or occular - eye
Otic - ear
Buccal - cheek
Nasal - nose
Oral - mouth
Mental - chin

Occipital - base of skull
Acromial - shoulder
Scapular - shoulder blade
Vertebral - spinal column
Dorsal - back
Olecranal or cubital - back of elbow
Lumbar - loin
Sacral - between hips
Coccygeal - tailbone
Gluteal - buttock
Perineal - area between anus and external genitals

Popliteal - back of knee
Sural - calf
Plantar - sole
Calcaneal - heel

Anterior view   *Posterior view*

anatomical position. Standard positioning of the body as standing; feet together; arms to the side; with head, eyes, and palms of hands forward.

ANATOMICAL POSITION

First, anatomical position describes the stance of an individual, and it gives a consistent frame of **reference** for the use of terminology. In anatomical position, the human body is erect and facing forward; arms are at the sides with palms forward. Feet are parallel, and arms and legs are slightly held away from the torso.

ANATOMICAL PLANES

Anatomical planes divide the body into two:

- Coronal or frontal plane is a front and back division.

- Transverse or cross-sectional plane is a top and bottom division.

- Sagittal or median indicates a left and right division.

These planes also apply to **organs**, which can also be divided along planes.

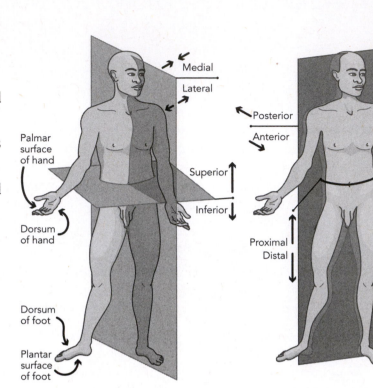

ANATOMICAL DIRECTION

Anatomical direction identifies the location of structures in relation to other structures. Commonly used terms include:

- "superior" and "inferior,"

- "anterior" and "posterior,"

- "lateral" and "medial."

Sometimes two **directional terms** can be combined, such as "posteroinferior."

The terms "distal" and "proximal" are used to indicate which structure is closer (proximal) to the structure or farther away (distal). For example, the fingers are distal to the wrist because the wrist is closer to the main body. "Lateral" and "medial" are used to determine which structure is closer to the medial line, which divides a body into right and left sides. The rib cage is lateral to the sternum (breastbone), whereas the sternum is medial to the ribcage.

Anatomical direction also includes "right" and "left." These terms reference the body's left and right rather than the viewer's position.

---

reference planes. Planes dividing the body to describe locations: sagittal, coronal, and transverse.

organ. A structure formed from various tissues that performs a specific function in an organism.

directional terminology. Words used to explain relationships of locations of anatomical elements (distal, posterior, medial, etc.).

ANATOMICAL REGIONS

The human body is compartmentalized into several regions that help with description. Principal regions include the head, neck, trunk, upper limbs, and lower limbs. Each region is further divided into multiple subregions. The diagram that follows shows regions and subregions labeled with both anatomical and common names.

Practice Problems

1. In the human body, which of the following body parts are in a superior position to the lungs? (Select all that apply.)

   A. Stomach

   B. Trachea

   C. Spleen

   D. Heart

   E. Brain

2. In two to three sentences, describe the part of the arm that is most distal to the shoulder of the human body.

3. Which terms add clarity to anatomical position relative to the coronal plane?

   A. "Superior" and "inferior"

   B. "Distal" and "proximal"

   C. "Anterior" and "posterior"

   D. "Lateral" and "medial"

4. Which two terms are likely to appear in the same discussion related to a part of the body?

   A. "Dorsal" and "lumbar"

   B. "Umbilical" and "crural"

   C. "Dorsal" and "orbital"

   D. "Lumbar" and "patellar"

5. Which of the statements below is/are accurate? (Select all that apply.)

   A. The axillary region is superior to the cephalic region.

   B. The oral, nasal, buccal, and ocular regions are all anterior to the occipital region

   C. Digital or phalangeal structures may be pedal or manual.

   D. The axillary, brachial, antecubital, antebrachial, popliteal, and sural subregions are all associated with the upper limbs.

S.1.2 — Describe the anatomy and physiology of the respiratory system

The respiratory system's main function is to perform the critical tasks involved in transporting oxygen from the atmosphere into the body's blood and removing carbon dioxide from the body's **cells**. The respiratory system is specifically structured to maximize surface area for the exchange of oxygen and carbon dioxide. In fact, the surface area of the **alveoli** in a human lung is equivalent to half the size of a basketball court! For the TEAS exam, you will need to know the various parts of the respiratory system and how they contribute to the function of the respiratory system. You will also want to be familiar with common respiratory problems and how they affect the system's function. Finally, the respiratory system works interdependently with the circulatory system, so you will need to understand how these **systems** interact.

Objectives

This objective includes, but is not limited to, the following examples of knowledge, skills, and abilities.

- Identify structures of the respiratory system.
- Explain the functions of the respiratory system.
- Explain the role of the respiratory system in gas exchange.
- Describe the relationship between the respiratory system and the cardiovascular system.

STRUCTURE OF THE RESPIRATORY SYSTEM

The respiratory system mediates the uptake of oxygen needed for metabolism and the release of carbon dioxide, which is a waste product of the human body, back into the atmosphere. The process of bringing oxygen into the lungs is known as breathing (inhaling and exhaling), and exchanging the gas oxygen with the gas carbon dioxide in the lungs is **ventilation**. Several structures shown in the following diagram cooperate to form the respiratory system. Air enters through nasal openings, moves into the nasal cavity, and travels past the pharynx (throat) and into the **trachea**, which is a large tube reinforced by cartilage rings that keep it from collapsing.

Anatomy: Respiratory System

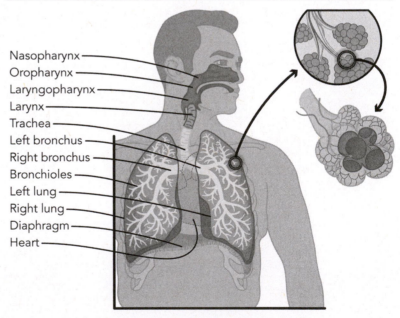

Nasopharynx
Oropharynx
Laryngopharynx
Larynx
Trachea
Left bronchus
Right bronchus
Bronchioles
Left lung
Right lung
Diaphragm
Heart

---

cells. The basic structural unit of an organism from which living things are created.

alveoli. Tiny air sacs in the lungs where exchange of oxygen and carbon dioxide takes place.

organ systems. Functional groups of organs that work together within the body: circulatory, integumentary, skeletal, reproductive digestive, urinary, respiratory, endocrine, lymphatic muscular, nervous.

ventilation. The exchange of oxygen with carbon dioxide in the lungs. .

trachea. The windpipe, which connects the larynx to the lungs.

Air continues to the first division of the trachea: the right and left primary **bronchi**. The air in the right bronchus continues to the right lung; the air directed to the left bronchus continues to the left lung. The right and left bronchi subdivide into smaller and smaller tubes called "**bronchioles**." Bronchioles terminate in alveoli, which are thin-walled (one cell thick) structures that organize to look like clusters of grapes. Alveoli are the sites of gas exchange. Besides the type I alveolar cells that make up the alveolar wall, alveoli have type II alveolar cells that release a lipoprotein called surfactant, a substance that reduces the surface tension.

INTERACTION OF THE CARDIOVASCULAR AND RESPIRATORY SYSTEMS

The **heart** is located in the **mediastinum** (the area between the two lungs), marginally on the left side. This allows the right lung more space, and as a result, it is a little larger than the left lung. The right lung has three lobes: the superior, middle, and inferior. The left lung has two lobes: the superior and inferior lobes. Each lobe is divided into bronchopulmonary segments. Each segment receives air from its own bronchus and receives blood from its own artery.

Each lung is contained within a tough, protective double membrane called the "**pleura**" and contains pleural fluid. The lungs are located in the thoracic cavity. Although the heart is not a part of the respiratory system, it has an important role when it comes to transporting oxygen and carbon dioxide throughout the body. The heart's pulmonary system sends blood low in oxygen and high in carbon dioxide to the lungs where oxygen is picked up and carbon dioxide is dropped off. This happens where **capillaries** of the circulatory system interact with alveoli of the lungs. This oxygenated blood is then returned to the heart where the systemic circulation sends it to all parts of the body. As oxygen is consumed by the cells, the blood becomes deoxygenated and is returned to the heart.

FUNCTION OF THE RESPIRATORY SYSTEM

The following diagram shows gas exchange in the lungs. Gas exchange in the lungs occurs by **diffusion**, which is a **passive transport** mechanism. The rate of diffusion is directly proportional to the surface area involved and the concentration gradient and is inversely proportional to the distance between the two solutions. For example, the rate of diffusion increases if the distance between the blood cells and the alveoli is decreased.

Gas Exchange in the Lungs

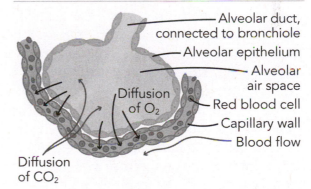

Alveolar duct, connected to bronchiole
Alveolar epithelium
Alveolar air space
Diffusion of O_2
Red blood cell
Capillary wall
Blood flow
Diffusion of CO_2

---

bronchi. The main passageways directly attached to the lungs.

bronchioles. Small passages in the lungs that connect bronchi to alveoli.

heart. Muscular organ that pumps blood throughout the body.

mediastinum. The area between the two lungs.

pleura. A membrane around the lungs and inside the chest cavity.

capillaries. Small vessels that connect smaller arteries, called arterioles, to smaller veins, called venules, and carry out gas exchange.

diffusion. The passive movement of a substance from an area of high concentration to an area of low concentration.

passive transport. Movement across a cell membrane that does not require energy input.

During diffusion, oxygen in the lungs moves into the blood, and carbon dioxide in the blood moves into the lungs. The lungs then exhale the carbon dioxide back to the atmosphere. When the heart's pulmonary vessels enter the lungs, the blood has a low concentration of oxygen, whereas the recently inhaled air in the alveoli has a high concentration of oxygen in comparison to the capillaries. Molecules move from regions of high concentration to regions of low concentration. The thin alveolar epithelium allows the diffusion. Concentration of carbon dioxide is reversed in their location compared to oxygen levels. Capillaries contain high levels of carbon dioxide, while alveoli contain high levels of oxygen and a low concentration of carbon dioxide; therefore, carbon dioxide diffuses into the alveoli and oxygen into the blood capillaries. Inhalation brings in oxygen, while exhalation releases carbon dioxide.

Ventilation occurs as a combination of **muscle** action and negative pressure. The diaphragm and the intercostal muscles between the ribs contract simultaneously to increase the volume of the lungs. This decreases the pressure in the lungs and draws air in. Subsequently, the diaphragm and the intercostal muscles relax, causing a reduction in lung volume and an increase in pressure in the lungs and causing air to be pushed out. Periodic inspiration (inhalation of air) and expiration (expulsion of air) from lungs clear out air rich in carbon dioxide and replaces it with air rich in oxygen. The amount of air breathed in and out of the lungs during a normal breath is called the "**tidal volume**." A small amount of air rich in carbon dioxide, called the "residual volume," remains trapped in alveoli after expiration and mixes with the air rich in oxygen brought in through inspiration. The breathing control centers of the brain's medulla oblongata control respiration through monitoring carbon dioxide levels and blood pH. If blood pH starts to decrease, then respiration rates will increase to balance carbon dioxide and oxygen levels.

FACTORS AFFECTING THE RESPIRATORY SYSTEM

Many environmental conditions, genetic factors, and pathogens affect lung function. For example, **asthma** is a condition in which the airways of respiratory system narrow. This results from the swelling of the airways or from mucus buildup. Asthma can make it difficult to inhale and exhale normal amounts of air. This can lead to shortness of breath, difficulty breathing, and wheezing. Be aware of the effect of environmental pollutants such as chemicals, pollen, and smoke, which can impede lung function by damaging cilia or causing emphysema, **allergies**, and **inflammation**. Genetic conditions such as lung surfactant insufficiency, asthma, and cystic fibrosis can seriously impede lung action. There are also several pathogens that affect lung function and cause **diseases** such as influenza, tuberculosis, and pneumonia. For example, influenza is an infection caused by a **virus** that affects many parts of the respiratory system, including the nasal cavity, trachea, bronchi, and lungs. The virus uses cells in the respiratory system to make new viruses. The body's **immune system** attacks these cells infected by the virus, causing some of the symptoms, including mucus, pain, and coughing.

---

muscle. Fibrous tissue that produces force and motion to move the body or produce movement in parts of the body.

tidal volume. The amount of air breathed in a normal inhalation or exhalation.

asthma. A lung disease characterized by inflamed, narrowed airways and difficulty breathing.

inflammation. The resulting redness, swelling, heat, and pain in an area of defense by innate immunity.

allergies. An immune response to a foreign agent that is not a pathogen.

disease. A condition that deteriorates the normal functioning of the cells, tissues, and/or organs.

virus. A noncellular entity that consists of a nucleic acid core (DNA or RNA) surrounded by a protein coat.

immune system. A system that protects the body from disease-causing agents known as pathogens by responding to substances on the surfaces of agents that the body perceives as foreign.

Practice Problems

1. Which of the following structures changes the volume of the lungs?

   A. Alveoli

   B. Heart

   C. Trachea

   D. Diaphragm

2. Which of the following statements best explains how the structure of alveoli relates to its function?

   A. Alveoli are large to maximize gas exchange.

   B. The walls the alveoli are thin to increase the rate of diffusion.

   C. The walls of the alveoli are thick to prevent pressure buildup.

   D. Alveoli are small to increase the transportation of cells.

3. Which of the following statements best describes the primary function of the respiratory system?

   A. It transports oxygen and carbon dioxide to cells all over the body.

   B. It involves the inhalation and exhalation of gases into the environment.

   C. It exchanges gases between the blood and the air in an environment.

   D. It maintains proper blood level pH.

4. Which of the following correctly describes the makeup of the lungs?

   A. Right lung, three lobes; left lung, two lobes

   B. Right lung, two lobes; left lung, two lobes

   C. Right lung, two lobes; left lung, three lobes

   D. Right lung, three lobes, left lung three lobes

5. In two to three sentences, describe what will occur in the blood if the tidal volume in the lungs increases.

S.1.3 — Describe the anatomy and physiology of the cardiovascular system

The cardiovascular, or circulatory, system is responsible for the movement of blood around the body. This system allows for nutrient distribution and waste removal. To be successful at meeting the objective, it is important to know not only the structure of these two systems but also the functional components of each.

PARTS OF THE CARDIOVASCULAR SYSTEM

The cardiovascular system includes the closed system of blood pumped around the body by the heart through a network of **arteries**, **veins**, and capillaries. The heart is made up of **cardiac muscle** and is split into four chambers. The upper chambers are called "atria" and the lower chambers are called "ventricles." The atria and ventricles are attached to veins and arteries that are connected to different parts of the body. One-way valves control the flow of blood into and out of the chambers of the heart. The Heart Anatomy diagram shows key parts of the heart.

FUNCTIONS OF THE CARDIOVASCULAR SYSTEM

The cardiovascular system performs the vital functions of transporting nutrients, **hormones**, and wastes. There are two well-integrated circulatory systems. The closed circulatory system is a double-loop system consisting of thick-walled arteries that transport blood away from the heart, thinner-walled veins that transport blood to the heart, and capillaries made of a single layer of endothelium that form a network that connect arteries to veins in **tissues**. The open lymphatic system circulates and filters interstitial fluid between cells and eventually drains into the circulatory system.

Heart Anatomy

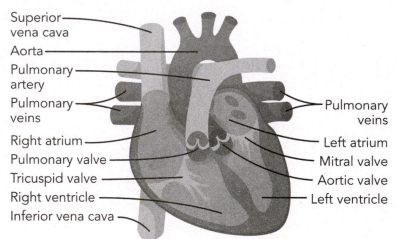

Superior vena cava
Aorta
Pulmonary artery
Pulmonary veins
Right atrium
Pulmonary valve
Tricuspid valve
Right ventricle
Inferior vena cava
Pulmonary veins
Left atrium
Mitral valve
Aortic valve
Left ventricle

---

arteries. Vessels that carry blood away from the heart toward other body parts.

veins. Vessels that carry blood toward the heart from other body parts.

cardiac muscle. Involuntary muscle found in the heart.cardiovascular system. The system comprised of the heart and blood vessels.

hormone. A chemical messenger produced by a gland and transported by the bloodstream that regulates specific processes in the body.

tissue. A group of cells with similar structure that function together as a unit, but at a lower level than organs.

The closed, double-loop system transports blood and hormones. There are two parts of this loop: the pulmonary and the systemic. The pulmonary loop carries deoxygenated blood from the right ventricle of the heart to the lungs where it is oxygenated and returns oxygenated blood to the left atrium. The systemic loop carries oxygenated blood from the left ventricle to the body, returning deoxygenated blood to the right atrium. The heart undergoes two cycles of contractions: **systole** and diastole. Systole indicates contraction of heart muscles, and diastole is **relaxation** of heart muscles. In a simplified overview of the heart cycle, the ventricles contract (i.e., ventricular systole), causing the atrioventricular valves (including the mitral and tricuspid valves) to close, making a "lub" sound. Subsequently, the empty ventricles are filled by blood pushed out during atrial systole. At the same time, the semilunar valves in the aorta and pulmonary trunk close, preventing blood from falling back into the ventricles, making a "dub" sound, and completing the "lub-dub" sound of the heart. These contractions are controlled by a "pacemaker" called the "sinoatrial node," which sends out electrical signals. Arteries have thick walls to withstand the pressure of blood pumped by the heart, whereas veins have walls with a thinner muscle layer and larger lumen.

Blood **plasma** contains nutrients, hormones, antibodies, and other immune proteins. Red blood cells contain **hemoglobin**, transport oxygen from the lungs to the rest of the body, and transport some of the carbon dioxide back to the lungs for removal. About 5 to 7% of carbon dioxide is dissolved in plasma, and 85% of carbon dioxide is used to maintain acid–base or pH balance in the blood through the bicarbonate **buffer** system. White blood cells are divided into two main lineages: granulocytes (basophils, eosinophils, and neutrophils) and agranulocytes (monocytes and **lymphocytes**). White blood cells defend against pathogens. Blood also contains cells called platelets, which are responsible for blood clotting.

The open circulatory system's capillaries drain interstitial fluid that fills the spaces between the cells and filter it through a system of **lymph** nodes that are enriched in lymphocytes and **macrophages** that provide surveillance by the immune system. Lymph (essentially plasma with the red blood cells removed) eventually drains into the large veins leading back to the heart. Large numbers of **leukocytes** and lymphocytes are enriched in lymph nodes, where they monitor and respond to foreign molecules washed into the system. Typically, lymph nodes are enriched in oral, nasal, and genital regions where foreign entities enter the body.

You should have a general understanding of pathologies of the circulatory system, such as heart attacks, stroke, aneurysms, atherosclerosis, arrhythmias, and hypertension.

---

systole. The portion of the cardiac cycle in which the heart expels blood.

relaxation. Release of tension in a muscle.

plasma. Clear pale yellow component of blood that carries red blood cells, white blood cells, and platelets throughout the body.

hemoglobin. Protein in red blood cells that carries oxygen from the lungs to the rest of the body.

buffer. A solution of a weak acid and its conjugate base or a weak base and its conjugate acid. Buffers maintain the proper pH of the body.

lymphocyte. A category of white blood cells that includes natural killer cells, B-cells, helper T-cells, and cytotoxic T-cells.

lymph. Clear fluid that moves throughout the lymphatic system to fight disease.

macrophage. A large white blood cell that ingests foreign material.

leukocyte. White blood cells, which protect the body against disease.

BLOOD FLOW THROUGH THE CARDIOVASCULAR SYSTEM

Blood flows throughout the cardiovascular system in a cyclic pattern as shown in the following diagram. Starting in the left ventricle, oxygenated blood is pumped to the body. As it flows through arteries to capillaries, it transports oxygen to tissues and picks up carbon dioxide. Then, the deoxygenated blood returns to the heart through veins. This blood is now deoxygenated and concentrated with carbon dioxide. It enters the heart through the right atrium and then flows into the right ventricle. The right ventricle pumps the blood toward the lungs through arteries, where it picks up oxygen and loses carbon dioxide. Then, it returns to the heart through the left atrium using veins and starts the cycle again.

Blood Cycle

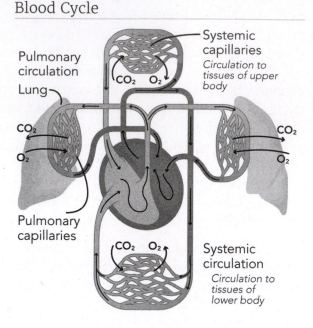

Practice Problems

1. Which of the following lists the primary parts of the heart?

    A. Blood cells

    B. Muscle tissue split into two chambers

    C. Muscle tissue split into four chambers

    D. Four ventricles

2. Which of the following blood components is responsible for transporting oxygen?

    A. Red blood cells

    B. Plasma

    C. Dissolved gases

    D. Leukocytes

3. Which of the following chambers pumps blood toward the lungs?

    A. Left atrium

    B. Right atrium

    C. Left ventricle

    D. Right ventricle

4. Which of the following statements best describes the function of veins?

    A. Veins carry deoxygenated blood.

    B. Veins carry oxygenated blood.

    C. Veins carry blood back to the heart.

    D. Veins carry blood away from the heart.

5. In two to three sentences, describe two chambers of the heart that have thicker walls. Why would these chambers be thicker?

S.1.4 — Describe the anatomy and physiology of the digestive system

The digestive system begins with the **mouth** and then proceeds throughout the abdominal cavity to the **anus**. Its function is to break down food for absorption and distribution of nutrients to the rest of the body. Specialized regions and **glands** perform both mechanical (physical) and **chemical (enzymatic) digestion**. The **smooth muscle** involved in mechanical digestion and movement of food through the digestive system is controlled by the parasympathetic **nervous system**. Blood vessels located along the **stomach** and small and **large intestines** absorb digested nutrients. Undigested food is stored in the **rectum** for elimination. For this task, you need to be able to describe the structure and function of the digestive system organs, as well as the secreted **enzymes** and hormones that control digestion.

Objectives

This objective includes, but is not limited to, the following examples of knowledge, skills, and abilities.

- Identify structures of the digestive system.

- Explain the functions of the digestive system.

- Distinguish between chemical and mechanical digestion.

- Describe the role of secretions in the digestive system.

STRUCTURE AND FUNCTION OF THE DIGESTIVE SYSTEM

The digestive system starts at the mouth and ends at the anus. Understanding the structure and function of the digestive system requires looking at specialized organs shown in the Digestion System diagram.

First, food is ingested through the mouth where mechanical digestion begins. Mechanical digestion is any physical breakdown of food. By chewing and grinding food in the mouth, food is broken down into smaller pieces, which increases the surface area. Mucus in **saliva** lubricates the food and provides the enzymes amylase and **lipase** to initiate chemical digestion of starch and **lipids**, respectively.

Chemical digestion is the process where enzymes break down food particles into simple chemicals that can be used by the body. Next, food is packaged into small parcels called a "**bolus**" and swallowed (deglutition). As the bolus passes through the pharynx, the epiglottis closes the tracheal opening so that food does not enter the respiratory system, and the food passes into the esophagus. **Peristalsis**, which is the contractions of muscle, moves the bolus through the gastric sphincter to the stomach. The esophageal (cardiac) sphincter prevents reflux of food back into the esophagus.

mouth. The oral cavity at the entry to the alimentary canal.

anus. The opening of the rectum from which solid waste is expelled.

gland. An organ that secretes a substance.

enzymatic digestion. The breakdown of food by enzymes for absorption.

smooth muscle. Muscle that can be found in the walls of hollow organs, such as the stomach and intestines.

nervous system. A complex system that controls and affects every part of the body in daily life functions and in the constant drive to maintain homeostasis

stomach. The organ between the esophagus and small intestine in which the major portion of digestion occurs.

large intestine. Comprised of the cecum, colon, rectum, and anal canal, it is where vitamins and water are absorbed before feces is stored prior to elimination.

rectum. The last section of the large intestine, ending with the anus.

enzyme. A substance produced by a living thing that acts as a catalyst. A catalyst that speeds up a chemical reaction by lowering the activation energy; in cells, most enzymes are proteins.

saliva. The clear liquid found in the mouth, also known as spit.

lipase. Pancreatic enzyme that breaks down fat.

lipids. Fatty acids and their derivatives that are insoluble in water.

bolus. A mass of food that has been chewed and swallowed.

peristalsis. A series of muscle contractions that move food through the digestive tract.

Once in the stomach, digestion continues. The stomach is a sac made up of smooth muscles. Stomach muscle contractions mechanically break down food even further and mix with secretions to form a substance called "*chyme*." There are three main secretions of the stomach: mucus, hydrochloric acid, and pepsinogen. Mucus lines the stomach, hydrochloric acid creates an acidic environment, and pepsinogen is converted into **pepsin**, which is an enzyme that helps chemically digest proteins in this acidic environment. Next, the chyme is pushed into the **small intestine**.

The first part of the small intestine is the duodenum. In the duodenum, chyme is neutralized by bicarbonate from pancreatic secretions. The duodenum receives alkaline bile juices from the gall-bladder, which helps neutralize acidic chyme. In addition, the duodenum produces a large number of "brush border" enzymes, including proteases, lactase and other disaccharidases, and bicarbonate. Villi and microvilli in the small intestine (largely the ileum) absorb water–soluble (polar, **hydrophilic**) digested nutrients into blood, lipids into lacteals as chylomicrons, and vitamin B12. Blood, carrying nutrients, passes from the small intestine to the **liver** through the hepatic portal duct, allowing liver enzymes to deaminate **amino acids**, convert ammonia to urea, metabolize consumed toxins, and store glucose as glycogen.

The digested material then passes into the cecum and into the large intestine or colon. The vermiform appendix projects from the cecum, which is located at the junction of the small and large intestines. A lot of water and nutrients are absorbed in the small intestine, and the large intestine absorbs remaining water and **salt** from digested food. The waste from the small intestine is exposed to **bacterial** fermentation in the colon. Vitamin K is absorbed in the large intestine. The waste accumulates in the rectum and is ejected through the anus.

HORMONES INVOLVED IN DIGESTION

Hormones regulate many aspects of nutrition. Ghrelin induces hunger, and leptin causes the sensation of satiety. Hormones induce secretions and speed up the movement of food through the small intestine. **Insulin** induces cellular uptake of glucose, and **glucagon** stimulates the breakdown of stored glycogen. Other hormones and **nerve** function modulate digestive action.

ENZYMES INVOLVED IN DIGESTION

Many enzymes play a role in digestion. Enzymes are proteins produced by the body that catalyze and speed up the breakdown of food so that nutrients are available for the body. Enzymes are involved in chemical digestion of foods in the five organs listed in the following table. For example, digestion of proteins is initiated in the stomach by the action of the enzyme pepsin, which is activated by hydrochloric acid. Bile contains chemicals that aid in digestion; it is not an enzyme. The liver makes and stores bile in the gall-bladder to be released later into the small intestine; bile is involved in the breakdown of lipids or fats.

chyme. The semifluid mass of partly digested food that moves from the stomach to the small intestine.

pepsin. A stomach enzyme that breaks down proteins.

small intestine. The part of the GI tract between the stomach and large intestine that includes the duodenum, jejunum, and ileum, where digestion and absorption of food occurs.

hydrophilic. Water loving.

liver. The organ that produces bile, regulates glycogen storage, and performs other bodily functions.

amino acids. The monomers that make up proteins.

salt. A chemical compound formed from the reaction of an acid with a base, with at least part of the hydrogen of the acid replaced by a cation.

bacteria. Unicellular organisms that are capable of causing disease.

insulin. A hormone that triggers the influx of glucose into cells, thus lowering blood glucose levels.

glucagon. A hormone secreted by the pancreas that stimulates its target cells in the liver to convert hepatic glycogen stores into glucose and release that glucose into the blood.

nerve. A long bundle of neuronal axons that transmits signals to and from the central nervous system.

Anatomy: Digestion System

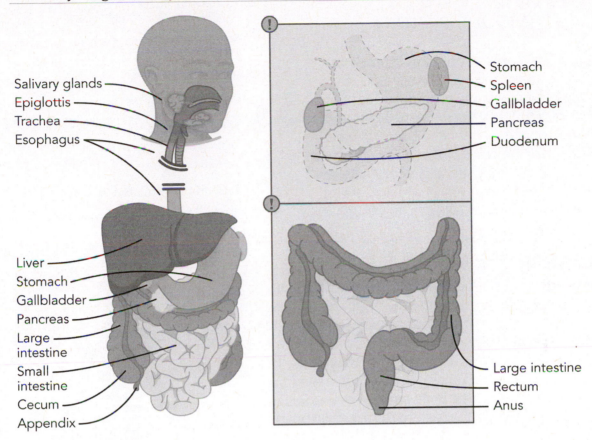

Salivary glands
Epiglottis
Trachea
Esophagus

Liver
Stomach
Gallbladder
Pancreas
Large intestine
Small intestine
Cecum
Appendix

Stomach
Spleen
Gallbladder
Pancreas
Duodenum

Large intestine
Rectum
Anus

Practice Problems

1. In which of the following organs does digestion begin?

   A. Mouth

   B. Stomach

   C. Small intestine

   D. Pancreas

2. In which of the following organs does the breakdown of proteins begin?

   A. Mouth

   B. Stomach

   C. Small intestine

   D. Pancreas

3. Which of the following structures absorbs nutrients in the small intestine?

   A. Mucus

   B. Microvilli

   C. Enzymes

   D. Hormones

4. Which of the following statements best describes peristalsis?

   A. The partly digested food moving from the stomach to the small intestine.

   B. The mechanical breakdown of food entering the stomach.

   C. Muscle contractions that move food through the digestive tract.

   D. Chemical digestion of food with the help of enzymes.

5. In a well-structured paragraph, describe the mechanical and chemical digestion of a starch or carbohydrate.

S.1.5 — Describe the anatomy and physiology of the nervous system

The nervous system is a complex system that affects every part of the body and is vital in controlling **involuntary** and **voluntary** movement. This TEAS task will ask questions about the specific parts of the nervous system and how those parts contribute to the function of the system. You will also be required to know the difference between the **central nervous system** (CNS) and **peripheral nervous system** (PNS).

Objectives

This objective includes, but is not limited to, the following examples of knowledge, skills, and abilities.

- Distinguish between the central and peripheral nervous system.

- Describe the structure of a neuron.

- Explain the functions of the nervous system.

DIVISIONS OF THE NERVOUS SYSTEM

The nervous system can be divided into two parts: the central nervous system (CNS) and the peripheral nervous system (PNS). The central nervous system consists of the brain and the spinal cord and acts as the central command for all communication and actions of the body. The peripheral nervous system includes all of the nerves that branch out to the rest of the body and ganglia. It allows the signals sent by the brain to reach their target destination in the body.

The Nervous System

PNS   CNS

STRUCTURE AND FUNCTION OF THE NEURON

Neurons, or nerve cells, comprise the nervous system. Nerves are long bundles of neuronal **axons** that transmit signals from the central nervous system. These signals start as graded electrical impulses generated at the **dendrites** of neurons. If strong enough, the impulse travels along the axon and causes chemical neurotransmitters to be secreted from the axon terminals into the **synapse**. In the synapse, these neurotransmitters will bind to either another neuron or a muscle cell.

The Neuron

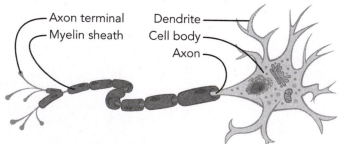

Axon terminal
Myelin sheath
Dendrite
Cell body
Axon

---

involuntary. Without intentional control.

voluntary. With intentional control.

central nervous system. The part of the nervous system that consists of the brain and the spinal cord and acts as the command center for all communication and actions of the body.

peripheral nervous system. The part of the nervous system that consists of all the nerves and ganglia that branch out from the brain and spinal cord to the rest of the body, allowing signals sent by the brain to reach their target destinations.

axon. A nerve fiber that carries a nerve impulse away from the neuron cell body.

dendrite. A nerve fiber that carries a nerve impulse towards the neuron cell body.

synapse. The structure that allows neurons to pass signals to other neurons, muscles, or glands.

Neurons send and receive signals in the nervous system. Sensory (afferent) neurons send messages to the central nervous system about sensory information, such as touch, smell, and pain. Motor (efferent) neurons send messages to muscle and can be subdivided into the autonomic (involuntary) motor nervous system and the somatic (voluntary) nervous system. The **autonomic nervous system** controls involuntary actions involving cardiac and smooth muscle, such as heart rhythm, digestion, and breathing. The **somatic nervous system** controls voluntary actions involving skeletal muscle, such as deliberate actions like walking, throwing, or typing. For these kinds of movement to take place, the nerves need to control muscles. Each muscle fiber is connected to a nerve fiber. For the entire muscle to move, it takes a concerted effort by many nerves and muscle fibers and the use of adenosine triphosphate (ATP) to power the contraction.

Practice Problems

1. Which of the following actions are controlled by voluntary nerve signals? (Select all that apply.)

   A. Walking

   B. Digestion

   C. Talking

   D. Heart beating

   E. Breathing

2. Which of the following best describes the function of a nerve synapse?

   A. It carries a nerve impulse away from the nerve body.

   B. It is responsible for involuntary muscle movements.

   C. It allows for the passing of signals between neurons and other neurons or between neurons and muscles.

   D. It contains a bundle of fibers that transmit electrical impulses.

3. Which of the following describes the role of the central nervous system?

   A. It transmits electrical signals to muscles.

   B. It transmits sensory information.

   C. It controls the regulation of body systems.

   D. It sends messages from the body to the spinal cord.

4. Which of the following types of nerves sends messages to the brain?

   A. Skeletal

   B. Smooth

   C. Sensory

   D. Motor

5. In three to five sentences, describe the differences between the central nervous system and the peripheral nervous system.

autonomic nervous system. The part of the peripheral nervous system that regulates unconscious body functions such as breathing and heart rate.

somatic nervous system. The part of the peripheral nervous system that controls conscious skeletal muscle function.

S.1.6 — Describe the anatomy and physiology of the muscular system

Along with the nervous system, the **muscular system** is an integrated system that affects every part of the body. It is also vital in controlling involuntary and voluntary movement. This TEAS task will ask you to identify the different types of muscle **tissue**. You will also be required to know the structure and functions of muscles.

TYPES OF MUSCLE TISSUE

There are three types of muscles: skeletal, cardiac, and smooth. Skeletal muscle often attaches to **bone** and is involved in the movement of bones. Skeletal muscle is striated and very strong. It is the only voluntary muscle tissue in the body. Cardiac muscle can be found in the heart and is also striated. Cardiac muscle tissue cannot be controlled consciously, making it involuntary muscle. Smooth muscle can be found in the walls of hollow organs, such as the stomach and intestines; in the walls of passageways, such as blood vessels; and elsewhere throughout the body, such as the eyes, the tracts of the reproductive system, and the **skin**. It is the weakest of all muscle tissues and is considered an involuntary muscle because it is controlled by the unconscious part of the brain.

Objectives

This objective includes, but is not limited to, the following examples of knowledge, skills, and abilities.

- Identify structures of the muscular system, including the three types of muscle tissue.
- Describe the functions of the muscular system.
- Describe how the nervous system controls the muscles.

Muscle Tissue

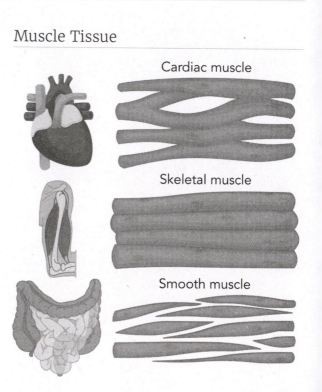

Cardiac muscle

Skeletal muscle

Smooth muscle

---

muscular system. An integrated system in the body that is vital for controlling involuntary and voluntary movement.

tissue. A group of cells with similar structure that function together as a unit, but at a lower level than organs.

bone. Hard, calcified material that makes up the skeleton.

skin. The thin layer of tissue that covers the body.

STRUCTURE AND FUNCTION OF MUSCLES

There are about 700 named muscles in the body that make up approximately half of person's total body weight. Most **skeletal muscles** are attached to bones by a tendon. **Tendons** are tough bands of connective tissue that have strong **collagen** fibers. These fibers firmly attach the muscle to the bone. Muscles move by contracting and shortening their length, which pulls on the tendons, moving one bone closer to another bone that is stationary.

Skeletal muscles are named based on many factors, such as their location, shape, and size. Skeletal muscles rarely work alone, but rather often work in groups to produce movements.

Muscles contain long myofibrils made of **sarcomere** units, each consisting of long strands of proteins called "actin" (thin filaments) and "myosin" (thick filaments).

Muscle Structure

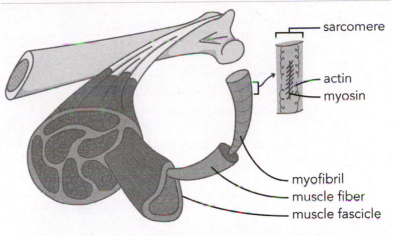

NERVES CONTROL MUSCLES IN THE NERVOUS SYSTEM

Each muscle fiber is connected to a nerve fiber. For the entire muscle to move, it takes a concerted effort by many nerves and fibers and the use of adenosine triphosphate (ATP) to power the **contraction** and relaxation. When a muscle is relaxed, myosin and actin filaments are not attached. When they contract, the filaments bind and are pulled together.

When the brain wants to send a message to a particular part of the body, the nervous system sends a signal to a muscle. Actin and myosin proteins in the muscle slide past each other, creating either a contraction or a relaxation of the muscle. These two basic motions are responsible for all muscle movement.

Ideally, muscles respond to nerve impulses in specific ways. Receptors in muscles allow them to receive a signal and respond with the appropriate magnitude and movement. This signal and response can be disrupted by disorders ranging from muscle strain to muscular dystrophy.

skeletal muscles. Muscles that attach to bones and are connected to and communicate with the central nervous system.

tendons. Tough connective tissue that attaches muscle to bone.

collagen. The primary structural protein of connective tissue.

sarcomere. Contracting unit of a muscle.

contraction. The process leading to shortening and/or development of tension in a muscle.

Anatomy: Muscles

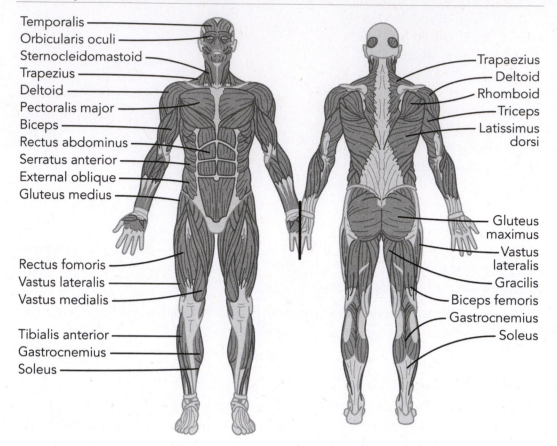

Temporalis
Orbicularis oculi
Sternocleidomastoid
Trapezius
Deltoid
Pectoralis major
Biceps
Rectus abdominus
Serratus anterior
External oblique
Gluteus medius

Rectus fomoris
Vastus lateralis
Vastus medialis

Tibialis anterior
Gastrocnemius
Soleus

Trapaezius
Deltoid
Rhomboid
Triceps
Latissimus dorsi

Gluteus maximus
Vastus lateralis
Gracilis
Biceps femoris
Gastrocnemius
Soleus

Practice Problems

1. Which of the following are the thick filaments in a muscle cell?

   A. Actin

   B. Myosin

   C. Myofibrils

   D. Sarcomere

2. Which of the following best describes the role of tendons?

   A. They connect muscle to bone.

   B. They connect bone to bone.

   C. They connect tendons to muscles.

   D. They connect cartilage to bone.

3. Which of the following types of muscle tissue is voluntary?

   A. Skeletal

   B. Smooth

   C. Cardiac

   D. Nervous

4. Which of the following muscles are located at the shoulder?

   A. Deltoids

   B. Pectorals

   C. Trapezius

   D. Abdominals

5. A person puts his hand on a hot stove but quickly removes it. In three to five sentences, describe the pathway of the signal and response through the nervous system.

S.1.7 — Describe the anatomy and physiology of the male and female reproductive system

The reproductive system includes physical structures, hormones, and secretions. The reproductive system works in tandem with the endocrine system to influence many other parts of the body. This TEAS task will ask questions about the various organs in the reproductive system and how they contribute to reproductive functions.

MALE REPRODUCTIVE SYSTEM

The purpose of the male reproductive system is to generate male gametes (**sperm**) and deliver them to the female reproductive system. The components of the male system include the **penis**, **vas deferens**, **urethra**, **prostate**, seminal vesicles, testis (plural: **testes**), and **scrotum**. The testes are the primary reproductive organs. Within the testes, there are lots of seminiferous tubules in which sperm are produced. The scrotum is a sac that houses the testes away from the body to lower their temperature during sperm production. The lower temperature provides the appropriate environment for sperm to mature. If they grow at body temperature or warmer, the sperm do not mature properly. The prostate and seminal vesicles produce the fluids necessary for lubricating and nourishing the sperm. The vas deferens, urethra, and penis form the conduit through which sperm is ejaculated. The vas deferens leads to the urethra, which leads sperm outside the body through the penis, which is the male copulatory organ.

Objectives

This objective includes, but is not limited to, the following examples of knowledge, skills, and abilities.

- Identify structures of the reproductive system.
- Explain the functions of the reproductive system.
- Describe the relationship between the reproductive system and the endocrine system.

Anatomy: Male Reproductive System

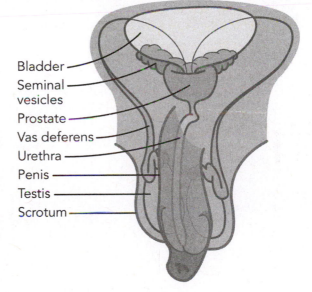

Bladder
Seminal vesicles
Prostate
Vas deferens
Urethra
Penis
Testis
Scrotum

---

sperm. Male gametes.

penis. Organ for elimination of urine and sperm from the male body.

vas deferens. The duct in which sperm moves from a testicle to the urethra.

urethra. The duct that delivers urine from the urinary bladder to the outside of the body.

prostate. The gland in males that controls the release of urine and secretes a portion of semen that enhances motility and fertility of sperm.

testes (testicles). The male gonads. The organs that produce sperm.

scrotum. The pouch of skin that contains the testicles.

FEMALE REPRODUCTIVE SYSTEM

The female reproductive system's primary roles include generating female gametes (*ova*, or eggs), *fertilization (conception)*, implantation (start of pregnancy), gestation (pregnancy), and parturition (birth). The components of the female reproductive system include the *ovaries*, *fallopian tubes* (also known as oviducts), *uterus*, cervix, *vagina*, labia minora and labia majora, and the clitoris. The labia majora and minora open into the vagina, which is a canal that serves as the female copulatory organ and the birth canal by connecting to the uterus through the cervix. The fallopian tubes connect the ovaries to the uterus. In response to changing *hormone* levels, a *follicle* in the ovary matures and releases an egg that then travels down the fallopian tubes to the uterus. Fertilization (or conception), which is the fusion of the egg and sperm, normally occurs in the Fallopian tubes.

Anatomy: Female Reproductive System

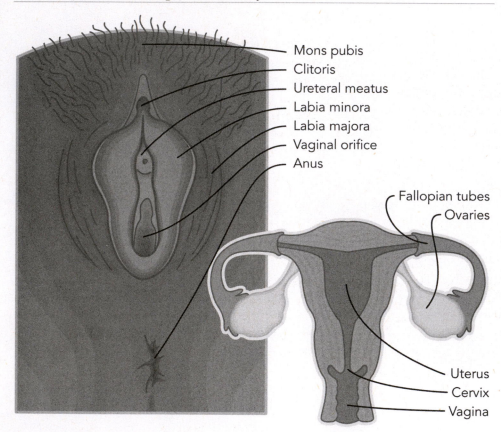

- Mons pubis
- Clitoris
- Ureteral meatus
- Labia minora
- Labia majora
- Vaginal orifice
- Anus
- Fallopian tubes
- Ovaries
- Uterus
- Cervix
- Vagina

If a released egg is fertilized by a sperm, it is then called a *zygote*. It undergoes several divisions into a ball of cells called a blastocyst, and it might undergo implantation. Implantation is the process by which a blastocyst implants itself in the uterine wall (endometrium). If the blastocyst successfully implants in the uterus, the blastocyst develops into an embryo and grows a placenta that allows the embryonic and maternal blood supplies into the network. The placenta nourishes the embryo as it grows into a fetus and removes wastes. Once the fetus is ready for birth, about 40 weeks after fertilization, the uterus contracts and the fetus is pushed out through the vagina.

ova (eggs). Female gametes.

fertilization (or conception). The fusion of the egg and sperm.

ovaries. The female gonads. Organs in which eggs are produced for reproduction.

fallopian tubes. Tubes that carry eggs from the ovaries to the uterus.

uterus. The womb.

vagina. The canal that connects the external genitals to the cervix in the female.

hormone. A chemical messenger produced by a gland and transported by the bloodstream that regulates specific processes in the body.

follicle. Saclike structure that contains and allows for maturation of the female ovum (egg) within the ovary.

zygote. Fertilized egg with full set of genetic material resulting from merging of egg and sperm nuclei.

RELATIONSHIP BETWEEN THE REPRODUCTIVE SYSTEM AND THE ENDOCRINE SYSTEM

Hormones are part of the endocrine system and allow for cell-to-cell communication. This communication controls many processes in the reproductive system. **Puberty** is initiated by the production of gonadotropin-releasing hormone from the **hypothalamus**, which triggers the release of **follicle-stimulating hormone** (FSH) and **luteinizing hormone** (LH) from the anterior **pituitary gland**. In males, LH is released and signals the testes to produce more **testosterone**. Testosterone and FSH stimulate the production of sperm cells. In females, FSH signals the ovaries to produce more **estrogen**. Release of estrogen causes some eggs (or ova, which is the plural for ovum) to mature in the ovary's follicles and the uterine endometrium to thicken. A surge of LH from the pituitary causes a developing egg that is most responsive to the LH surge to be released. The empty mature follicle is now called the "corpus luteum" and produces large amounts of progesterone to prepare the endometrium for implantation of the fertilized egg. If implantation does not occur, the uterine lining sheds. This cycle of maturation and shedding of endometrium is called the menstrual cycle. In males, testosterone production is not cyclical, so sperm, unlike eggs, are constantly produced and mature. Reproductive hormones also manage the development of secondary sexual characteristics, such as production of mammary glands, axial and facial hair, fat deposition patterns, and muscle growth.

Practice Problems

1. Which of the following organs produce female gametes?

   A. Ovary

   B. Testes

   C. Prostate

   D. Uterus

2. Which is the location where fertilization typically takes place?

   A. Vagina

   B. Penis

   C. Vas deferens

   D. Fallopian tubes

3. Which of the following best describes one function of estrogen?

   A. Production of sperm cells

   B. Maturation of eggs

   C. Implantation

   D. Fertilization

4. Which of the following result from the production of luteinizing hormone (LH) in males? (Select all that apply.)

   A. Heart growth

   B. Facial hair growth

   C. Testosterone production

   D. Sperm production

5. In three to five sentences, describe how the production of male and female gametes differs.

---

puberty. A physiological period in which changes in hormone levels cause a general "growth spurt" and development of secondary sex characteristics.

hypothalamus. A location in the brain that integrates the endocrine and nervous systems.

follicle-stimulating hormone. A hormone secreted by the anterior pituitary that stimulates development of eggs in ovaries and sperm in testes.

luteinizing hormone. A hormone secreted by the anterior pituitary that is responsible for triggering ovulation in ovaries and the production of testosterone by testes.

pituitary gland. The endocrine gland at the base of the brain that controls growth and development.

testosterone. The hormone that stimulates male secondary sexual characteristics.

estrogen. A female sex hormone released by the ovaries.

S.1.8 — Describe the anatomy and physiology of the integumentary system

The **integumentary system** refers to the body's largest organ, the skin. The integumentary system contains organs and glands that are vital to protecting the body and regulating temperature. This TEAS task requires knowledge of the structures of the integumentary system and its function in both **excretion** and **homeostasis**.

STRUCTURE OF THE INTEGUMENTARY SYSTEM

The integumentary system consists of skin, hair, and nails, as well as the **sebaceous**, sudoriferous, and **ceruminous glands**. Within the skin, there are **hair follicles**, **sweat glands**, and blood vessels.

Objectives

This objective includes, but is not limited to, the following examples of knowledge, skills, and abilities.

- Identify structures of the integumentary system.

- Explain the functions of the integumentary system.

- Describe the role of the integumentary system in homeostasis.

Anatomy: Skin

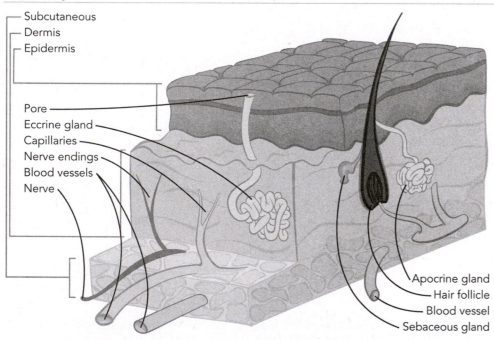

- Subcutaneous
- Dermis
- Epidermis

- Pore
- Eccrine gland
- Capillaries
- Nerve endings
- Blood vessels
- Nerve

- Apocrine gland
- Hair follicle
- Blood vessel
- Sebaceous gland

The skin can be divided into the **epidermis** (outer layer), **dermis** (middle layer), and **subcutaneous** or **hypodermis** (inner layer), as shown in the following diagram. The epidermis is made up of dead cells on the outside, and it has an inner layer of living cells. The epidermis also includes cells known as "melanocytes." Melanocytes produce and distribute melanin, which is a skin pigment. Beneath the epidermis is the dermis. The dermis contains collagen, blood vessels, glands, hair follicles, and nerve endings. The innermost layer is the hypodermis.

integumentary system. An organ system comprised of skin and its associated organs.

excretion. Elimination of metabolic waste from the body.

homeostasis. The maintenance of a constant internal environment.

sebaceous glands. Accessory structures originating in the dermis that secrete sebum onto hair emerging from the hair follicle.

ceruminous glands. Accessory structures that produce ear wax. They are found only in the dermis of the ear canal.

hair follicles. Tubes arising from the dermis surrounded by invaginations of epithelial tissue, from which hair growth occurs.

apocrine sweat gland. Accessory structures of the dermis that are in physical association with hair follicles, producing a secretion with an odor (possibly a sex pheromone to humans).

eccrine sweat glands. Accessory structures originating throughout the dermis of the human body that secrete sweat, used primarily for regulation of body temperature.

epidermis. The outer layer of the skin.

dermis. The middle layer of skin.

subcutaneous. Under the dermis.

hypodermis. The deepest layer of the skin.

FUNCTIONS OF THE INTEGUMENTARY SYSTEM

There are many functions of the integumentary system. The first is protection. The epidermis provides a barrier between the body and outside pathogens, such as bacteria. It also prevents the body from drying out. The inner cells of the epidermis divide quickly, pushing older cells toward the surface. These old cells die and create a tough, waterproof outer surface. Melanocytes in the epidermis produce melanin, which helps to protect the body from ultraviolet radiation from the sun. Skin cells also produce nails that protect the tips of fingers and toes.

Another function of the integumentary system is excretion. Along with water, minerals, including sodium, chloride, and magnesium, are excreted by glands. When these minerals build up in the body, they are excreted in higher amounts. *Sweat* can also contain trace amounts of urea, lactic acid, and alcohol.

The skin allows for the interaction between the body and the environment. The skin contains sensory nerve endings that allow the body to detect touch, change in temperature, and pain. These nerve endings are found in the skin's dermis layer. Skin also produces *vitamin D* when ultraviolet light hits the skin.

HOMEOSTASIS AND THE INTEGUMENTARY SYSTEM

The integumentary system plays a vital role in homeostasis. When the body becomes too warm, sweat glands produce sweat. The evaporation of sweat on the skin creates a cooling effect. Blood vessels in the skin can also dilate when the body is warm. The dilated blood vessels carry more blood closer to the skin's surface, and this can appear as flushed cheeks. The blood is then cooled and returned to deeper tissue at a cooler temperature. If the body is too cold, blood vessels *constrict* so that less blood is carried to the skin surface.

Practice Problems

1. Which of the following is the layer of skin that forms a protective, waterproof barrier?

   A. Dermis

   B. Sudoriferous

   C. Sebaceous

   D. Epidermis

2. Which of the following best describes the function of melanocytes?

   A. Secretion of substances like minerals and alcohol

   B. Production of melanin

   C. Absorption of vitamin D

   D. Sensing the environment

3. Which of the following layers of the skin contains hair follicles?

   A. Dermis

   B. Sudoriferous

   C. Sebaceous

   D. Epidermis

4. Which of the following layers of the skin contains a layer of dead cells?

   A. Dermis

   B. Hypodermis

   C. Sudoriferous

   D. Epidermis

5. In two to three sentences, describe how the integumentary system reacts to a rise in body temperature.

sweat. Perspiration excreted by sweat glands through the skin.

vitamin D. A vitamin made by the skin that helps the intestine absorb dietary calcium.

cutaneous vasoconstriction. A decrease in the diameter of blood vessels in the dermis that reduces blood flow through the skin.

S.1.9 — Describe the anatomy and physiology of the endocrine system

The endocrine system is a set of organs that secrete hormones directly into the circulatory system. Hormones are the chemicals released into the blood and act as signals to target organs to perform various functions. Hormones are involved in regulating many functions in the human body, so understanding the endocrine system helps in understanding how the human body works. The TEAS task will require you to know about the parts of the endocrine system, hormones, and the regulatory functions provided by the endocrine system. In particular, you will need to be familiar with homeostasis, positive and **negative feedback** mechanisms, and the relationship between the endocrine system and the central nervous system.

Objectives

This objective includes, but is not limited to, the following examples of knowledge, skills, and abilities.

- Identify structures of the endocrine system.

- Explain the functions of the endocrine system.

- Describe the role of the endocrine system in homeostasis.

- Recognize examples of positive and negative feedback mechanisms.

- Describe the relationship between the endocrine system and the nervous system.

GLANDS OF THE ENDOCRINE SYSTEM

The endocrine system is a complex network of glands and organs. A gland is a specific type of organ that secretes hormones into the blood to target and affect other organs. The following diagram shows the major glands in the endocrine system: pineal, pituitary, **thyroid**, **parathyroid**, **thymus**, and **adrenal**. Organs that contain endocrine tissue and produce hormones are the **pancreas** and the ovaries or testes.

The hypothalamus is a part of the brain involved in the endocrine system, and it controls the pituitary gland that is found just below it. The **pineal gland** is located in the middle of the brain. The thyroid and parathyroid glands are found in the neck, and the two adrenal glands are located on the top of each kidney.

Anatomy: Glands

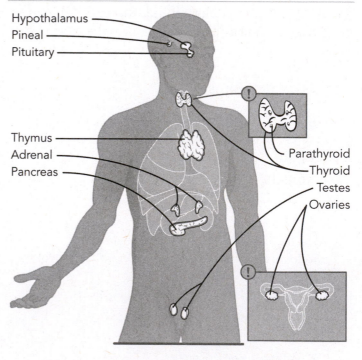

---

negative feedback. A mechanism that includes the monitoring for specific homeostatic levels and a signal to a gland. This signal stimulates or inhibits the gland's secretion in order to maintain homeostasis or cause compensations that returns the level to homeostasis.

thyroid gland. The gland in the neck that secretes hormones that regulate growth, development, and metabolic rate.

parathyroid. An endocrine gland in the neck that produces parathyroid hormone.

thymus. The lymphoid organ that produces T-cells.

adrenal. A gland above the kidney that produces hormones to regulate heart rate, blood pressure, and other functions.

pancreas. The gland of the digestive and endocrine systems that produces insulin and secretes pancreatic juices.

pineal gland. A small gland near the center of the brain that secretes melatonin.

FUNCTIONS OF THE ENDOCRINE SYSTEM

The endocrine system regulates many body functions by controlling the amount of hormones released. All body systems are regulated by the endocrine system in some way. Examples include the regulation of blood production, appetite, reproduction, brain function, sleep cycle, electrolyte balance, growth, sexual development, and response to stress and injury. Glands and organs secrete hormones into the blood to be transported to target organs and tissues to control their function. For example, the pancreas releases the hormone insulin, which signals cells to uptake *sugar*. The pineal gland releases the hormone melatonin, which is involved in regulating sleep cycles.

Endocrine glands produce hormones that have different chemical structures. Lipid-based hormones can enter a cell and regulate DNA. Some nonpolar, fat-soluble hormones, such as estrogen and progesterone, are released in a pattern set by age and development, and their effects are long lasting. Reproductive hormones are responsible for gamete production. For example, estrogen production increases at puberty and leads to the development of secondary sex characteristics.

Other polar, water-soluble hormones, such as **epinephrine**, are released in response to stress, and their actions are short lived. Hormone receptors on the cell membrane cause cellular changes to regulate and control body functions. When the adrenal glands secrete epinephrine into the bloodstream, heart rate, blood pressure, muscle strength, and metabolism increase. This response is called "the fight-or-flight" response. Hormone imbalance can cause metabolic diseases such as **diabetes**, **hyperthyroidism**, and **gigantism**. For example, in people with hyperthyroidism, the thyroid gland releases too much thyroxine. This can lead to an increase in both weight loss and heartbeat. To diagnose hyperthyroidism, doctors look for elevated levels of thyroxine in the blood. Gigantism occurs when the pituitary gland makes too much **growth hormone**, causing excessive growth. Hormone levels are often measured to determine if an endocrine-related disease is present. Gigantism is too much GH in children, too much GH in adults is acromegaly.

HOMEOSTASIS

Homeostasis is the maintenance of a constant internal environment. It helps the cells to work as efficiently as possible. Most homeostatic mechanisms work through feedback systems, and they are mainly controlled by endocrine glands. Feedback systems bring about physiological and behavioral changes, which help to maintain the internal constancy. Some examples of homeostasis include the following

- Maintaining the constant concentration of glucose in the blood, which is controlled by the hormones insulin and glucagon.

- Maintaining the right amount of water in the blood, which is under the control of **antidiuretic hormone** (ADH) secreted by the pituitary gland.

---

sugars. The monomers used to build polysaccharides; also molecules made of two or a few monosaccharide units that are used for fuel in the body.

endocrine gland. A gland that secretes hormones. A duct-less gland.

epinephrine. A polar, water-soluble hormone released by the adrenals in response to stress. Also known as adrenaline.

diabetes. Pathologically high blood sugar levels that result from a pancreatic hormone regulation malfunction.

hyperthyroidism. A malfunction of regulatory feedback loops leading to the overproduction of thyroid hormone.

gigantism. Excessive growth resulting from overproduction of growth hormone.

growth hormone. A secretion of the anterior pituitary that stimulates tissue growth. Also known as somatotropin.

antidiuretic hormone. A secretion from the pituitary gland that increases the amount of water able to be reabsorbed from a collecting duct.

POSITIVE AND NEGATIVE FEEDBACK MECHANISMS

Positive feedback causes an increase in the secretion of a hormone. An example of positive feedback is the secretion of the hormone *oxytocin*. During childbirth, the cervical stretching from fetal pressure triggers a release of oxytocin from the posterior pituitary. Oxytocin stimulates uterine contractions that, in turn, cause the fetus to push against and stretch the *cervix* even more. This positive feedback continues until the fetus is expelled through the cervix.

Most hormone levels in the body are regulated through negative feedback and are influenced by the production of a releasing hormone or an inhibiting hormone. Negative feedback helps to maintain homeostasis. The cells of the pancreas are able to adjust the amount of hormone they secrete in proportion to the amount of blood glucose they detect. When the blood sugar levels are too high, the beta cells of the pancreas release the hormone insulin. This signals the cells to uptake sugar, which lowers the blood sugar levels. When blood glucose levels are too low, alpha cells secrete a different hormone, glucagon. This hormone promotes the breakdown of glycogen, which is stored in the liver and in muscle cells, into glucose, which raises blood sugar levels. The hormone secretion is stopped when a homeostatic level of blood glucose is detected.

THE CENTRAL NERVOUS SYSTEM AND THE ENDOCRINE SYSTEM

The nervous system is involved in rapid communication within the body as it detects stimuli and coordinates responses quickly. The endocrine system is generally involved with comparatively slower and more long-lasting responses to stimuli than the nervous system. The integration of these two systems is called the "activation of the neuroendocrine system." For example, the hypothalamus of the brain directs the activities of the pituitary gland. Certain biochemical levels send messages to the hypothalamus, which either stimulates or turns off messages to the pituitary gland, which is located just below the brain. Specialized cells in the hypothalamus secrete hormones called "*releasing hormones*" or "*inhibiting hormones*" to the pituitary. The pituitary gland then makes and sends specific hormones to target organs. For example, the pituitary gland secretes follicle-stimulating hormone (FSH), which functions in egg development in the ovaries.

Another example of the activation of the neuroendocrine system occurs in childbirth. During labor, the pressure of the fetus on the cervix sends signals through the nervous system to the hypothalamus, which results in oxytocin being secreted by the posterior pituitary gland.

---

positive feedback. A mechanism that stimulates glandular secretions to continue to increase, temporarily pushing levels further out of homeostasis, until a particular biological effect is reached (e.g., expulsion of the fetus during childbirth).

oxytocin. A hormone made by the hypothalamus and stored in the posterior pituitary. One of its functions is to stimulate uterine contractions during childbirth.

cervix. The passage that forms the lower part of the uterus.

releasing hormones. Chemical messengers that stimulate the production of certain hormones.

inhibiting hormones. Chemical messengers that restrict the production of certain hormones.

Practice Problems

1. Which of the following best describes the kind of message sent in the endocrine system?

   A. Electrical signals between axons

   B. Chemical signals that travel through the bloodstream

   C. Physical sensory signals received through the integumentary system

   D. Audiovisual signals processed through the brain

2. Which of the following structures secretes releasing hormones?

   A. Hypothalamus

   B. Pituitary

   C. Pancreas

   D. Liver

3. Which of the following is a function of the pineal gland?

   A. Releasing growth hormone

   B. Releasing melatonin

   C. Releasing insulin and glucagon

   D. Releasing luteinizing hormone

4. Which of the following glands releases epinephrine during stress?

   A. Hypothalamus

   B. Adrenal glands

   C. Pancreas

   D. Pituitary gland

5. In three to five sentences, explain what happens to the levels of blood glucose and hormones after eating.

S.1.10 — Describe the anatomy and physiology of the urinary system

The organs in the urinary, or urogenital, system function in the excretory process. Some structures, such as the urethra and penis in the male, are also used by the reproductive system. This section of the TEAS will focus on the excretion process and its associated structures. Excretion is a necessary function for salt and water homeostasis and getting rid of wastes. It is important to know how the structures function and their contributions to the process of excretion and reproduction. It is also important to understand the relationship between the **urinary system** and the cardiovascular system.

Objectives

This objective includes, but is not limited to, the following examples of knowledge, skills, and abilities.

- Identify structures of the urinary system.
- Explain the functions of the urinary system.
- Describe the relationship between the urinary system and the cardiovascular system.

PARTS OF THE URINARY SYSTEM

The urinary system is composed of the kidneys, ureters, **urinary bladder**, and urethra. The **kidneys** lie against the dorsal body wall above the waist, superior to the lumbar region. Kidneys have two main regions or layers: the **renal cortex** and the **renal medulla**. The cortex is the outer layer of the kidney where blood vessels are located. The cortex also produces erythropoietin, a hormone that stimulates the production of new red blood cells. The renal medulla is the inner region of the kidney where the concentration of **urine** is regulated.

Kidneys have a **renal artery**, which allows oxygenated blood to enter the kidney, and renal veins, which allow filtered, deoxygenated blood to leave the kidney. Kidneys manufacture urine, which travels through the ureters to the urinary bladder where it is stored until it is excreted through the urethra.

The ureters, urinary bladder, and urethra are parts of the excretory system. The ureters (one for each kidney) are small tubes that carry urine from the kidney to the urinary bladder, which holds the urine until elimination. In males, the urethra passes through the penis and also carries sperm. Females have a much shorter urethra and are therefore more prone to UTIs as compared to males.

Anatomy: Urinary System

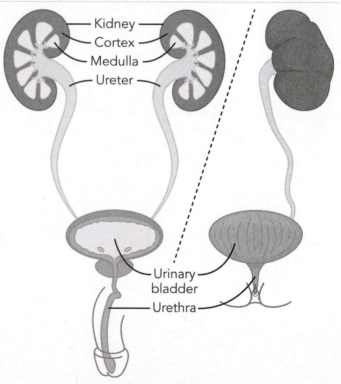

- Kidney
- Cortex
- Medulla
- Ureter
- Urinary bladder
- Urethra

urinary system. Is composed of the kidneys, ureters, urinary bladder, and urethra and function in the excretory process

urinary bladder. The structure that stores urine in the body until elimination.

kidneys. The pair of organs that regulate fluid balance and filter waste from the blood.

renal cortex. The outer layer of the kidney.

renal medulla. The innermost part of the kidney.

urine. Liquid waste excreted by the kidneys.

renal arteries. The two branches of the abdominal aorta that supply the kidneys.

FUNCTIONS OF THE URINARY SYSTEM

In the human body, it is important to maintain homeostasis. The urinary system is responsible in helping to maintain this balance by getting rid of wastes. Nitrogenous waste from protein digestion is toxic and must be removed because it will form ammonia. Kidneys, a major organ in this system, are primarily responsible for filtering blood, creating urine, stabilizing water balance, maintaining blood pressure, and producing the active form of vitamin D. The endocrine system also plays a vital role in several of these functions.

The structural and functional unit of the kidney is the **nephron**. Nephrons are a system of microscopic tubes that use various pressure levels to remove wastes and reabsorb important molecules and water. Blood enters the kidney full of waste from metabolism, especially of protein metabolism. It enters a nephron capillary connected to the renal artery. It then flows to the **glomerulus**, a small, dense group of capillaries in the nephron. Here, material is filtered from the blood. This material is called "**filtrate**" and includes water, urea, glucose, salts, and other small molecules. Then, the filtrate moves through the **proximal tubule**. Water and other important substances to the body are reabsorbed through the capillaries back into the blood.

Finally, what remains in the tubule, urine, is emptied into a cavity in the kidney and drains from there to the **ureter**. It is then stored in the urinary bladder. The urinary bladder is a hollow, muscular organ that holds 400 to 800 mL of liquid and has sensors that communicate with the central nervous system. For excretion to occur, both the internal and external sphincters of the bladder must relax. From the bladder, the urine is released through the urethra. Released urine is a waste product composed of 95% water, with urea, salts, and excess **organic molecules**.

Anatomy: Nephron

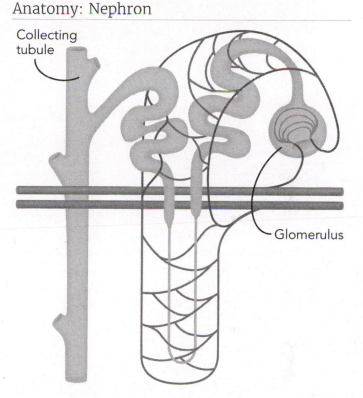

Collecting tubule

Glomerulus

---

nephron. A system of microscopic tubes in the kidneys that use various pressure levels to remove wastes and reabsorb important molecules and water.

glomerulus. A network of capillaries from which blood pressure pushes water, salt, glucose, amino acids, and urea from the blood.

filtrate. Materials, including water, that leave the blood through the walls of the glomerular capillaries to enter the Bowman's capsule.

proximal tubule. The first location where glucose and other useful solutes are reabsorbed back into the blood through the walls of surrounding capillaries. It connects the Bowman's capsule to the Loop of Henle.

ureter. The duct that delivers urine from the kidney to the bladder.

organic molecule. A molecule found in a living thing that contains carbon.

RELATIONSHIP BETWEEN THE URINARY SYSTEM AND THE CARDIOVASCULAR SYSTEM

Kidneys play a vital role in maintaining blood pressure by controlling the volume of the blood. Secreted hormones of the kidneys constrict or dilate blood vessels, causing the needed increase or decrease in blood pressure. Kidneys also help to control the production of red blood cells. The cardiovascular system pumps blood into the kidneys through the renal artery. The pressure of the blood helps the glomerulus filter out wastes and return vital nutrients through the **renal vein** to the blood. The kidneys also produce **renin**, a hormone that regulates blood pressure by retaining or removing water and salt.

Practice Problems

1. Which of the following parts of the male urinary system also transports sperm?

   A. Ureter

   B. Urethra

   C. Uterus

   D. Urinary bladder

2. Which of the following waste products from digestion does the kidney remove?

   A. Nitrogen

   B. Sodium chloride

   C. Protein

   D. Carbon

3. Which of the following best describes the outcome if the kidneys stopped functioning?

   A. Blood would increase its carbon dioxide concentration.

   B. Blood would fill with waste and the human body would not be able to maintain homeostasis.

   C. The kidneys would fill with urine.

   D. The frequency in which a human excretes urine would increase.

4. Which of the following structures is the structural and functional unit of the kidney?

   A. Renal capillaries

   B. Glomerulus

   C. Nephron

   D. Cortex

5. In two to three sentences, explain the role of blood pressure and the kidney.

---

renal vein. A vein carrying blood from a kidney to the inferior vena cava.

renin. An enzyme released by the kidney when reduced blood pressure is detected by baroreceptors in aorta and carotid arteries.

S.1.11 — Describe the anatomy and physiology of the immune system

The immune system functions like soldiers and forti-fications in a battle to protect the body. For this TEAS task, you will need to be familiar with the various parts of the immune system and how they contribute to that protection scheme. In particular, you will need to understand how the immune system relates to the other body systems.

PARTS OF THE IMMUNE SYSTEM

The immune system protects the body from disease-causing agents known as pathogens. The immune system is composed of both **innate defense** and **adaptive defense** systems. Innate defense is considered a nonspecific response to pathogens, and adaptive defense is considered specific to a given pathogen. The **innate immune system** has three lines of defense: The first (skin, mucus, secretions) keeps pathogens from entering the body, the second (phagocytes, specific proteins, inflammatory response) fights pathogens that have entered the body, and the third is the **adaptive immune system**. Lymphocytes such as **B cells** and various types of **T cells** not only fight the pathogen but also retain a memory of the specific pathogen.

FUNCTIONS OF THE IMMUNE SYSTEM

The immune system prevents entry of pathogens through the presence of barriers (much like walls and moats) composed of the skin and secretions such as acid, enzymes, and salt. If the external barriers are breached, there are cells and chemicals that act as soldiers to attack the pathogens. If that barrier fails, then the adaptive immune system specifically identifies, targets, and remembers the pathogen. Visualize the immune system as layers of protection that include barriers to prevent entry, signaling, and targeting. The ultimate function is to protect the body from a pathogen attack while allowing harmless molecules to enter the body.

The immune system functions through interactions with several others through which pathogens can enter the body. Pathogens enter through body openings of the digestive, urinary, and reproductive systems; injuries can also create ways for pathogens to enter. The lymph system is critical to the functioning of the immune system because pathogens from the blood also circulate through the lymph. B cells and T cells reside in the lymph nodes and are activated when a pathogen is encountered.

innate defense. A nonspecific response to pathogens by the immune system
adaptive defense. A specific response by the immune system to a given pathogen.
innate immune system. A collection of nonspecific barriers and cellular responses that serve as an inborn first and second line of defense against pathogens.
adaptive immune system. A kind of passive or active immunity in which antibodies to a particular antigen are present in the body.
B cells. Lymphocytes that mature in bone marrow and make antibodies in response to antigens.
T cells. White blood cells that mature in the thymus and participate in an immune response.

THE INNATE IMMUNE SYSTEM

The innate immune system is a series of nonspecific barriers—physical, cellular, and soluble components—that impede pathogens from entering the body or from multiplying. External barriers include the physical barrier of the skin and mucus secretions; chemical barriers, such as low pH, salt, enzymes; and cellular barriers of **commensal microorganisms**. If the pathogen breaches the barriers and enters the blood or tissues, a second line of defense is activated. For example, when a pathogen makes it into your body through a cut in the skin, mechanisms will go into effect to prevent the pathogens from affecting your body. One of the first responses is called the "inflammatory response." In an inflammatory response, **histamines** are released, increasing not only blood flow to the area but also the number of white blood cells known as phagocytes to the area. These phagocytes destroy bacteria. **Interferons**, which are proteins that interfere with the production of new viruses, are released if a virus enters the body. Fever is also sometimes used by the body to speed up the immune response. Other internal barriers include **antimicrobial** peptides and "natural killer" (NK) lymphocyte cells that attack host cells that harbor intracellular pathogens.

THE ADAPTIVE IMMUNE SYSTEM

The adaptive immune system has two general responses to specific pathogens: cellular or humoral. A cellular response destroys the infected cell, and the humoral response destroys pathogens found in body fluids using antibodies secreted by B cells.

The adaptive immune system responds by remembering signature molecules, called "**antigens**," from pathogens to which the body has previously been exposed. The adaptive immune system's functional cells are lymphocytes called "T cells" and "B cells." **Antigen-presenting cells** (APCs) such as macrophages digest pathogens and present the pathogen's antigen signature to "helper" T cells. Depending on the type of antigen presented to the **helper T cell**, either a B cell or a **cytotoxic T cell** is activated. Helper T cells produce **cytokines** to activate a cytotoxic T cell. The cytotoxic T cell then searches out and destroys any cell that contains the pathogen's antigen signature. The helper T cell can also activate B cells in response to a specific antigen. The helper T cell induces the B cell to multiply rapidly into secretory cells called "plasma cells." These plasma cells will then produce large amounts of an **antibody** that can bind the antigen. B cells also clone into **memory cells** at the same time. This allows the body to remember a specific antigen. When that antigen appears again in the body, this triggers the memory cells to form plasma cells, which quickly produces the specific antibody to the antigen.

---

commensal microorganisms. Microscopic organisms that live in or on the human body without causing it harm.

histamine. A white blood cell secretion that triggers capillary permeability and vasodilatation.

interferons. Proteins secreted by leukocytes when they are infected with viruses.

antimicrobial. A substance that kills or inhibits growth of microorganisms with minimal damage to the host.

antigens. Substances on the surfaces of agents that act to identify them, to the body, as being native or foreign.

antigen-presenting cell. A cell that displays foreign antigens with major histocompatibility complexes on their surfaces.

helper T-cell. A type of lymphocyte that secretes interleukins, a protein that triggers the action of other cells, including the attack of foreign cells by the cytotoxic T cell.

cytotoxic T cells. The category of lymphocyte that attacks foreign cells.

cytokines. Cell signaling molecules released primarily by helper T-cells and macrophages. Certain cytokines activate cytotoxic T-cells.

antibody. A blood protein that counteracts a specific antigen.

memory cell. A lymphocyte that responds to an antigen upon reintroduction.

PASSIVE AND ACTIVE IMMUNITY

Passive and *active immunity* are the two ways to protect the body through either passive introduction of antibodies as a protective agent or its active production by the body. Both passive and active immunity can be induced artificially. Vaccinations introduce antigens, which are weakened or killed, to elicit an immune response. *Passive immunity* introduces antibodies from another source that can rapidly neutralize toxins. Rapid treatment for a snakebite is an example of passive immunity.

Many diseases are caused by a malfunction of the immune system. Underactivity of the immune system can cause components to be ineffective. Acquired immune deficiency syndrome (AIDS) is caused by the human immunodeficiency virus (HIV), which infects helper T cells and prevents them from activating cytotoxic T cells and B cells and prevents the adaptive immune system from operating. Conversely, overactive immune systems can target innocuous foreign particles like pollen, causing the body to overproduce huge amounts of antibodies that trigger a histamine release from mast cells, which results in allergy symptoms, such as sneezing and mucus secretion. Alternately, the immune system can mistakenly target a host molecule as a foreign antigen, leading to *autoimmune diseases*, conditions in which the immune system mistakenly attacks the body. Examples include type I diabetes, *rheumatoid arthritis*, and multiple sclerosis.

THE IMMUNE SYSTEM AND OTHER BODY SYSTEMS

The immune system works hand in hand with other body systems to transport immune cells, signaling molecules, and antibodies throughout the body. For example, the circulatory system transports white blood cells throughout the body. The lymphatic system produces white blood cells or lymphocytes. The vessels in the lymph system drain fluid from body tissues and deliver foreign material to the lymph nodes to be processed by lymphocytes. Red *bone marrow*, found in many bones of the *skeletal system*, also produce white blood cells. In addition, the integumentary system functions as the first line of defense for most of the body.

---

active immunity. Protection against a specific pathogen resulting from the production of antibodies in response to the presence of specific antigens.

passive immunity. Temporary immunity gained by a body that has acquired antibodies from an outside source.

autoimmune disease. A pathology that results from the immune system mistaking part of the body as a pathogen.

rheumatoid arthritis. A progressive autoimmune disease that causes joint inflammation and pain.

bone marrow. A soft material within spongy bone and medullary cavity of long bones.

skeletal system. The system of bones in the body that provides protection for delicate organs and serves as the scaffold against which muscles pull for movement. It has three main functions: movement, protection, and storage of minerals and fat.

Practice Problems

1. Which of the following is a barrier that helps prevent pathogens from invading the body?

   A. Histamines

   B. Mucus

   C. T cells

   D. Macrophages

2. A bacteria cell enters the body through a cut in the skin. Which of the following describes the immune response that would occur next?

   A. Cytotoxic T cells form.

   B. Histamines are released.

   C. Antigens are released.

   D. Helper T cells are activated.

3. Which of the following types of cells produce antibodies?

   A. T cells

   B. Plasma cells

   C. Memory cells

   D. Macrophages

4. Which of the following best describes the purpose of a vaccine?

   A. To produce extra inflammatory responses such as the release of histamines

   B. To practice passive immunity

   C. To produce antibodies in case of future infection

   D. To increase macrophage production

5. In three to five sentences, describe what occurs in the immune system when it encounters an allergen.

S.1.12 — Describe the anatomy and physiology of the skeletal system

The skeletal system has three main functions: movement, protection, and storage of minerals and fat. To be successful at this task, you should know the names of the major bones of the human body, particularly those that help with movement, protection, and synthesis of blood cells. Study the structure of bone, including cells involved in bone synthesis and breakdown. You will also want to be familiar with diseases of the skeletal system, such as **osteoporosis** and **osteoarthritis**.

> ### Objectives
>
> This objective includes, but is not limited to, the following examples of knowledge, skills, and abilities.
>
> - Identify structures of the skeletal system.
> - Explain the functions of the skeletal system.
> - Describe the relationship between the skeletal system and the muscular system.

STRUCTURE AND FUNCTION OF THE SKELETAL SYSTEM

The skeletal system is the scaffold against which muscles pull for movement, and it provides protection for delicate organs. For example, the brain is protected by the skull. Bones also provide support and shape for the human body. Bones have other functions that you may not think of right away. They synthesize blood and immune cells, as well as store calcium, phosphate, and lipids. Bone is a dynamic tissue that is made and broken down according to need.

Bones come in four major types: long, short, flat, and irregular. **Long bones** have longer lengths than widths and make up most of the bones in the arms and legs. The femur, or upper leg bone, is an example of a long bone. Other examples of long bones are the humerus, ulna, radius, tibia, and fibula.

Anatomy: Skeleton

RJHARDY/BEYHES/ATI/ADAPTED FROM GETTY IMAGES/ISTOCKPHOTO

---

osteoporosis. A disease that causes brittle, fragile bones.
osteoarthritis. Degenerative joint disease.
long bones. Bones that have a pronounced longitudinal axis.

The marrow in a long bone is called "yellow marrow" and stores lipids (fat). Red bone marrow is found at the ends of long bones and is the site of blood cell production (RBCs, WBCs, and platelets). The ends of long bones have **growth plates**, and this is where the bone lengthens if it is growing.

Short bones have the same length and width. Examples of short bones are the square bones of the wrist and ankle. **Flat bones** are thin and flat and are used to protect vital organs. For example, ribs are flat bones that protect the heart and lungs. Flat bones also contain red bone marrow and produce blood cells. **Irregular bones**, such as the hip bones and vertebrae, have other shapes.

Joints are places where bones meet other bones. Some joints are movable, like the **ball-and-socket joint** of the hips and shoulders. There are other joints, such as those in the skull, that are **immovable** because the bones are fused together. Typically, bones are attached to other bones through **ligaments**. The hyoid bone, which supports the tongue, is the only bone in the body that is not connected to other bones and is held in place only by suprahyoid and infrahyoid muscles. The articulating surfaces of bones are covered in **hyaline cartilage**, which prevents them from grinding against each other. Synovial joints, such as the pivot, ball-and-socket, and **hinge**, also contain lubricating synovial fluid and are usually capable of movement.

Bone is synthesized in tubular structures called "**osteons**," which are composed of calcium and phosphate-rich hydroxyapatite embedded in a collagen matrix and are the functional units of **compact bone**. Osteons are also called "Haversian systems." The osteon includes the matrix that forms in a concentric ring and the **osteocytes** that are in small cave-like spaces in the matrix, called "**lacunae**." The matrix forms around the central canal that contains blood vessels and nerves. Bone is covered by a fibrous sheath called the "**periosteum**," which contains nerves and blood vessels. Just like other cells of the body, bone cells need to be supplied with oxygen and nutrients and need to communicate with other body systems.

---

growth plate. Hyaline cartilage in long bones where bone elongation happens. Also known as the epiphyseal plate.

short bones. Bones that are similar in both length and width, such as those found in the wrist. They have limited articulation with each other as gliding joints.

flat bones. Thin bones that have a plate-like shape, such as bones of the cranium.

irregular bones. Bones that do not fit into the three bone shape categories: flat bone, long bone, short bone.

joints. Places in the skeletal system where bones meet other bones. Some joints are movable, and some are immovable because the bones are fused together.

ball and socket joints. Point of articulation that allows for abduction, adduction, circumduction, and rotation. The hip socket is one example of a ball and socket joint.

sutures. Joints, such as those between the plates of the skull, that do not allow motion.

ligaments. A tough connective tissue that attaches bone to bone.

hyaline cartilage. The kind of connective tissue that protects bone in articulating joints.

cartilage. The primary structural protein of connective tissue.

hinge joint. A joint that allows for flexion and extension of the more distal bone along only one plane.

osteons. Tubular structures that make up compact bone.

compact (dense) bone. Bone containing densely packed osteons that make up the peripheral layer of bone.

osteocytes. Osteocytes are star-shaped cells that maintain bone and are able to sense physical stresses.

lacunae. Microscopic pits in bones that contain osteocytes and connect to each other within an osteon by way of canaliculi.

periosteum. A thin layer that surrounds bone and is the surface for attachment of tendons and ligaments.

There are two main types of bone cells: multinucleate **osteoclasts** and mononucleate **osteoblasts**. Osteoblasts replace cartilage and secrete mineral deposits that form the matrix, the nonliving substance of the bone. Osteoblasts also develop into osteocytes, which strengthen bone tissue and carry out metabolic functions. Osteoclasts break down bone minerals of the matrix. This building up and breaking down of bone is important for strengthening bones. However, this can sometimes lead to problems. If osteoclasts break down bone faster than osteoblasts deposit minerals, the bones become weak and brittle. This is what happens in osteoporosis.

Bone Composition

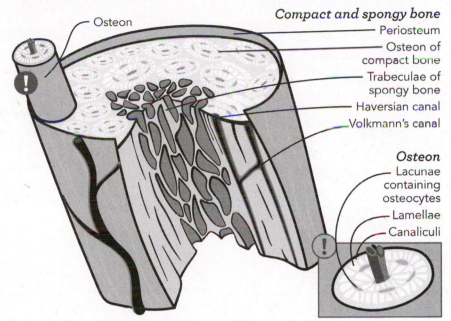

There are several common diseases of bone. Excessive withdrawal of minerals from bone can cause the bone's rigidity to be lost and lead to osteoporosis. Arthritis damages the cartilage that articulates between joints. **Brittle bone disease** (**osteogenesis imperfecta**) results from a genetic defect in the collagen matrix. In osteogenesis imperfecta, the gene that codes for a collagen needed to form the matrix of the bone is missing and causes bones to break easily.

THE SKELETAL SYSTEM AND MUSCULAR SYSTEM

The skeletal muscles of the muscular system and the bones involved in movement must work together in the body. Skeletal muscles attach to bones, and these muscles are connected to and communicate with the central nervous system. When the muscle receives a signal to contract from the central nervous system, the muscle contracts, moving the bone to which it is connected. Muscles connect to bones with tendons, which are made of connective tissue. For example, triceps and biceps muscles control the movement of the elbow. Biceps and triceps connect to the arm bones, and when contracted, they move the arm bones into different positions. Muscles work in tandem. As one of the pair relaxes, the other contracts for one type of movement as shown in the following diagram. The contracting muscle is called the "**prime mover**," and the relaxed muscle in the pair is called the "**antagonist**."

Anatomy: Muscles in the Arm

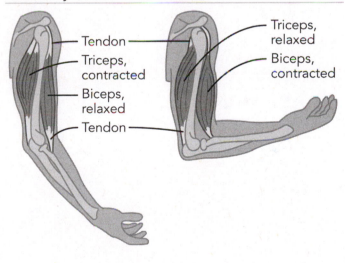

---

osteoclasts. Cells that remove bone.

osteoblasts. Osteocytes are star-shaped cells that maintain bone and are able to sense physical stresses. Their long projections connect to each other through the canaliculi of bones.

brittle bone disease. A group of diseases that affect collagen and result in fragile bones.

prime mover. The contracting muscle in the pair of muscles that is involved in a given movement; also called the agonist.

antagonist. The relaxed muscle in the pair of muscles that is involved in a given movement.

Practice Problems

1. Which of the following breaks down bone material?

   A. Osteoclasts

   B. Osteoblasts

   C. Canaliculi

   D. Osteocytes

2. Which of the following are considered short bones?

   A. Skull bones

   B. Radius and ulna

   C. Carpals and tarsals

   D. Humerus and scapula

3. Which of the following best describes the purpose of hyaline cartilage in the skeletal system?

   A. It forms the matrix of a bone.

   B. It develops into osteocytes.

   C. It strengthens the entire skeletal system.

   D. It reduces friction at joints.

4. Which of the following best explains the cause of osteoporosis?

   A. Pathogens eat away at bone tissue.

   B. Ligaments degrade, causing joints to malfunction.

   C. Osteoclasts break down bone faster than osteoblasts deposit minerals.

   D. Osteoclasts break down bone slower than osteoblasts build up bone.

5. In three to five sentences, describe how the skeletal and muscular system work together.

Life and Physical Sciences

S.2.1 — Describe cell structure, function, and organization.

This TEAS task requires an understanding of the general anatomy and physiology of the human body. It is first important to understand the hierarchy of structures and functions within the human body. You will need a general knowledge of cell parts and their functions and how cells form structures. You will also need to explain and differentiate between **mitosis** and **meiosis**. There are many resources available on this subject, including print textbooks, online content and quizzes, and free online textbooks. These are excellent for both learning the concepts and committing them to memory.

BIOLOGICAL HIERARCHY OF THE BODY

Biological hierarchy is a way to organize structures in living things, classifying structures from the most basic components to the most complex, as shown in the diagram.

Chemicals build cells. **Macromolecules** are large chemicals that are important to living things and include **carbohydrates**, **proteins**, lipids, and **nucleic acids**.

The cell is the fundamental unit of life because all life functions can take place there. More than 250 different types of cells enable the human body to carry out life processes.

Cells with shared functions form larger collective groups called tissues. The four basic types of tissues are epithelial, connective, nervous, and muscular.

Tissues of different types can then join to form organs, which carry out a single task. For example, lungs are an organ whose task is to deliver oxygen to the bloodstream.

Organs work together in an organ system that performs coordinated, large-scale functions. In the nervous system, the nerves and brain work together to collect and process information. The nervous system then works with other systems in the body. For example, the nervous system sends signals to the muscular system to coordinate movement. Together, coordinated organ systems allow an organism to function.

Objectives

This objective includes, but is not limited to, the following examples of knowledge, skills, and abilities.

- Describe the levels of hierarchical organization of the body (e.g., how cells are organized into tissues).

- Identify the components of a cell.

- Describe the functions of cell components (e.g., obtaining and using energy, cell reproduction, cell growth and metabolism).

- Distinguish between processes and functions of mitosis and meiosis.

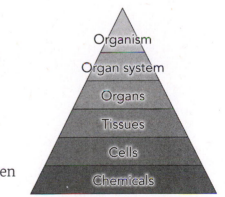

Organism
Organ system
Organs
Tissues
Cells
Chemicals

---

mitosis. Cell division in eukaryotes that produces two daughter cells, each with the same chromosome number as the parent cell.

meiosis. Specialized cell division used to create haploid gametes in diploid organisms.

macromolecules. Very large molecules, four major types of which are important to living things: carbohydrates, proteins, lipids, and nucleic acids.

carbohydrates. Sugars and starches, which the body breaks down into glucose.

proteins. Molecules composed of amino acids joined by peptide bonds.

nucleic acids. Long molecules made of nucleotides; DNA and RNA.

CELL STRUCTURE AND FUNCTION

The cell is the building block of all living organisms. The basic parts of a cell are the **nucleus**, **plasma membrane**, and **cytoplasm**. Structures called "**organelles**" are found in a cell's cytoplasm. The diagram shows the key organelles found in most animal cells.

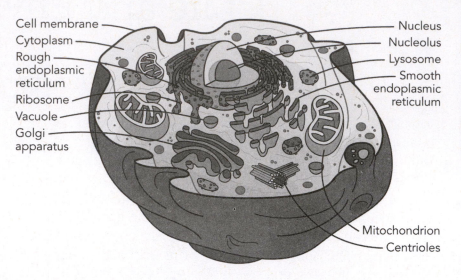

Each type of organelle performs a specific function. For example, the **mitochondrion** is the site of energy production. Although certain organelles are found in all cell types, the number and type of organelles vary depending on the cell type. Skeletal muscle cells, for example, contain high numbers of mitochondria because of the energy needed for movement.

Organelles coordinate with other organelles to perform a cell's basic functions, such as energy processing, waste excretion, or protein synthesis. For example, several organelles, such as ribosomes, the **endoplasmic reticulum**, and the **Golgi apparatus**, work together to build proteins.

---

nucleus. A large organelle within a cell that houses the chromosomes and regulates the activities of the cell.

cell (plasma) membrane. A membrane that surrounds the cell and maintains its internal environment through the property of selective permeability.

cytoplasm. The material within a eukaryotic cell that supports and suspends structures inside the cell membrane and transfers materials required for cellular processes.

organelle. A specialized part of a cell that has a specific function and is found in the cell's cytoplasm.

mitochondrion. The site of energy production in a cell.

smooth endoplasmic reticulum. A cell organelle that synthesizes and concentrates lipids in the cell; does not contain ribosomes.

Golgi apparatus. A cell organelle that processes proteins and lipid molecules.

The following chart lists the functions of key organelles in the cell.

Organelle	Function	Image
Cell (plasma) membrane	Maintains cells' environment through the process of selective permeability	
Cytoplasm	Supports and suspends structures inside the cell membrane; transfers materials required for cellular processes	
Golgi Apparatus	Processes proteins and lipid *molecules*	
Lysosome	Aids in digestion and recycling of old cell materials; may help destroy invading viruses and bacteria	
Mitochondrion	Generates chemical energy in the form of ATP molecules	
Nucleus	Holds genes that carry hereditary information; regulates the activity of the cell Nucleolus assembles RNA and proteins into ribosomes.	 Nucleolus
Ribosome	Synthesizes proteins (many are found on the surface of the *rough endoplasmic reticulum* although some can be free-floating in the cytoplasm)	

molecule. An arrangement of two or more atoms bonded together.

lysosome. A cell organelle that aids in digestion and the recycling of old cell materials.

ribosome. A protein-RNA complex that is the site of protein synthesis.

rough endoplasmic reticulum. A cell organelle containing ribosomes that synthesizes and processes proteins in the cell.

Organelle	Function	Image
Rough Endoplasmic Reticulum	Contains ribosomes; synthesizes and processes proteins in the cell	
Smooth Endoplasmic Reticulum	Does not contain ribosomes; synthesizes and concentrates lipids in the cell Inactivates toxins and harmful metabolic products.	
Vacuole	Serves as storage for a variety of elements, such as water, toxins and carbohydrates.	

MITOSIS AND MEIOSIS

Via the process of mitosis, cells duplicate for tissue growth and repair. In mitosis, one cell reproduces two genetically identical daughter cells. The events of mitosis are shown in the diagram below.

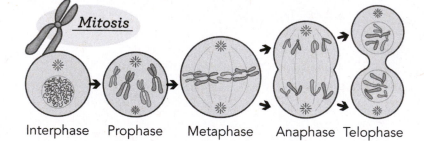

- **Interphase.** DNA replicates.

- **Prophase.** *Chromosomes* condense and visible chromosomes appear.

- **Metaphase.** Chromosomes line up.

- **Anaphase.** Chromosomes are pulled apart to the poles. Cell division begins.

- **Telophase.** Two nuclei form. Daughter cells separate in cytokinesis.

interphase. The stage in mitosis or meiosis in which DNA replicates.

prophase. The stage in mitosis in which chromosomes condense in preparation for being pulled apart.

chromosome. A structure made of protein and one molecule of DNA that contains genetic information.

metaphase. The stage in mitosis in which chromosomes align.

anaphase. The stage in mitosis in which the chromosomes are pulled apart to the poles and cell division begins.

telophase. The stage in mitosis in which two nuclei form and the daughter cells separate.

vacuole. A cell organelle that serves as storage for a variety of substances, including water, toxins, and carbohydrates.

In the process of meiosis, the nucleus of a germ cell divides, and then each part divides again (two fissions), producing four **gametes**, or sex cells. Each sex cell has half the genetic information of the original germ cell and supplies half the genetic information for sexual reproduction. The events of meiosis are shown in the diagram that follows.

- Interphase: DNA replicates.

- Meiosis I

  - **Prophase I**: Homologous chromosomes pair and cross over.

  - **Metaphase I:** Homologous chromosomes line up in pairs.

  - **Anaphase I:** One chromosome from each homologous pair is pulled towards each pole.

  - **Telophase I:** Nuclear membranes form as the cell separates into two.

- Meiosis II

  - **Prophase II:** Daughter cells contain half the chromosomes of the original cell.

  - **Metaphase II:** Chromosomes align.

  - **Anaphase II**: Sister **chromatids** separate and move to opposite ends of the cells.

  - **Telophase II:** Nuclear membranes form as the two cells separate into four haploid daughter cells.

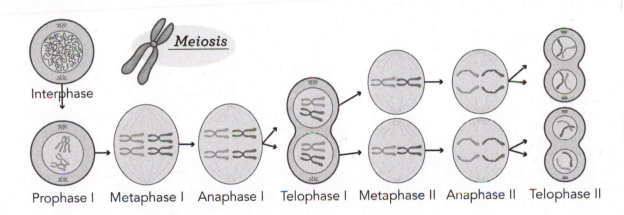

gamete. Sex cell; in males the sperm, in females the eggs (ova).

prophase I. The stage in meiosis I in which chromosomes condense and form homologous pairs.

metaphase I. The stage in meiosis I in which pairs of homologous chromosomes align.

anaphase I. The stage in meiosis I in which homologous chromosomes move to opposite ends of the cell.

telophase I. The stage in meiosis I in which nuclear membranes form as the cell separates into two haploid daughter cells with chromosomes consisting of two sister chromatids.

telophase II. The stage in meiosis II in which nuclear membranes form as the two daughter cells from meiosis I separate into four haploid daughter cells with chromosomes consisting of a single chromatid each.

prophase II. The stage in meiosis II in which chromosomes in the haploid daughter cells condense.

metaphase II. The stage in meiosis II in which individual chromosomes align.

anaphase II. The stage in meiosis II in which sister chromatids separate and move to opposite ends of the cell.

chromatid. One of the two duplicates of a chromosome formed during the cell cycle.

Practice Problems

1. List the six components of the biological hierarchy of the body, from least to most complex.

2. Which of the following describes the function of the ribosome?

   A. Protein synthesis

   B. Energy production

   C. Cell movement

   D. Storage of molecules

3. Because muscle cells require large amounts of energy to function correctly, which organelles would be abundant in those types of cells?

   A. Ribosomes

   B. Mitochondria

   C. Cytoskeleton

   D. Cell membrane

4. Which of the following organelles houses the genetic material?

   A. Nucleus

   B. Ribosomes

   C. Cell membrane

   D. Lysosomes

5. Write two or three sentences to define and differentiate mitosis and meiosis.

S.2.2 — Describe the relationship between genetic material and the structure of proteins

The hereditary material of most organisms is contained in DNA molecules. DNA is also responsible for directing protein synthesis in living organisms. RNA controls the intermediate steps involved in protein synthesis. **Genes** are segments of DNA which can code for specific proteins. Genes are located on larger structures called chromosomes. Offspring inherit traits encoded by genes present within their parents' DNA. In this TEAS task, you will explain the structure and function of DNA, RNA, genes, and chromosomes.

Objectives

This objective includes, but is not limited to, the following examples of knowledge, skills, and abilities.

- Explain the relationship between the structures and functions of chromosomes, genes, DNA, and RNA.

- Describe the processes of transcription and translation.

- Explain DNA replication.

- Explain the effects of genetic mutations on amino acid sequence.

CHROMOSOMES

Genetic information is contained in structures called "chromosomes." Chromosomes consist of tightly coiled DNA that winds around histone proteins as shown in the following figure. The winding process condenses the DNA and allows regulation of genes located on the particular chromosome. Each species of living things has a particular number of chromosomes. Prokaryotic organisms like bacteria have a single circular chromosome, whereas organisms that are eukaryotic (cells with nuclei) have many linear chromosomes. For example, humans have 46 chromosomes, and dogs have 78 chromosomes.

GENES

Genes are made up of DNA and are the basic physical and functional unit of heredity. Specifically, a gene is the length of DNA that contains instructions to make a protein or regulate the making of proteins. Interestingly, genes tend to be clustered in areas in between regions of DNA with unknown function. Genes vary in size from a few hundred DNA bases to more than a million bases. Researchers estimate that humans have about 25,000 genes.

Genes can have structural or regulatory functions. Structural genes are converted into a short-lived RNA message (mRNA) that is decoded by the ribosomes and assembled into proteins that build structures in living things. Regulatory genes control the expression of protein-coding genes by turning on or off activity, either directly or through a protein intermediate. In this way, regulatory genes control the expression of different subsets of structural genes in different cell types.

Genetic code in DNA and chromosomes within the nucleus

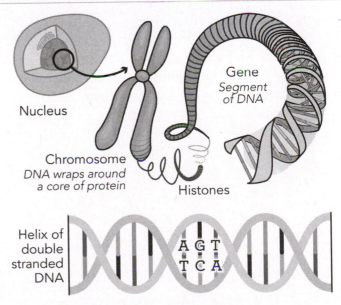

Nucleus

Chromosome
DNA wraps around a core of protein

Gene
Segment of DNA

Histones

Helix of double stranded DNA

gene. A sequence of DNA that is the basic unit of heredity.

Not all cells will express the same genes; therefore, they will make different proteins. For example, skin cells produce the protein **keratin**. Other cell types may not need keratin. Regulatory genes in these other cell types will "turn off" the genes that code for keratin. In this way, only the genes coding for needed proteins in a given cell are "turned on" or expressed.

DNA

Deoxyribonucleic acid (DNA) is a macromolecule that contains genes that are the coded instructions for a cell to produce proteins. The structure of DNA is a twisted ladder, or double helix. The sides of the ladder are made of phosphate and **deoxyribose sugar** molecules. The rungs of the ladder are composed of four nucleotide bases.

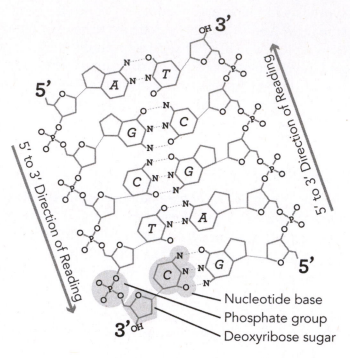

The four nucleotide bases are represented by letters: A (adenine), T (thymine), G (guanine), and C (cytosine). A "codon" is a sequence of three **nucleotides** that codes for a specific amino acid or stop signal during protein synthesis. A gene for a specific protein can be thousands of **codons** long. The gene will end with a "stop signal" codon. Ribosomes are the organelles that assemble proteins. They assemble proteins from amino acids in the order specified by the codons of the gene.

The DNA molecule is composed of two strands (or two sides of the ladder). The two strands of DNA are **complementary**. This means that the nucleotide bases of the two strands are paired correctly and specifically. The base A (adenosine) always pairs with T (thymine) on the other strand, and G (guanine) always pairs with C (cytosine). Thus A–T and G–C are referred to as complementary base pairs. Complementary bases are linked by two **hydrogen bonds** between A and T and three hydrogen bonds between G and C. Although an individual hydrogen bond is weak, these bonds are strong in DNA because they occur in large numbers and maintain DNA's integrity. However, these bonds are easier to break than covalent bonds. This allows the two strands to be separated for DNA replication and **transcription**. Before a cell replicates, chromosomes containing DNA must be copied to make two identical copies called "chromatids." Chromatids can then be separated, and the two new cells will have identical copies of DNA.

---

keratin. A tough protein made by epithelial keratinocytes.

deoxyribonucleic acid (DNA). The material that contains genetic information and is responsible for directing protein synthesis in living organisms.

deoxyribose sugar. The sugar portion of a deoxyribose nucleotide.

nucleotides. The monomers used to build DNA and RNA.

codons. Triplets of nucleotides that code for amino acids.

complementary strand. A molecule of RNA (or a strand of DNA) synthesized from a complementary template strand.

hydrogen bond. A type of non-covalent bond; a weak attraction between a hydrogen atom bound to an electronegative atom and a second highly electronegative atom.

transcription. The synthesis of RNA from a DNA template.

The two strands of DNA "run" in opposite directions as shown in the following figure. This makes the strands anti-parallel. Information is coded in DNA in the 5' to 3' direction, so this strand is called the "sense strand." The other strand going in the 3' to 5' direction is called the "anti-sense strand." The anti-sense strand is used as the template in DNA replication and transcription.

A **mutation**, which may arise during replication, is a permanent change in the nucleotide sequence of DNA. These mutations can occur either by substitution, deletion, or insertion of base pairs. Mutations, for the most part, are harmless except when they lead to cell death or tumor formation. Cells have evolved mechanisms for repairing damaged DNA.

RNA

Ribonucleic acid's (RNA) principal role is to act as a messenger carrying instructions from DNA for controlling the synthesis of proteins. Protein synthesis requires three types of RNA: messenger RNA (mRNA), transfer RNA (tRNA), and ribosomal RNA (rRNA). RNA is a single chain of ribose sugar-containing nucleotides. The nucleotides are adenine, uracil (uracil replaces thymine), guanine, and cytosine. The base pairing is A–U and G–C.

TRANSCRIPTION AND TRANSLATION

Protein synthesis can be described in two stages: transcription and **translation**. Transcription is the synthesis of RNA from a DNA template. The word transcription means "to copy" or "to rewrite," and this is a fitting term. DNA is too big to leave the nucleus of the cell; therefore, it "copies" the code for the instructions for a gene to mRNA. This form of RNA is smaller and can leave the nucleus and carry the information to the cytoplasm, where protein synthesis takes place. Recall that the DNA is double stranded; mRNA is an exact copy of the **template strand** (5' to 3') of DNA, except that thymine is replaced with uracil.

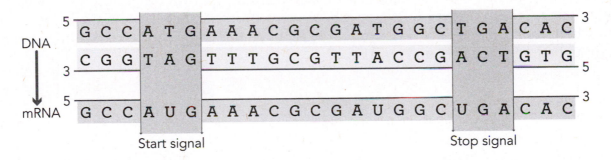

mutation. A permanent change in the nucleotide sequence of DNA that may arise during replication.

translation. Protein synthesis that takes place after mRNA exits the nucleus and binds to a ribosome.

template strand. A sequence of bases on a strand of DNA that is used to form a complementary mRNA molecule.

Once mRNA has entered the cytoplasm through the nuclear pores, rRNA in ribosomes attaches to the mRNA strand and begins to "transcribe" the instructions. Each mRNA codon designates a particular amino acid to be inserted into a protein (peptide) chain. The amino acids are "transferred" (tRNA) to the ribosome subunit and deliver the anticodon (codon

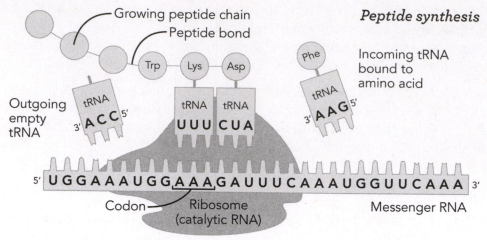

complement). Once a match is made, the tRNA releases the amino acid and catalytic rRNA binds the match together via a **peptide bond**. The result is the desired protein.

DNA, RNA, GENES, AND CHROMOSOMES

Understanding the relationship among DNA, RNA, genes, and chromosomes can be confusing. Let's use the human **genome** as an example. Humans have 23 pairs of chromosomes, for a total of 46 chromosomes. Chromosomes are composed of DNA wrapped around a histone protein. Specific regions of the DNA molecule are called "genes." Genes contain the instructions for proteins or other regulatory molecules. RNA controls the steps of protein synthesis. Genes are made of codons that are three DNA nucleotide bases long. A gene can be thousands of codons long.

Human chromosomes vary in length, and each chromosome has a DNA molecule that has a specific number of genes. For example, the eighth human chromosome has DNA composed of billions of nucleotide bases. Certain regions of DNA on this chromosome make up genes. On the eighth chromosome, there are hundreds of genes. Some of the genes on this chromosome code for proteins important to brain development and function.

---

peptide bond. The link between amino acids in a protein.

genome. The complete set of genetic information in a cell.

Practice Problems

1. Which of the following nucleotides pairs with adenine in DNA?

   A. Guanine

   B. Adenine

   C. Cytosine

   D. Thymine

2. Which of the following is the number of chromosomes found in a human cell?

   A. 1 circular chromosome

   B. 22 (11 pairs)

   C. 46 (23 pairs)

   D. 50 (25 pairs)

3. Which of the following statements about nucleotides and genes is correct?

   A. A gene contains thousands of chromosomes.

   B. A nucleotide contains many genes and chromosomes.

   C. Nucleotides form strings of DNA that make up genes.

   D. Nucleotides form strings of chromosomes that make up DNA.

4. Which of the following is the name for a segment of DNA that codes for a protein?

   A. Nucleotide

   B. Gene

   C. Chromosome

   D. DNA

5. In your own words, explain the relationship among chromosomes, DNA, RNA, and genes.

S.2.3 — Apply concepts underlying Mendel's laws of inheritance.

Inheritance refers to the principles regarding how traits are passed on to offspring. Mendel's three Laws of Heredity refer to Gregor Mendel's generalizations about how traits are inherited. Mendel was a 19th-century monk who grew and studied pea plants to determine how their characteristics were passed onto the next generation of plants. By crossing pea plants with different characteristics, Mendel was able to discern patterns in the inheritance of traits. In this TEAS task, you will need to explain Mendel's laws and describe differences in how traits are inherited. You will also need to explain how cell division through meiosis helps to create genetic variety. You will use a chart, called a "***Punnett Square***," to make predictions about the likelihood of a trait being passed from parent to offspring.

Objectives

This objective includes, but is not limited to, the following examples of knowledge, skills, and abilities.

- Distinguish between genotype and phenotype.

- Describe the differences between dominant and recessive traits.

- Explain how alleles are inherited from parents.

- Explain how meiosis results in genetic variation.

- Use a Punnett square to predict traits of offspring.

DOMINANT AND RECESSIVE TRAITS

One of Mendel's observations was that there are differences in the prevalence of traits. This means that some traits are more likely to be passed on than others. He hypothesized that offspring inherit "factors" from their parents. Today we know that Mendel's factors are genes. Each gene for a trait comes in varieties, called "***alleles***." For example, the gene for seed color in pea plants has an allele for green and another for yellow. Mendel found that for two alleles for a gene, the ***dominant*** trait is always expressed or shown by the organism if it is present, because it masks the ***recessive*** allele. The recessive allele is only expressed when both alleles are recessive. This is Mendel's third law, The Law of Dominance. For seed color, the green allele is dominant, and the yellow allele is recessive.

---

inheritance. Transmission of characteristics to offspring.

Punnett square. A square diagram used to determine the various genotype combinations that may be passed from parent to offspring and their likelihood of occurring.

Mendelian inheritance. Inheritance of traits that follow Gregor Mendel's two laws and the principle of dominance.

allele. A specific copy of a gene.

dominant. Refers to the most powerful trait or the allele for that trait.

recessive. Refers to traits that are masked if dominant alleles are also present; also refers to the allele for that trait.

INHERITANCE OF GENE PAIRS

Most living things inherit one of each pair of chromosomes from each parent. For example, humans have 23 pairs of chromosomes for a total of 46 chromosomes. Each parent contributed 23 chromosomes. Therefore, offspring inherit two copies of each gene, one from each parent. They will have two alleles for each gene. This combination of two alleles is called a "***genotype***." If a chromosome contains two alleles that are the same, that genotype is called "***homozygous***." If the chromosome contains two different alleles, that genotype is called "***heterozygous***." The alleles that are present in an organism determine the ***phenotype*** of the organism; a "phenotype" is the expression of the genes for that trait. Phenotypes are visible traits such as seed color and unseen traits such as blood type.

Offspring express either a dominant or recessive phenotype based on the two alleles inherited for a trait. Only inherited traits are determined this way. Inherited traits are passed from parent to offspring through gametes (eggs or sperm). Each gamete carries 1 chromosome of the chromosome pair (and only one copy of each gene). For example, human gametes contain 23 chromosomes. When an egg and sperm fuse together (fertilization), a cell with two copies of each chromosome (and two copies of each gene) results. For humans, the zygote contains 46 chromosomes. Traits, such as culturally influenced behavior, are not inherited as part of the genome. These are nonheritable traits not coded for in genes. Mendel's Laws of Heredity focus on inherited traits.

USING PUNNETT SQUARES

One way to predict the likelihood of traits in offspring is to use a Punnett square. A Punnett square is a chart that can be used to determine the ratios of the genotypes of offspring from a reproductive cross. To use a Punnett square, you must know the genotypes of the parents. Genotypes are represented by two letters. Capital letters will represent dominant alleles, and lowercase letters will represent recessive alleles. In pea plants, purple (P) is the dominant flower color and white (p) is recessive.

The following graphic shows the genotypes of two parent pea plants. The first parent plant has a genotype of "PP," which means two dominant alleles. This plant would express the dominant trait or phenotype of purple flowers. This parent is homozygous dominant for this trait. The second individual has the genotype "pp." This second parent plant would express the recessive phenotype of white flowers because there is no dominant allele present. This parent is homozygous recessive for this trait.

When these two parents (the P1 generation) are crossed, each parent contributes one allele. The "PP" parent can only contribute a "P" or dominant allele. The "pp" parent can only contribute a "p" or recessive allele. All offspring of this cross (the F1 generation) will have the heterozygous genotype "Pp." They will all have the phenotype of purple because they contain a dominant allele.

Pea Plant Genotypes

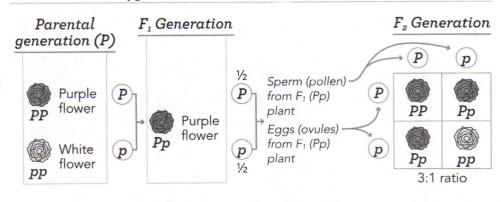

3:1 ratio

---

genotype. The genetic makeup of an individual.

homozygous. The state of carrying a pair of identical alleles of a gene; e.g., AA or aa.

heterozygous. The state of carrying different alleles of a gene; e.g., Aa.

phenotype. Physical appearance of a trait formed by genetics and environment.

Now consider a cross between two heterozygous flowers (F2 generation) using a Punnett square. The genotype of the sperm (pollen) from one plant, "Pp," is placed at the top of the square. The genotype of an egg (ovules) from another plant, "Pp," is placed on the side. The F2 genotypes can then be calculated. The Punnett square helps us to predict that 25% of offspring will be PP, 50% of offspring will be Pp, and 25% will be pp. This means that it is likely that 75% of the offspring will have purple flowers, and 25% will be homozygous recessive and have white flowers.

These results hold true only if parental genes for a trait must segregate or separate equally and randomly into haploid gametes (sperm or eggs) during meiosis. That way offspring have an equal chance of inheriting either allele. Offspring inherit one allele from each parent for a trait, and no allele is favored or has an advantage over the others. This is Mendel's Law of Segregation.

The inheritance of two traits can also be studied using a Punnett square. This is called a "**dihybrid cross**," as shown in the following image. A dihybrid cross illustrates Mendel's Law of Independent Assortment.

A dihybrid cross tracks the inheritance of two different traits and starts with a parental cross of two true-breeding or homozygous organisms. One parent is homozygous dominant for both traits, and the other parent is homozygous recessive for both traits. The offspring (F1 generation) are all heterozygous (YyRr) and show only two dominant traits—in this case round, yellow seeds. When an F1 cross is performed, the F2 generation shows both dominant and recessive traits. The result is a ratio of 9:3:3:1.

This illustrates Mendel's Law of Independent Assortment because it shows that alleles are not inherited together. Each allele (Y, y, R, and r) is inherited separately, or independently assorted. This is supported by the fact that four phenotypes appear, rather than only the two phenotypes of the parental generation.

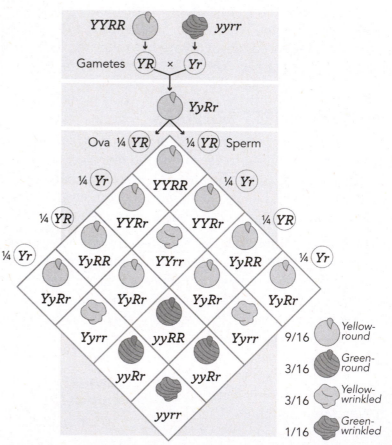

dihybrid cross. A cross between parents heterozygous at two specific genes.

The gametes that are produced from meiosis are all slightly different from one another and from the starting cell that went through meiosis. No two are identical, and each has a unique combination of genetic material. Crossing over and the random assortment of homologous chromosomes both help to bring about the shuffling of genetic material during the formation of gametes.

Finally, **non-Mendelian inheritance** occurs when there are factors other than dominant and recessive alleles in play. Mendelian ratios occur when a simple dominant–recessive relationship exists between two alleles. Non-Mendelian inheritance results from factors such as multiple alleles (e.g., blood groups A, B, and O), incomplete dominant–recessive relationships that lead to an intermediate (e.g., red and white alleles making pink flowers), co-dominance (AB blood group express both A and B proteins), interactions between genes, called "epistasis," and when the gene is carried on one of the sex chromosomes, X or Y, differential expression is seen in males (XY) versus females (XX). If the 3:1 or 9:3:3:1 relationship is not obtained when the F2 phenotypes are analyzed, it is indicative of non-Mendelian inheritance.

Practice Problems

1. A pea plant has a dominant homozygous genotype. Which of the following letters best represent this genotype?

   A. WW

   B. Ww

   C. ww

   D. WX

2. Pea plants have seeds that are either green or yellow. Green seeds are dominant to yellow seeds. Two pea plants that are heterozygous for seed color are crossed. What percentage of their offspring will have green seeds?

3. Which of the following best describes the expression of alleles?

   A. Heritable trait

   B. Genotype

   C. Phenotype

   D. P generation

4. Which of the following best describes non-Mendelian inheritance patterns?

   A. They occur when there are factors other than dominant and recessive traits.

   B. Each trait has one dominant and one recessive allele.

   C. Heterozygous monohybrid crosses result in a 3:1 ratio of dominant-to-recessive phenotypes.

   D. Traits are only inherited on the somatic chromosomes.

5. Use a Punnett square to show the likely phenotypes of crossing two heterozygous tall pea plants. The allele for tall plants is dominant.

non-Mendelian inheritance. Inheritance of traits that do not follow Mendelian patterns of inheritance.

S.2.4 — Describe structure and function of the basic macromolecules in a biological system

Living organisms are composed of carbon and other **elements** bonded together to form organic macromolecules. **Monomers** from food are used to build these macromolecules in biological systems. Monomers are broken down, and the energy is extracted and stored in adenosine triphosphate (ATP) bonds to fuel the cell's energy needs. In this TEAS task, you will identify the structure of each type of macromolecule and explain how the chemical structure of each macromolecule is related to its function. You will also recognize how reversible chemical reactions build macromolecules and break them down into their monomers. Finally, you should be able to recognize the macromolecule category of familiar food items.

Objectives

This objective includes, but is not limited to, the following examples of knowledge, skills, and abilities.

- Describe basic structure of carbohydrates, lipids, proteins, and nucleic acids.

- Describe how macromolecules are synthesized and broken down.

- Describe how basic macromolecules function in a biological system.

MACROMOLECULES

Macromolecules are large polymers. A "**polymer**" is a chemical compound formed when covalent bonds link monomers in long, repeating chains. Covalent bonds in macromolecules are formed by an endergonic removal of a water molecule. This chemical reaction is known as "**dehydration**" or "condensation synthesis." This reaction requires energy. Conversely, these bonds can be broken by an exergonic addition of water, which is known as "**hydrolysis**." Hydrolysis releases energy as bonds break between monomers.

The structures of macromolecules give them unique properties that allow them to perform different functions in biological systems. Macromolecules are classified into four groups: carbohydrates, lipids, proteins, and nucleic acids. The figure here shows the monomers that are joined by dehydration synthesis to form each type of macromolecule.

Monomers Joined by Dehydration

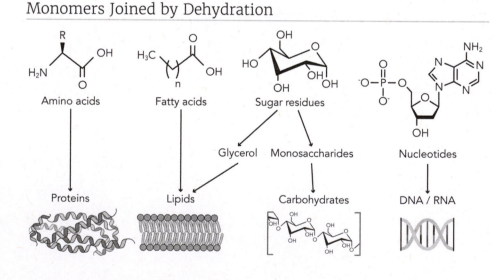

Amino acids → Proteins

Fatty acids, Glycerol → Lipids

Sugar residues → Monosaccharides → Carbohydrates

Nucleotides → DNA / RNA

---

element. Pure substances that cannot be broken into simpler substances.

monomers. Molecules that can bond to similar or identical molecules to form a polymer.

polymer. A substance composed of similar units bonded together.

dehydration reaction. A chemical reaction between two molecules in which a water molecule is released and a covalent bond forms; often requires an input of energy; polymers are built as a result of this reaction.

hydrolysis reaction. A chemical reaction in which a water molecule cleaves a covalent bond to form two products; monomeric subunits of polymers are cleaved from a polymer by this reaction.

CARBOHYDRATES

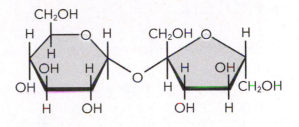

Carbohydrates, also known as "sugars" or "starch," are found in all living organisms. The monomers that join together to form carbohydrates have the general formula $C_nH_{2n}O_n$. Carbohydrate monomers are typically 3, 4, 5, or 6 carbons long. They are also known as "monosaccharides," or "simple sugars." For example, $C_6H_{12}O_6$ is a common monosaccharide known as "glucose." Two monosaccharides join by dehydration synthesis to form disaccharides. Sucrose is a common disaccharide shown in the figure. Sucrose is made up of two monosaccharides joined together: one glucose monosaccharide and one fructose monosaccharide.

Polysaccharides are carbohydrate molecules formed by large numbers of linked monosaccharides. Animals store the monosaccharide glucose in the form of polysaccharide glycogen. Glycogen is formed by dehydration synthesis and is stored mainly in the liver and the muscles. When glucose is needed for energy production by a cell, glycogen is hydrolyzed into glucose. Plants store carbohydrates as the polysaccharide starch. Oligosaccharides contain a small number of monosaccharides. They are found on the surface of the cell membrane and function in cell recognition.

Carbohydrates can take many forms and perform a variety of functions. They can be linear, branched, or helix shaped. Linear carbohydrates such as cellulose and chitin often form structures. Cellulose is a major component in the rigid cell walls in plants. Branched carbohydrates such as glycogen and amylopectin function in energy storage. Glycoproteins and glycolipids are molecules that contain carbohydrates and other macromolecules, and they function in cell recognition.

LIPIDS

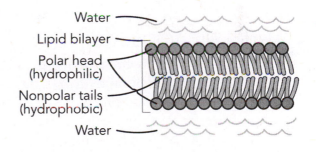

Lipids are important structural, energy-storage, and hormone macromolecules. Familiar lipids like oils and fats are not true polymers because they are not formed from one type of repeated monomer. Instead, lipids are formed from a linear arrangement of carbon atoms and hydrogen atoms called "fatty-acid chains" that are attached to a **glycerol** molecule. Lipids tend to be **hydrophobic** and nonpolar.

Lipids are subdivided into four groups: fats and oils, waxes, phospholipids, and steroids, and all are insoluble in water. Each group of lipids has unique characteristics and functions. A fat molecule consists a glycerol backbone and three **fatty acid** chains. The human body uses fats for energy storage, cushioning, and insulation. Fats are a dietary component found in oils, butter, and meat. Waxes usually contain long fatty acid chains connected to alcohols. Waxes are hydrophobic and are used by living things to stay dry. Waxes cover the feathers of some birds and the leaves of many plants. Phospholipids are two fatty-acid chains attached to a phosphate molecule. One function of phospholipids is to form a semi-permeable membrane around cells. Phospholipids help to separate aqueous compartments in living things. Steroids have a four-ring structure and include cholesterol, sex hormones, and hormones of the adrenal cortex. Steroids often function as chemical messengers.

---

polysaccharides. Carbohydrate polymers made of many sugar molecules.

glycerol. A sugar compound that serves as the backbone for triglycerides and phospholipids.

hydrophobic. Water fearing.

fatty acid. A molecule composed of a long hydrocarbon chain with a carboxylic acid group on one end.

PROTEINS

Proteins are polymers of long chains of amino acid monomers. Amino acids are composed of a central carbon, an amine group, a carboxylic acid, and a side group. The side group shown as the R side chain in the following diagram provides the variation that creates the 20 different types of amino acids. Each amino acid has different properties because of its different side group. In proteins, the link between amino acids is a covalent bond called a "peptide bond."

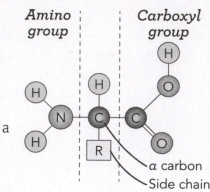

Proteins have a variety of shapes and functions. Fibrous, hydrophobic proteins like keratin and collagen have hydrophobic amino acids on their surface and are not soluble in water. They function as structural molecules in hair and nails. Globular proteins have hydrophilic surface amino acids and are soluble in water. They function as carrier molecules like hemoglobin, as antibodies, and as enzymes. Proteins associated with the cell membrane have a layer of hydrophobic amino acids sandwiched between layers of hydrophilic amino acids. Proteins are also embedded in membranes where they function in transport or signal transfer. Proteins can be found in foods such as eggs, meat, and beans.

Enzymes are an important class of proteins that catalyze biochemical reactions without being consumed in the reaction. Enzymes speed up reactions by lowering the energy required by the system to initiate the reaction. Reactions can be exergonic (release energy) or endergonic (require energy). Energy in living organisms is typically supplied and released as ATP. Different cell types have a different enzymes present based on the metabolic function of the cell. Enzyme activity is affected by environmental conditions such as temperature and pH level. Enzymes typically have an active site into which the substrate or molecule being acted on fits. The active site is where catalysis occurs. One example of an enzyme is pepsin. Pepsin is produced and secreted by stomach cells and initiates protein digestion in the stomach.

NUCLEIC ACIDS

Nucleic acids are polymers made of linked nucleotides that contain hydrogen, carbon, oxygen, nitrogen, and phosphorus. Nucleotides have three components: a nitrogenous base, a sugar, and a **phosphate group**. The adenine nucleotide is shown in the following figure. The two nucleic acids in living systems are deoxyribonucleic acid (DNA) and **ribonucleic acid (RNA)**.

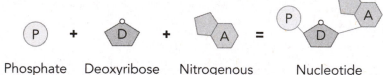

DNA is a double-stranded helix that stores genetic information. Genes are made up of DNA. Some genes provide the instructions to make molecules called "proteins." In humans, genes can contain a few hundred DNA bases to more than a million bases. Genes made of DNA are located on larger structures called "chromosomes." Chromosomes made of DNA and proteins are located in the nucleus of the cell. DNA contains nucleotides composed of a deoxyribose sugar, one of four nitrogenous bases (adenine, guanine, cytosine, or thymine), and a phosphate molecule.

---

phosphate group. A phosphorus atom bound to four oxygen atoms.

ribonucleic acid (RNA). An important biological macromolecule that is present in all cells and controls the intermediate steps involved in protein synthesis.

RNA consists of ribonucleotides containing a ribose sugar, a nitrogenous base (adenine, guanine, cytosine, or uracil), and is typically a single–stranded molecule. RNA helps to convert information stored in the genes composed of DNA into the proteins. There are three types of RNA molecules. Messenger RNA (mRNA) located in the nucleus of the cell transcribes the *genetic code* for a protein from the DNA template. It then carries the genetic code out of the nucleus to ribosomal RNA (rRNA) located in the ribosomes in the cell's cytoplasm. The transfer RNA (tRNA) brings the amino acid dictated by the mRNA's code to the ribosome. The ribosome provides the catalytic environment necessary for peptide bonds to form. Ribosomes are the site of protein synthesis from amino acid monomers.

The sequence of nucleotides in a nucleic acid is important in the process of building proteins. The sequence of nucleotides determines the specific protein synthesized. Errors in the precise sequence of nucleotides are referred to as mutations that typically interfere with protein structure and function. Nucleic acids can be found in small amounts in all foods that contain cells.

Practice Problems

1. Which of the following groups is synthesized from mono-saccharides like glucose?

   A. Carbohydrates

   B. Lipids

   C. Protein

   D. Nucleic acid

2. Which of the following macromolecules stores genetic information?

   A. Carbohydrates

   B. Lipids

   C. Protein

   D. Deoxyribonucleic acid

3. Which of the following monomers form enzymes?

   A. Glucose and fructose

   B. Amino acids

   C. Nucleotides

   D. Fatty acids

4. Which of the following foods contain mostly lipids?

   A. Potatoes

   B. Oil

   C. Chicken

   D. Lettuce

5. In 8 to 10 sentences, explain why each type of macromolecule is important to the human body.

---

genetic code. The set of 64 codons that specify the 20 amino acids.

S.2.5 — Describe the role of microorganisms in disease.

Microbes are organisms that cannot be seen with the naked eye. They can be classified as bacteria, viruses, **fungi**, protozoa, or animals. The nature of microorganisms makes them both easy and difficult to study. Many reproduce quickly and establish large populations that can be easily studied in a laboratory. Due to their small sizes, they can be difficult to study. Special techniques and equipment, such as microscopes, are needed. To be successful at meeting the objective, it is important to know the types of microorganisms, the difference between **infectious** and **non-infectious disease** caused by microbes, and the types of microscopes used to study them.

Objectives

This objective includes, but is not limited to, the following examples of knowledge, skills, and abilities.

- Define a microorganism.
- Distinguish between the main groups of pathogenic microbes (e.g., viruses, bacteria, protozoans, fungi, animals).
- Distinguish between infectious and non-infectious disease.
- Identify the microbial causes of common infectious diseases.
- Identify types of microscopes and their uses.

MICROORGANISMS

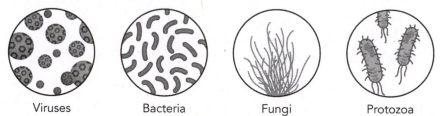

| Viruses | Bacteria | Fungi | Protozoa |

Microorganisms, also called microbes, are living things that are too small to be seen without magnification. Microorganisms are beneficial in producing oxygen, decomposing organic material, providing nutrients for plants, and maintaining human health. However, some can be pathogenic and cause diseases in plants and humans. Microbes are characterized based on cellular components, morphology (size & shape), means of locomotion and reproduction. They can be divided into several types: bacteria, viruses, **protozoans**, fungi and animals. Microbes are typically free-living and gain all they need from the surrounding environment. **Parasites** live in or on the body of a larger organism called the **host** and derive most of its sustenance from that host. A parasite's actions generally damage the host through infection and disease. This type of microbe is considered a **pathogen**.

microbes/microorganisms. Organisms that cannot be seen with the naked eye and may be classified as bacteria, viruses, fungi, protozoa (including algae), or animals.

fungi. Eukaryotic organisms that obtain nutrients by absorbing organic material from their environment (decomposers) through symbiotic relationships with plants or harmful relationships with a host.

infectious/communicable diseases. Diseases that spread from one person to another.

noninfectious diseases. Diseases that cannot be transmitted directly from one person to another.

protozoans/protists. Unicellular eukaryotes. They are the largest group of organisms in the world in terms of numbers, biomass, and diversity.

parasites. Microbes that are not free-living and must find a host from which to gain nutrients.

host. A larger organism on/in whose body a parasite lives.

pathogen. An infectious agent.

Bacteria are unicellular organisms capable of causing disease such as tuberculosis, meningitis, food poisoning, and more. Bacterial cells are described as prokaryotic because they lack a nucleus. The difference in their cell wall structure is a major feature used in classifying these organisms. Not all bacteria are pathogenic. In the body there are many types of harmless bacteria, and some may even support essential bodily functions.

Viruses are noncellular entities that consist of a nucleic acid core (DNA or RNA) surrounded by a protein coat. Although viruses are classified as microorganisms, they are not considered living things. Viruses invade and multiply inside healthy prokaryotic and eukaryotic cells causing diseases. Examples of viral diseases include influenza, measles, mumps, HIV, and COVID-19 virus.

Protozoans, or protists, are unicellular eukaryotes. They make up the largest group of organisms in the world in terms of numbers, biomass, and diversity. Protozoa feed on other cells and have been traditionally divided based on their mode of locomotion. Protist diseases include dysentery, malaria and sleeping sickness (African trypanosomiasis).

Fungi include mushrooms, molds, and yeast. All are eukaryotic cells means they have a true nucleus. They obtain nutrients by absorbing organic material from their environment (decomposers), through symbiotic relationships with plants or harmful relationships with a host (parasites). There are thousands of species of fungi, some of which cause disease in humans. Fungi can be the cause of many different types of illnesses, such as asthma, some common fungal skin conditions (athlete's foot and ringworm), lung infections and even bloodstream infections.

Animals such as parasitic worms, also known as helminths, are large enough for people to see with the naked eye, and they can live in many areas of the body. Some parasitic worms include flatworms (tapeworms) which can live in the intestines, and roundworms that can survive in the gastrointestinal tract and lymphatic system.

INFECTIOUS VS. NON-INFECTIOUS DISEASES

A disease is a condition that deteriorates the normal functioning of the cells, tissues, and organs. The two disease categories are infectious diseases and non-infectious diseases. Infectious diseases are diseases that spread from one person to another and are commonly called communicable diseases. They are caused by pathogenic microorganisms such as bacteria, protozoans, virus and other such microbes. Some examples of infectious diseases are cholera, chickenpox, and COVID-19 virus.

Non-infectious diseases do not spread to others and they remain within a person who has contracted them. These diseases are not caused by pathogens, but by other factors such as age, nutritional deficiency, gender, and lifestyle. Some examples of non-infectious diseases are diabetes, cancer, and asthma.

MICROBES AND INFECTIOUS DISEASES

Infectious diseases spread in multiple ways. In many cases, direct contact with a sick individual, either by skin-to-skin contact (including sexual contact) or by touching common surfaces, can transmit the disease to a new host. Contact with body fluids, such as blood and saliva, also spreads infectious diseases.

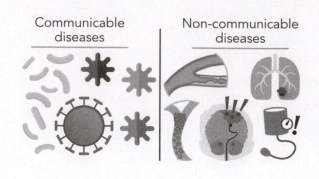

Some diseases spread through droplets discharged from a sick person's body when they cough or sneeze. These droplets linger in the air for a short period of time, landing on a healthy person's skin or being inhaled into their lungs.

In some cases, infectious diseases travel through the air for long periods of time as small particles. Healthy people inhale these particles and can become sick.

MICROSCOPES

The microscope is one of the most important tools of the microbiologist. It was invented in the 1600s when Anton Van Leeuwenhoek built a simple model consisting of a tube, magnifying lens, and a stage to make the first visual discoveries of microbes and circulating blood cells. In 1665 Robert Hooke used a compound microscope, meaning it contained two sets of lenses for magnification: the ocular lens next to the eye and the objective lens next to the specimen or object.

Nowadays, microscopy is essential in the medical field to make new cellular discoveries, and the types of microscopes can be classified based on the physical principles they use to generate an image. Some of the most common categories of microscopes include light microscopes and electron microscopes. Resolution is inversely dependent upon the wavelength of illumination being used. Electrons have a wavelength of 0.5 nanometers, and resolve small structures better than light, whose wavelength is 1000 times larger (~0.5 micrometers).

Light microscopes are dependent on a light source. There are six types of light microscopes: bright-field microscope, dark-field microscope, phase contrast microscope, fluorescence microscope, confocal scanning laser microscope (CSLM), and differential interference contrast (DIC).

Electron microscopes are microscopes that replace light with electrons for visualization. The magnification can reach 150,000 times the size of the specimen and can achieve a greater resolution than light microscopes. The drawback of electron magnification is that it must be contained in a vacuum, which eliminates the possibility of working with live cells. Two types of electron microscopes include the transmission electron microscope (TEM) and the scanning electron microscope (SEM).

---

electron microscope. A magnification instrument that forms an image using a beam of electrons that travel at high speeds and form a wavelike pattern.

Practice Problems

1. What term is used to describe all disease-causing micro-organisms?

   A. Decompose

   B. Prokaryote

   C. Pathogen

   D. Eukaryotes

2. Which if the following is at the core of every virus particle?

   A. DNA or RNA

   B. Enzymes

   C. DNA and RNA

3. Which microscope achieves the greatest resolution and highest magnification?

   A. Bright-field

   B. Dark-field

   C. Fluorescence

   D. Electron

4. Which of the following are considered microorganisms? (Select all that apply.)

   A. Mosquitoes

   B. Protozoa

   C. Bacteria

   D. Fungi

5. In your own words, explain the differences between infectious and non-infectious diseases.

Chemistry

S.3.1 — Recognize basic atomic structure.

The **atom** is the fundamental constituent of matter that retains the properties of an element. As such, the atom is the smallest unit that has a unique identity. There are 118 elements arranged in the **periodic table**, starting with hydrogen (which has one **proton**) and increasing proton numbers for each subsequent element. Although atoms have distinct properties, all are composed of the same three subatomic particles: protons, **neutrons**, and **electrons**.

To be successful in this TEAS topic, it is important to understand the structure of an atom and the arrangement of electrons that determine an atom's chemical properties. Atoms undergo chemical reactions by gaining or losing electrons to achieve stability. An atom's properties can be inferred by its position on the periodic table. These properties relate to the number of valence electrons in the atom's outermost shell.

> ### Objectives
>
> This objective includes, but is not limited to, the following examples of knowledge, skills, and abilities.
>
> - Describe the structure of an atom.
>
> - Identify the number of electrons, protons, and neutrons in an atom or ion.
>
> - Use the periodic table to explain and predict the properties of elements.

Atoms can lose, gain, or share electrons to make a variety of chemical bonds of varying strengths and properties. Familiarize yourself with the periodic table, get comfortable with identifying the valence of an atom based on its position, and infer the number and type of bonds that an atom would make.

PARTS OF AN ATOM

Atoms have a structure consisting of a central **nucleus** containing positively charged protons and neutral neutrons. Surrounding the nucleus are negatively charged electrons. Electrons exist in an electron cloud surrounding the nucleus. The negative electrons are held in shells—or energy levels—by their attraction to the positively charged protons in the nucleus and increase in energy with distance from the nucleus. Each type of atom will always have the same number of protons. For example, carbon has 6 protons.

The number of neutrons in different atoms of the same element can vary, and these atoms are called **isotopes**. The **atomic mass** of an atom is determined by the number of protons and neutrons found in the nucleus. Electrons are so small that their mass does not significantly add to the mass of the atom.

Carbon atom
6 protons + 6 neutrons

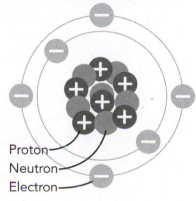

Proton
Neutron
Electron

---

atom. The fundamental constituent of matter that retains the properties of an element. It is the smallest unit that has a unique identity.

periodic table. The table of elements expressed as columns and rows.

proton. A positively charged atomic particle.

neutron. An atomic particle with no electric charge.

electron. A negatively charged atomic particle.

nucleus (atom). The central part of an atom that contains the protons and neutrons.

isotopes. Atoms of the same element that have different numbers of neutrons but the same numbers of protons and electrons.

atomic mass. The sum of the masses of protons and neutrons in one atom of an element.

For the carbon atom in the figure, the atomic mass is determined by adding the protons and neutrons: 6 protons + 6 neutrons = 12 atomic mass units (or amu). Another isotope of carbon might have 7 neutrons. All carbon atoms have 6 protons. This isotope would have an atomic mass of 13 amu (6 protons + 7 neutrons).

Subatomic particles have masses and charges related to their identity. The number of protons gives the **atomic number** of an atom. The number of protons plus neutrons equals the atomic mass of the atom. Neutral atoms have equal numbers of protons and electrons. The carbon atom illustrated previously would have a charge of 0 (neutral) because it has six positively charged protons and six negatively charged electrons. Neutrons do not change the charge because they are not charged particles.

Subatomic Particles	Charge	Mass (Atomic Mass Units)
Proton	+1	1
Neutron	0	1
Electron	-1	0

IONS

Ions are atoms with a positive or a negative charge. A sodium (Na) atom is made up of 11 protons and 12 neutrons in its nucleus and 11 electrons surrounding the nucleus. Because it has a single electron in its outer shell, sodium is likely to lose an electron. A sodium atom that has lost an electron becomes a charged sodium ion and is written Na+. It has a positive charge because it now has more protons than electrons. A chlorine atom has 17 protons and either 18 or 20 neutrons in its nucleus, and 17 electrons in the cloud around its nucleus. Because a chlorine atom has a nearly full outer shell, it is likely to gain an electron. A chlorine atom that has gained an electron becomes a charged chlorine ion and is written Cl-.

USING THE PERIODIC TABLE

The periodic table arranges atoms from left to right by increasing atomic number (number of protons). Atoms are neutral, so the number of protons equals the number of orbiting electrons. The atomic number is shown as an integer in the periodic table. To identify the number of electrons and protons, look at the integer shown with the element. Atomic masses on the periodic table are shown in decimal form to account for the natural abundance of the element's various isotopes. The atomic mass shown on the periodic table is determined by the percentage of each isotope found in nature for that particular atom.

The periodic table puts elements with similar properties in the same vertical columns, called **groups**. This grouping of atoms by properties reflects the fact that the elements in each group have the same number of valence (bonding) electrons. The rows in the periodic table are referred to as **periods**, and they indicate the outermost shell of an atom. Depending on the number of the period, there are different numbers of **orbitals** that can accommodate different electron numbers. Note that an s orbital can accommodate a maximum of two electrons at a time. The s orbital is closest to the nucleus. Hydrogen and helium only have an s orbital that can hold a total of two electrons.

---

atomic number. The number of protons in the nucleus of an atom.

ion. A positively or negatively charged atom or molecule.

group. A column of elements in the periodic table.

period. One of seven horizontal rows in the periodic tables.

orbital. An area around the nucleus where an electron can be found.

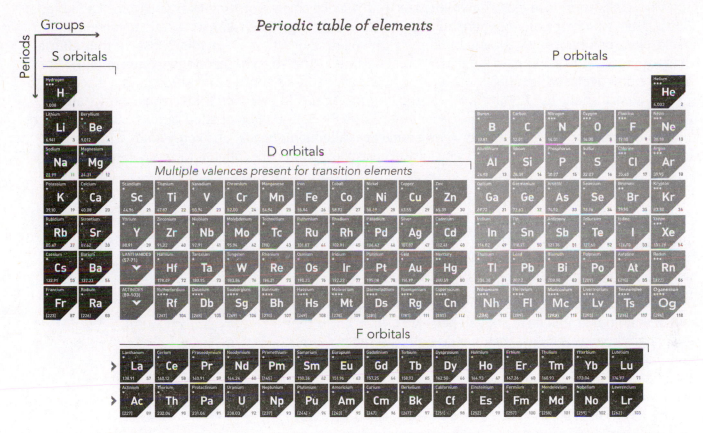

Periodic table of elements

Periods represent large electron "highways" with multiple orbital "lanes." For example, the lower-energy Period 1 has one s orbital with a maximum of two electrons allowed. Period 2 has two orbitals: s and p. The s orbital can only accommodate two electrons, but p can accommodate six electrons. Therefore, Period 2 can contain a maximum of eight electrons. Study the following chart and periodic table to familiarize yourself with atomic mass, atomic number, orbitals, and periods.

Relationship among periods, orbitals, and electrons			
Period Number	1	2	3	4
Orbital Names	s	s, p	s, p, d	s, p, d, f
Maximum Number of Electrons	s = 2	s = 2, p = 6	s = 2, p = 6, d = 10	s = 2, p = 6, d = 10, f = 14

Valence electrons are in the outermost shell of an atom and participate in chemical reactions (or bonding). Because atoms are most stable when they have a full valence shell, atoms are most likely to move toward stability. Noble gases, like helium and neon, have full valence shells and are quite stable. They do not react with other atoms because they are so stable. Because they are stable, they are also called inert gases.

Other atoms gain or lose electrons to achieve full valence shells, forming charged atoms called ions. Gaining electrons typically happens in atoms with valences greater than 4 (usually **nonmetals**), and losing electrons typically happens in atoms with valences less than 4 (**metals**). Observe that all the elements in group 15 will gain 3 electrons and become negatively charged ions (called **anions**). For example, nitrogen—which has 7 protons and 7 electrons in a neutral atom—will gain 3 electrons to fill its valence shell. It will have a –3 charge (7 protons and 10 electrons). Electrons are donated by atoms that prefer to lose electrons, becoming positively charged ions (called **cations**). Bonds that are formed by transfer of electrons between atoms are called **ionic bonds**, and **compounds** with ionic bonds are soluble in water and conduct electricity. These compounds are called ionic compounds.

Let's look at an example. Sodium loses 1 electron to fill its outer shell, giving it a +1 charge. Chlorine gains an electron to fill its outer shell (taking 1 electron from sodium) giving it a –1 charge. The now positively charged sodium ion is attracted to the positively charged chloride ion.

Ionic Bond Example

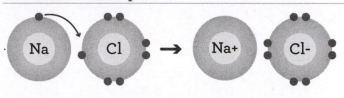

Atoms can also share electrons to achieve stability. For example, two oxygen (O) atoms have six valence electrons each. If they each shared two electrons, they would both resemble neon in their electron number. This is simpler to understand when visualized. It takes two electrons to make one bond, so there are two bonds between the O atoms in O_2. These shared bonds are known as **covalent bonds**. They are typically formed between two p–block elements. The following diagram shows four electrons creating two bonds between oxygen atoms.

Covalent Bond Example

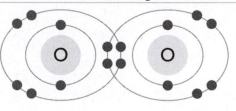

---

nonmetal. Any element or substance that is not a metal.

metal. A substance that is a good conductor of electricity and heat, forms cations by loss of electrons, and yields basic oxides and hydroxides.

anion. A negatively charged ion.

cation. A positively charged ion.

ionic bond. The bond between two oppositely charged ions.

compound. A substance made of two or more elements.

covalent bond. A chemical bond in which electron pairs are shared between atoms.

Practice Problems

1. Which of the following neutral atoms would have 10 protons, 11 neutrons, and 10 electrons?

   A. Neon

   B. Sodium

   C. Calcium

   D. Boron

2. Two isotopes of carbon are found, one with an atomic mass of 12 and the other 14. Which of the following best describes how these isotopes differ?

   A. The number of protons and electrons is different.

   B. Carbon 12 has fewer protons than carbon 14.

   C. Carbon 14 has more neutrons than carbon 12.

   D. Carbon 12 has two fewer electrons than carbon 14.

3. A neutral atom of calcium has two electrons in its outer shell. Which of the following will occur when calcium forms an ion?

   A. Calcium will lose two electrons to have a full valence shell.

   B. Calcium will gain two electrons to have a full valence shell.

   C. Calcium will add two protons to become neutral.

   D. Calcium will add six electrons to have a full valence shell.

4. Which of the following best describes an oxygen atom with 8 protons and 10 electrons?

   A. An anion with a −2 charge

   B. A cation with a +2 charge

   C. An anion with an atomic mass of 18

   D. A cation with a positive charge of +2

5. Use information in the periodic table to complete the following chart.

Element name	Element symbol	Proton number	Neutron number	Electron number	Atomic number	Atomic mass (amu)
Hydrogen						
	N	7				14
		78	117			
Chlorine						35
	K			19		39
	He				2	4

S.3.2 — Physical properties and changes of matter.

Matter can exist in different states determined by environmental conditions. This TEAS task requires a proficient understanding of the relationship between mass, volume, and **density**. In this task, you will need to distinguish between states of matter. You also need to be able to explain how the movement of the molecules is related to the state of matter, as well as the transition between different phases of matter. The TEAS test uses examples of substances changing between states of matter, so knowing how the processes work is important

PHYSICAL PROPERTIES OF MATTER: MASS, VOLUME, AND DENSITY

Physical properties refer to observed properties of the substance and those that can change the state without changing the identity of the substance. An example is boiling liquid water. The steam (vapor) that is produced is a gaseous state of water with the same molecular formula as liquid water. The molecules in liquid water and vapor are both made up of two hydrogen atoms and one oxygen—its identity has not changed. The vapor can be condensed to form liquid water again. Intensive physical properties (e.g., density, boiling point) do not depend on the amount of the substance present. Extensive physical properties (e.g., mass, volume) can change depending on the amount of matter present.

Mass is the specific number of molecules, while volume is the amount of space taken up by that number of molecules. Density is the ratio of mass to volume. This ratio is not dependent on the size of the sample but rather the unique structure of the substance. This means that a sample of liquid water has a density of 1 **gram** per cubic centimeter (1 g/cm3) independent of the sample size. Denser substances will sink, whereas less dense substances will float. For example, solid water (ice) is less dense than liquid water. That is why ice, like icebergs and ice cubes, floats in liquid water. Density can be used to identify a substance. For example, a 100 g sample of an unidentified metal takes up about 187 cm^3. The density of this sample is 100 g/187 cm^3, or about 0.534 g/cm^3. This is the density of lithium, so based on this density, this unknown sample can be identified as lithium metal.

---

density. The ratio of mass to volume.
gram. Metric unit of mass.

STATES OF MATTER

Molecules make up all matter. Matter exists in four phases: solid, liquid, gas, and plasma. Above absolute zero (0 K or −273° C), molecules are in constant motion. According to the **Kinetic Molecular Theory**, molecular motion changes as heat is added or removed. Heat overcomes the forces that hold matter together. As the temperature of a substance increases, the intermolecular forces that hold the molecules together are broken, causing the molecules to move away from each other. The amount of heat required for a phase change will not break the bonds within a molecule.

In solids, the molecules are packed together in a tight, orderly pattern; there is vibrational motion but no translational motion experienced by the molecules. The molecules in liquids are less ordered and exhibit both translational and vibrational motion. Gas molecules are rapidly moving and spread far apart.

The phase of a substance depends on two conditions: temperature and pressure. Increasing temperature has a tendency to move the particles of matter apart, and increasing pressure has a tendency to pack them closer together. In the phase diagram for carbon dioxide, the temperature and pressures for solid, liquid, and gaseous carbon dioxide are shown. At the triple point, solid, liquid, and gas coexist; above the critical point, liquid and gas coexist.

Solid matter has definite volume and shape. Think about a solid block of ice. It has a specific number of molecules (matter) and takes up a specific amount of space. Liquid matter has definite volume but no definite shape, meaning that it will conform to the shape of the container. Gas has no definite volume or shape. Gases are highly compressible and subject to changes in volume, but liquids and solids are generally non-compressible.

Effect of Pressure and Temperature upon Phase

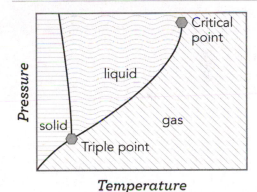

CHANGES BETWEEN STATES OF MATTER

A change from solid to liquid (melting) requires an addition of heat, which causes the molecules to become more energized. This increases their vibrational and translational motion. Adding heat (energy) causes the forces holding particles together in a solid state to break. Adding heat is also required to change matter from liquid to gas. Boiling and evaporation are examples of a liquid changing to a gas. Removing heat from matter is required to change gas to liquid (condensation) or liquid to solid (freezing). An unusual phase change called **sublimation** directly converts solids to gas. For example, solid carbon dioxide (also known as dry ice) will change directly from a solid to gas at room temperature through sublimation. Deposition is the opposite of sublimation, in which a gas directly converts to a solid. For example, in cold temperatures, water vapor can directly become solid ice crystals (causing the formation of frost on windows).

kinetic molecular theory. A theory stating that the molecules that make up all matter are in constant motion, and the temperature of a substance is directly proportional to the average kinetic energy of its molecules.

sublimation. The transition of a substance from solid to gas without passing through the liquid state.

Practice Problems

1. Which of the following phase changes requires the loss of heat?

   A. Melting

   B. Evaporation

   C. Freezing

   D. Sublimation

2. Which of the following is true of liquids?

   A. They have definite shape and volume.

   B. They have no definite shape, but they have definite volume.

   C. They have a definite shape but no definite volume.

   D. They have no definite shape and no definite volume.

3. What is the density in grams per cubic centimeter of a substance that has a mass of 22.5 g and a volume of 5 cm^3?

4. Which of the following best describes the triple point?

   A. Point where temperature, pressure, and volume all equal one another

   B. Point where a substance can exist as a solid, liquid, and gas

   C. Point where no more energy can be absorbed by a substance

   D. Point where a substance starts to lose its shape

5. On a hot summer day, you place a cup of ice water outside. Using your knowledge of states of matter, describe what will likely happen in three to five sentences.

S.3.3 — Describe chemical reactions

Chemical reactions occur constantly to create and break bonds between elements and compounds. Elements in the same group in the periodic table undergo similar chemical reactions due to shared **valence electron** number. For this TEAS task, you need to be able to describe chemical bonding and reactions, recognize the role of valence electrons in bonding, know how to balance a chemical reaction, and understand how quantities of **reactants** and **products** are represented in a chemical reaction.

VALENCE ELECTRONS

The electrons of the outermost shell of an atom are called valence electrons, and they have the highest energy. These outer electrons are more readily transferred or shared during chemical reactions than those in an atom's interior. Transfer of the electron to another atom or sharing these electrons with another atom allows the atom to achieve the noble gas electron configuration by having eight electrons in the outermost shell and become stable. Because of this, valence electrons play an important role in chemical reactions. The number of valence electrons an element has can be determined based on its group in the periodic table. Although the periodic table was originally assembled based on chemical behavior of the elements before their atomic structure was known, it turned out that elements in the same group in the periodic table have the same chemical behavior because they have the same number of valence electrons.

Group IA elements—such as sodium and potassium—have one valence electron. The elements in the neighboring group, IIA—such as magnesium and calcium—have two valence electrons. Typically, elements on the left side of the periodic table have relatively low ionization energies (the energy required to remove the most loosely held electron) and low electronegativity (the tendency to attract electrons). These elements are classified as metals and usually lose electrons to another atom during a chemical reaction. Group IA elements lose one valence electron, leaving an imbalance between the number of positive protons in the nucleus and electrons, resulting in positive cations with a +1 charge, with an outermost shell similar to a noble gas. For example, sodium (Na) loses the only electron in its valence shell, so now the Na^+ ion has the same number of electrons as neon (Ne) and therefore is more stable. Magnesium (Mg) can lose 2 valence electrons, forming Mg^{2+}, which also has the same number and configuration of electrons as Ne.

The elements in the upper right side of the periodic table, such as those in groups VIA and VIIA, tend to gain electrons in chemical reactions. These elements have high ionization energies and a significant ability to draw valence electrons from other atoms toward themselves. Elements in Group VIIA—such as fluorine (F), chlorine (Cl), and bromine (Br)—gain one electron and thus end up with more electrons than the number of protons in the nucleus, becoming negative anions with a –1 charge (F^-, Cl^-, and Br^-). Because they end up with the same number of electrons as the neighboring noble gas, they achieve stability. Group VIA elements oxygen (O) and sulfur (S) gain 2 electrons, forming O^{2-} and S^{2-} ions and noble gas valence electron configurations for stability.

---

valence electron. An electron in an outer orbital that can form bonds with other atoms.

reactants. In a chemical equation, the substances on the left side of the equation; the starting materials in a chemical reaction.

products. In a chemical equation, the substances on the right side of the equation; the substances that are formed in a chemical reaction.

Based on an element's group and placement in the periodic table, a trend can be observed to determine whether an element will gain, lose, or share valence electrons. Elements on the left side of the periodic table with low ionization energies and low electronegativity are metals, which will tend to lose electrons and become cations. The electrons lost by metals are gained by elements on the right side of the periodic table, which have high electronegativities—that is, a high affinity for them—and are nonmetals. Nonmetals gain electrons to become negatively charged anions. Reactions between elements with similar tendencies to gain or lose electrons will tend to share electrons with each other. For example, when two or more nonmetals react, they become stable by sharing valence electrons.

COVALENT AND IONIC BONDS

Chemical bonds occur when two or more atoms have interactions between their valence electrons. Ionic bonds can only form when the elements involved have a large difference in electronegativity, such as exists between metals and nonmetals. This difference allows for the transfer of electrons from the metal to the nonmetal. These elements then become ions or charged atoms. As mentioned earlier, metals tend to become positively charged cations, and nonmetals become negatively charged anions. For example, sodium (Na) is a metal that easily transfers one electron to the nonmetal fluorine (F). Na becomes positively charged (Na^+) because it has lost an electron, and F becomes negatively charged (F^-). These oppositely charged ions attract one another, forming an ionic bond and making sodium fluoride (NaF). Metals are found on the left side of the periodic table, and nonmetals are found on the right.

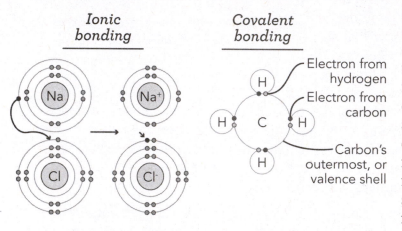

Sometimes elements share electrons instead of transferring electrons, forming a different type of bond. Covalent bonds require the sharing of electrons and occur between two nonmetals. In covalent bonds, there is not a sufficient difference in electronegativity to gain or lose electrons. However, differences in electronegativity within a covalently bonded molecule cause them to be polar or nonpolar. Polar covalent compounds have a negatively charged side and a positively charged side. Water is a polar molecule; the hydrogen side of the molecule is partially positively charged, and the oxygen side is partially negatively charged. This is a result of the strong electronegativity of oxygen pulling at the shared electrons. These polar covalently bonded molecules are still neutral in overall charge.

CHEMICAL REACTIONS

Chemical reactions are represented by **chemical equations**. Chemical equations have a basic layout going from left to right: reactants, reaction sign showing the direction of the reaction ($\rightarrow$), and products.

Reactants → Products

The formation of table salt is an example of a chemical equation: $2Na + Cl_2 \rightarrow 2NaCl$. In this reaction, sodium and chlorine are the reactants and the ionic compound sodium chloride is the product.

Take a look at an example of a combustion reaction.

$CH_4 + 2O_2 \rightarrow CO_2 + 2H_2O$

Methane (CH_4) and oxygen (O_2) are the reactants. The products are water (H_2O) and carbon dioxide (CO_2).

Looking at the two sample reactions shown above, you can see there are numbers in front of some of the formulas. These are coefficients, and they help to adjust the quantities in the reaction so that equal numbers of atoms of each element in the reactants are also in the product and the reaction is balanced.

BALANCING CHEMICAL REACTIONS

During a chemical reaction, there is a change in the bonding between atoms that occurs, but the total mass of the elements entering and exiting the reaction does not change. Chemical equations must be shown as balanced equations, meaning there must be the same numbers of each element on both sides. Looking at the combustion reaction again, the equation could have simply shown the identities but not the quantities of the reactants and products, like this:

$CH_4 + O_2 \rightarrow CO_2 + H_2O$

The reaction now suggests that two hydrogen atoms are destroyed and an oxygen atom is created going from reactants to products, and so the equation is said to be unbalanced.

If a coefficient of 2 is placed in front of the oxygen (O_2), we are now indicating that two oxygen molecules react with methane (CH_4). The coefficient of 2 in front of the water (H_2O) molecule in the product means the reaction forms two water molecules instead of one.

$CH_4 + 2O_2 \rightarrow CO_2 + 2H_2O$

The equation for this chemical reaction is now balanced, and the same number of atoms for each element are present on both sides.

---

chemical equation. Mathematical representation of a chemical reaction.

Take a look at another unbalanced equation. The reaction of sodium iodide (NaI) with lead nitrate $Pb(NO_3)_2$ produces sodium nitrate ($NaNO_3$) and lead iodide PbI_2.

$NaI + Pb(NO_3)_2 \rightarrow NaNO_3 + PbI_2$

Count the atoms of each element on both sides.

- Reactant side: 1 Na, 1 I, 1 Pb, 2 N, and 6 O

- Product side: 1 Na, 2 I, 1 Pb, 1 N, and 3 O

In order to balance the reaction, we add the smallest coefficient that will give the same number of each atom on either side of the reaction.

$2NaI + Pb(NO_3)_2 \rightarrow 2NaNO_3 + PbI_2$

Now the reaction has 2 Na, 2 I, 1 Pb, 2 N, and 6 O on each side. It is balanced.

MOLES IN CHEMICAL REACTIONS

In order to perform a chemical reaction efficiently, it is important to know the quantities of the reactants that will be mixed together to determine the amount of products formed. One convenient way to measure amounts of a substance is using a balance to measure out the mass of the reactants. A mole is the atomic mass (measured in grams) of a substance. For example, carbon has an atomic mass of 12 amu, so 12 g of carbon is 1 mole of carbon. One molecule of NaCl has a molecular mass of 36.5 amu, so 36.5 g of NaCl is 1 mole of table salt. This can be translated to atom or molecule numbers, because one mole of anything (carbon atoms, table salt, apples, pennies) contains exactly 6.022×10^{23} particles (Avogadro's number).

In the equation $2NaI + Pb(NO_3)_2 \rightarrow 2NaNO_3 + PbI_2$, the coefficients represent **moles**. This means that 2 moles of NaI react with 1 mole of $Pb(NO_3)_2$ to make 2 moles of $NaNO_3$ and 1 mole of PbI_2. To translate this to grams, the molecular mass of each compound has to be calculated using the periodic table. NaI has a molecular mass of 149.9 amu (Na = 23.0 amu; I = 126.9 amu). $Pb(NO_3)_2$ has a molecular mass of 331.2 amu (Pb = 207.2 amu; N = 14.0 amu; O = 16.0 amu). In the reaction, the reactants have to be mixed in a proportion that results in the appropriate molar quantities: 2 moles of NaI are equal to 299.8 g, and 1 mole of $Pb(NO_3)_2$ weighs 331.2 g. You can see that mixing 2 g of NaI and 1 g of $Pb(NO_3)_2$ would not be equimolar quantities.

---

mole. A unit of a substance that is equal to exactly $6.02214076 \times 10^{23}$ particles of that substance.

Practice Problems

1. Which of these elements have the same number of valence electrons and similar chemical properties as strontium (Sr)? Use the periodic table to help you answer the question.

   A. Magnesium (Mg)

   B. Rubidium (Rb)

   C. Oxygen (O)

   D. Neon (Ne)

2. Which of the following substances are ionic compounds? (Select all that apply.)

   A. H_2O

   B. CO_2

   C. NH_3

   D. KCl

   E. NaCl

3. Which of the following sets of coefficients balances the following chemical reaction? $\_N_2 + \_H_2 \rightarrow \_NH_3$

   A. 1, 3, 2

   B. 1, 1, 1

   C. 2, 3, 1

   D. 3, 2. 1

4. How many oxygen atoms are present on each side of the following reaction? $2C_2H_{18}+25O_2 \rightarrow 16CO_2+18H_2O$

   A. 25

   B. 34

   C. 50

   D. 32

5. In the reaction $2AgCl \rightarrow 2Ag + Cl_2$, assuming you started with 4 moles of AgCl, how many moles of Ag could be produced?

S.3.4 — Demonstrate how conditions affect chemical reactions.

Chemical reactions occur at varying rates with changing conditions. Some chemical reaction go to completion, while others are **equilibrium** reactions. For this TEAS task, you need to be able to describe the factors that influence reactions rates and how perturbing an equilibrium impacts the reactions.

FACTORS THAT INFLUENCE REACTION RATES

Reaction rates can be altered by changing the conditions of a reaction. Changing factors—such as pressure, concentrations of reactants and products, temperature, and the presence of **catalysts**—will change the speed of a reaction. All of these conditions can be applied to an equation to assess the rate of reaction. For example, when temperature rises, the rate of an **endothermic** reaction (where heat is required) will increase. However, when temperature rises, an **exothermic** reaction (where heat is released) will slow down.

Increasing the pressure surrounding a gas phase reaction increases the chance of collisions between atoms and molecules. This will increase the reaction rate. Increasing the concentration of reactants increases the probability that reactants will come in contact with each other, thus increasing the likelihood of breaking or creating a bond. If product concentration is increased, the reaction will slow down.

CHEMICAL EQUILIBRIA

Not all chemical reactions go to completion. Look at the usual way we write a chemical reaction.

$$ZnS + 2HCl \rightarrow ZnCl_2 + H_2S$$

Reactions written this way are assumed to go to completion. In other words, 1 mole of ZnS would react with 2 moles of HCl. When the reaction stops, there is no remaining reactant. Only the two products are present. However, many reactions are reversible and go to equilibrium, not completion. At equilibrium, both reactants and products are present and their concentrations no longer change.

$$CO + 3H_2 \rightleftarrows CH_4 + H_2O$$

The equilibrium is dynamic, and once reached, the rate of the formation of CH_4 and H_2O equals the rate of formation of CO and $3H_2$.

---

equilibrium. The stage of a chemical reaction in which both reactants and products are present and their concentrations no longer change.

catalyst. A substance that increases the rate of a chemical reaction without undergoing permanent chemical change by lowering the activation energy required for the reaction to occur.

endothermic. Involving absorption of heat.

exothermic. Involving release of heat.

Many biological process, like the binding of oxygen (O_2) to hemoglobin, are equilibrium reactions or processes. In the lungs, where oxygen levels are high, O_2 binds to hemoglobin. In tissues, where oxygen is consumed by metabolism, O_2 levels are low.

$$Hb + 4O_2 \rightleftarrows HB(O_2)_4$$

Levels or concentrations of reactants and products, along with temperature and pressure, are some of the factors that affect the equilibrium.

When a chemical reaction at equilibrium is perturbed, it responds by going in a direction in order to restore the equilibrium. This is known as **Le Chatelier's principle**. For the hemoglobin example above, inhalation causes O_2 blood concentration to rise, driving the reaction to the right. In tissue that is undergoing metabolism, O_2 is consumed; thus a reactant for this process is disappearing and the reaction shifts to the left in response. Endothermic reactions absorb heat and shift to the right as temperature rises. Exothermic reactions shift to the left upon a temperature increase.

Endothermic reaction: $A + B + heat \rightleftarrows C + D$

Exothermic reaction: $A + B \rightleftarrows C + D + heat$

CATALYSTS

Catalysts are chemicals that lower the **activation energy** required for a chemical reaction to occur. The activation energy is the minimum energy needed to initiate the reaction. Thus, catalysts speed up reactions that would otherwise be extremely slow to occur. The catalyst does not change during the reaction and can be reused. In biological systems, catalysts are mostly proteins called enzymes, which speed up chemical reactions within the body. For example, the enzyme amylase is a catalyst for the breakdown of starch polymers to glucose monomers. This enzyme helps the body digest starches.

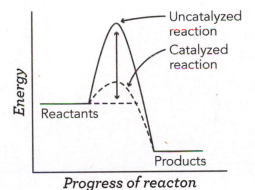

Progress of reacton

---

le Chatelier's principle. A principle stating that when a chemical reaction at equilibrium is perturbed, it responds by proceeding in a direction that will restore the equilibrium.

activation energy. The minimum energy needed to initiate a chemical reaction.

Practice Problems

1. For the reaction $CO + H_2 \rightleftarrows CH_4 + H_2O + heat$, equilibrium would favor the reactant side if which of the following occurs?

   A. H_2O is added

   B. The temperature decreases

   C. CO is added

   D. CH_4 is removed

2. Which of the following would increase the forward rate of this gas phase reaction?

   $CO + H_2 \rightleftarrows CH_4 + H_2O + heat$

   A. Adding CO

   B. Increasing the temperature

   C. Adding H_2O

   D. Increasing the pressure

3. A substance that lowers the activation energy is which of the following?

   A. Reactant

   B. Product

   C. Catalyst

   D. Time

4. Which of the following would slow down a reaction rate?

   A. Increasing the temperature

   B. Adding enzymes

   C. Decreasing the pressure

   D. Decreasing the reactants

5. An enzyme does which of the following to a chemical reaction?

   A. Shifts the reaction to the right

   B. Shifts the reaction to the left

   C. Speeds up both the forward and reverse reactions

   D. Changes the reaction from one that is at equilibrium to one that goes to completion

S.3.5 — Understand properties of solutions

Solutions are homogeneous mixtures of two or more substances whose components are uniformly distributed on a microscopic scale. This task requires a proficient understanding of solutes, solvents, and the unique properties of water. You will also learn about the different ways to express concentration and how **osmosis** and diffusion help in the transport of molecules.

POLARITY OF WATER

Water has several unique properties. It is a polar molecule, which means it has negatively charged (oxygen end) and positively charged (hydrogen end) sides. The polarity of water allows it to form hydrogen bonds and demonstrate both cohesive and adhesive properties. **Cohesion** is a measure of how well similar molecules stick to each other or group together. Water molecules are cohesive because they are attracted to other water molecules. The cohesiveness of water allows it to travel through small capillaries without using energy. Cohesiveness also creates surface tension by creating a tight-knit layer of water molecules on the surface of any body of water. Breaking up the multitude of hydrogen bonds between water molecules requires a lot of energy, so water is said to have high specific heat and high heat of vaporization. Water boils at 100°C (212°F). Ice floats on water because it has lower density than liquid water. Most substances have greater densities in solid form. **Adhesiveness** is a measure of how well dissimilar particles or surfaces cling to one another. The adhesiveness of water allows it to stick to other molecules because of water's polarity. Water is also considered the universal **solvent**, meaning many substances dissolve in water.

SOLVENTS AND SOLUTES

The formation of a **solution** from a **solute** and a solvent is a physical process, and it does not involve any chemical transformation. A solution is formed when a liquid mixture consisting of one or more solutes dissolves in a solvent. The solvent constitutes a greater proportion of the solution than the solute. Solutions exist as gases, liquids, and solids. The overall phase of the solution is the same phase as the solvent. So if the solvent is a liquid and the solute is a solid, then the solution will be a liquid. The solubility of a substance is determined by intermolecular interactions. Solutes can be classified as hydrophilic (water-loving) or hydrophobic (water-fearing).

---

osmosis. A specific type of diffusion in which water moves across a semipermeable membrane from an area of high concentration to an area of low concentration.

cohesion. The tendency of similar molecules to stick to each other or group together.

adhesiveness. A measure of how well dissimilar particles or surfaces cling to one another.

solvent. The substance in which a solute is dissolved to form a solution.

solution. A homogeneous mixture of two or more substances whose components are uniformly distributed on a microscopic scale.

solute. The substance that dissolves in a solvent to form a solution.

The difference between hydrophilic and hydrophobic solutes has substantial consequences in biological systems. Vitamins with hydrophilic structures are water-soluble, whereas those with hydrophobic structures are fat-soluble. The solubility of most solid and liquid solutes increases with increasing temperature. The solubility of a gas decreases with increasing temperature. A *saturated solution* has the maximum possible amount of solute. When less than the maximum amount of solute is dissolved, the solution is unsaturated. A *supersaturated solution* can be produced at higher temperatures, allowing more solute to dissolve than at lower temperatures.

CONCENTRATION AND DILUTION OF SOLUTIONS

The *concentration of a solution* is the quantity of solute in a given quantity of solution. **Dilution** is the addition of solvent, which decreases the concentration of the solute in the solution. Different units are used to express the concentrations of a solution depending on the application.

- Molarity = moles of solute ÷ liters of solution (mol/L)
- Mole fraction = moles of solute ÷ total moles present (mol/mol)
- Molality = moles of solute / kg of solvent (mol/kg)
- Mass percentage = (mass of solute [g] ÷ mass of solution [g]) × 100
- Parts per thousand (ppt) = g solute ÷ kg solution
- Parts per million (ppm) = mg solute ÷ kg solution
- Parts per billion (ppb) = mcg solute ÷ kg solution

Units of ppb or ppm are used to express very low concentrations, such as those of residual impurities in foods or of pollutants in environmental studies. The molarity of a solution is temperature dependent, but the other units are independent of temperature.

OSMOSIS AND DIFFUSION

Diffusion and osmosis are key processes for the transport of molecules through substrates and across membranes. Diffusion is the movement of any substance from areas of high concentration to areas of low concentration. One example of this is when perfume is sprayed in a room. The molecules of perfume will at first be concentrated in the area where it was sprayed. However, over time, the molecules of perfume will spread out until the concentration of perfume molecules is the same in all areas of the room. Another example is the molecules in the capillaries of the lungs. The blood in the capillaries moving from the heart to the lungs has a high concentration of carbon dioxide. This carbon dioxide will move out of the capillaries and diffuses across the respiratory membrane into the air of the lung alveoli. This decreases the carbon dioxide in the blood. The air in the lungs, which is rich in carbon dioxide, is then exhaled.

saturated solution. A solution containing the maximum possible amount of solute.

supersaturated solution. A solution that has been raised to a higher temperature in order to dissolve more solute than would be possible at room temperature.

concentration of a solution. The quantity of solute in a given quantity of solution.

dilution. The addition of solvent to decrease the concentration of solute in a solution.

Osmosis is a specific type of diffusion referring to water moving from an area of high concentration to low concentration. Water moves passively across a membrane through pores made of proteins called aquaporins. Remember that water is a solvent, meaning substances (solutes) dissolve in it. Water moves from regions where solvent concentration is high to areas where solvent concentration is low. One example of osmosis is how plants take in water through their roots. Root cells contain minerals, sugars, and salts dissolved in water. So, when water is available in soil, osmosis causes water to flow through the cell walls to the root interior where there is a lower concentration of water. Diffusion and osmosis do not require energy, other than the kinetic energy of moving molecules. This is called passive transport.

However, sometimes cells need substances to move from areas of low to high concentrations. To move from regions of low to high concentrations, energy must be used. Movement against the concentration gradient that requires energy is called **active transport**.

Practice Problems

1. A solution has a concentration of 0.05 kg/L of glucose. What is its concentration in ppm?

2. Which of the following statements is true?

   A. In a solution, solutes constitute a greater proportion.

   B. The solubility of solid solutes increases with increase in temperature.

   C. Vitamins with hydrophobic structures are water soluble.

   D. The solubility of gas increases with increase in temperature.

3. Which of the following describes the process of diffusion?

   A. It is the movement of substances from a solid to liquid state.

   B. It is the movement of a substance from areas of high concentration to low concentration.

   C. It requires a large amount of energy.

   D. It is specific to the movement of water only.

4. Concentrations of sodium dissolved in water are higher inside the cell than outside. Which of the following best predicts which way the water will flow?

   A. Water will remain in equal concentrations on both sides of the cell membrane.

   B. Water will move from its low concentration (outside the cell) to the higher concentration (inside the cell).

   C. Water will move from its high concentration (outside the cell) to the lower concentration (inside the cell).

   D. Water will increase in concentration inside and outside the cell.

5. In two or three sentences, explain why water has high specific heat and high heat of vaporization.

active transport. Movement across a cell membrane that travels against the concentration gradient and thus requires energy.

S.3.6 — Describe concepts of acids and bases.

Many chemical reactions that occur in nature involve *acids* and *bases* or are sensitive to the presence of these compounds. For this TEAS task, you need to be able to describe acids, bases, and the reactions that occur when they are mixed. You also need to understand what a buffer is and describe how buffers help maintain *pH* in the body.

Objectives

This objective includes, but is not limited to, the following examples of knowledge, skills, and abilities.

- Define acid, base, and pH scale.
- Describe the role of biological buffers in resisting pH change.
- Describe neutralization reactions.

ACIDS AND BASES

An acid produces hydrogen ions, H^+, in aqueous solution. Hydrochloric acid (HCl) is a strong acid and completely dissociates in water.

$$HCl \rightarrow H^+ + Cl^-$$

Each H^+ ion released is very reactive, and in aqueous solution it bonds to a water molecule. The product is known as the hydronium ion.

$$H^+ + H_2O \rightarrow H_3O^+$$

The two reactions can be combined, giving the following reaction.

$$HCl + H_2O \rightarrow H_3O^+ + Cl^-$$

In this overall equation, hydrochloric acid is donating a H^+ to water. An acid can also be called a proton or hydrogen ion donor.

We experience many acids in our everyday life. The sour taste in fruits such as lemons is due to citric acid. Vinegar is an aqueous solution of acetic acid. Acetic acid is a weak acid because it does not fully dissociate or donate all of its hydrogen ions. Human stomachs use hydrochloric acid to aid in digestion of proteins. Hydrochloric acid is strong acid because it fully dissociates in water.

A base produces hydroxide ions, OH^-, in aqueous solution. Strong bases such as sodium hydroxide (NaOH) completely dissociate in water. One of the products of this dissociation is the hydroxide ion.

$$NaOH \rightarrow Na^+ + OH^-$$

A base can also be thought of as a proton acceptor.

$$NH_3 + H_2O \rightleftarrows NH_4^+ + OH^-$$

In the reaction of ammonia (NH_3) with water, ammonia accepts a proton from water. Ammonia is acting as a base. The products of this reaction are the ammonium ion (NH_4^+) and OH^-. Ammonia is a weak base because not every ammonia molecule present accepts protons, and therefore—as is indicated by the double arrow—this reaction is reversible.

---

acid. A substance with a pH less than 7.

base. A substance with a pH greater than 7.

pH. A logarithmic scale based on the amount or concentration of hydrogen ions (H^+) in a solution, calculated as pH = $-\log[H^+]$ and used to express acidity or basicity.

Bases taste bitter and feel slippery because they react with oils in skin, forming a soap–like compound. Many drain cleaners contain the base sodium hydroxide. Baking soda is a base used for cooking. Bicarbonate in pancreatic juice neutralizes stomach acid before the acidic chyme passes into the small intestine.

pH

pH is a logarithmic scale based on the amount or concentration of hydrogen ions ($pH = -\log[H^+]$) in a solution and is used to express acidity or basicity. The pH scale goes from 0 to 14.

- pH < 7: acidic
- pH = 7: neutral
- pH > 7: basic

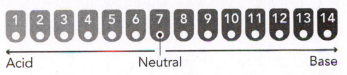

A neutral solution has a pH of 7, and the concentrations of H^+ and OH^- are equal to each other. Solutions with a pH less than 7 are acidic and have a greater concentration of hydrogen ions (H^+) than hydroxide ions (OH^-). Solutions with a pH greater than 7 are basic and have a greater concentration of hydroxide ions (OH^-) than hydrogen ions (H^+). Adding a base to a solution will raise the pH of that solution, whereas adding an acid will lower the pH. Human blood has a pH close to neutral (pH = 7.4). The pH of blood is maintained by the use of buffers.

BUFFERS

Most solutions will rapidly become more acidic (lower pH) upon addition of acid or more basic upon addition of base. A buffer can help to resist the change in pH by neutralizing the added acid or base. Cells function in a narrow pH range. The human body uses chemicals called buffers to regulate blood pH. Buffers can absorb excess H^+ or OH^-. A buffer is a solution of a weak acid and its conjugate base or a weak base and its conjugate acid. Buffers maintain the proper pH of the body. The pH of human blood is maintained by a buffer system of carbonic acid and bicarbonate. One of the products of cellular metabolism is carbon dioxide. This CO_2 reacts with water, forming carbonic acid (H_2CO_3).

$$CO_2 + H_2O \rightleftharpoons H_2CO_3$$

Carbonic acid then dissociates, forming H^+ and bicarbonate ions (HCO_3^-).

$$H_2CO_3 \rightleftharpoons H^+ + HCO_3^-$$

This buffer system works by H_2CO_3 (the weak acid) acting as a H^+ donor in the presence of a base. Bicarbonate (the conjugate base), on the other hand, acts as a proton acceptor, neutralizing any added acid. Here is an alternate way of looking at this buffer system: The dissociation reaction of carbonic acid forming H^+ and HCO_3^- is reversible. If a base is added, the reaction will run from right to left, providing H^+ to neutralize the base. However, the addition of acid will cause the reaction to run in reverse, and the acid will be neutralized. The concentration of H^+ in the system is maintained constant due to the equilibrium of the reaction, thus the pH of the solution is also maintained constant. The cytoplasm of cells is also buffered by a similar system using a phosphate (PO_4^-) buffer system.

NEUTRALIZATION REACTIONS

Upon mixing an acid with a base, the H^+ from the acid combines with the OH^- from the base, forming water. The formation of water from hydrogen ions and hydroxide ions is the heart of a **neutralization reaction**. An example of this reaction occurs when NaOH is mixed with HCl.

$$HCl + NaOH \rightarrow H_2O + NaCl$$

The products of this acid–base neutralization reaction are water and sodium chloride (a salt or ionic compound). Acid–base reactions typically form water and some type of ionic compound. When equal moles of acid and base are used, the system becomes neutral, with a pH of 7.

Practice Problems

1. Which of the following substances is an example of an acid?

   A. HI

   B. CO_2

   C. NH_3

   D. KCl

2. Which of the following substances are examples of a base? (Select all that apply.)

   A. KOH

   B. HCl

   C. NH_3

   D. HI

   E. NaOH

3. Orange juice, stomach acid, and coffee are all acids. Which of the following is the pH level for these substances?

   A. A pH less than 2

   B. A pH less than 7

   C. A pH at about 7

   D. A pH above 7

4. Which of the following statements for this reaction is false?
   $H_2PO_4^- \rightleftarrows H^+ + HPO_4^{2-}$

   A. The reaction is reversible.

   B. $H_2PO_4^-$ is acting as an acid.

   C. $H_2PO_4^-$ and HPO_4^{2-} could be used to make a buffer.

   D. This is a neutralization reaction.

5. Predict the outcome of the neutralization reaction:
   $H_2SO_4 + Ca(OH)_2 \rightarrow$

---

neutralization reaction. A chemical reaction in which mixing an acid with a base causes the H^+ from the acid to combine with the OH^- from the base, forming water.

Scientific Reasoning

S.4.1 — Use basic scientific measurements and measurement tools.

Accuracy in measuring, recording, and diagramming data are important skills. This TEAS task focuses on scientific measurements, scale, and tools. You will need to identify measurement tools and be able to measure **volume**, **mass**, and **length**. You will also need to understand and convert units involved in measuring large and small quantities of objects and substances.

UNITS OF MEASUREMENT

Scientists use the metric system, or Système Internationale (SI), to measure and record data. This system uses base units and prefixes to increase or decrease size. The SI base units for mass, length, and time are kilogram, meter, and second, respectively. **SI units** are also used to measure volume. The volume of a three-dimensional object has length, width, and height, all of which are measured in length units. Thus, the volume of a container 10 cm × 10 cm × 10 cm is 1,000 cm³. This SI base unit for volume is more familiarly called a "**liter**."

The SI system also uses prefixes to indicate the size of units. For example, the prefix "kilo" means 1,000, so 1 kilometer is 1,000 meters. The prefix "centi" means 0.01, so 1 centimeter is 0.01 meters. The prefixes can be used with any base. One kilogram is 1,000 grams, and 1 centigram is 0.01 grams. The TEAS will cover prefixes including kilo, hecta, deca, deci, centi, and milli.

Dimensional analysis is used to convert measurements from one unit size to another. A conversion factor expresses the relationship between units that is used to change the quantity without altering the value of the measurement. For example, to convert 5 liters to milliliters, we can multiply 5 L by 1,000 mL/1 L.

Objectives

This objective includes, but is not limited to, the following examples of knowledge, skills, and abilities.

- Describe concepts of the metric system, including units of measurement and conversions.
- Identify the unit of measurement in a model (e.g., diagram, illustration, photograph, graph).
- Identify the numerical value of a measurement of an object.
- Select the tool necessary to measure volume, mass, or length of an object.
- Choose a scale unit appropriate for the object being measured.

Common Prefixes

Prefix	Meaning
kilo	1000
hecta	100
deca	10
	1
deci	0.1
centi	0.01
milli	0.001
micro	0.0001

volume. The amount of space something takes up.

mass. A measurement of inertia, commonly considered the amount of material contained by an object and causing it to have weight in a gravitational field.

length. Measurement of distance from end to end.

SI units (Système Internationale). International System of Units based on meters, kilograms, seconds, amperes, Kelvin, candela, and mole. Commonly known as the metric system.

liter. Measurement of liquid volume.

When measuring, it is important to identify the numerical value correctly. Consider the ruler shown here. Each number represents a centimeter (cm). The smaller lines between the centimeter represent 1/10 of a centimeter, or a millimeter. If we were measuring to the first small line after the 2, the length would be 2.1 cm or 21 millimeters (mm).

SELECTING A MEASUREMENT TOOL

Tool selection will also be part of this section of the TEAS. Length is typically measured with a ruler or meterstick. Length is the distance from end to end of an object and is used to describe width, height, and length. Be sure to always start measuring length from the 0 point on your measurement tool. Volume can be measured in different ways, depending on the state of matter. Volume is the amount of space an object takes up. The volume of solids can be calculated by multiplying the measurements of length, width, and height, as seen in the following figure. The sides can be measured using rulers or metersticks.

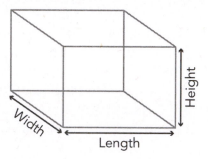

Several types of glassware can be used to measure the volume of liquids. The most accurate tool in measuring large volumes is a volumetric flask, and small volumes are best measured using a **volumetric pipette**. **Graduated cylinders** can also be used to measure a range of volumes in the laboratory, but they are less accurate than volumetric flasks or pipettes. Remember that liquids form a meniscus in a measuring tool. A "meniscus" is the curve formed at the top of a liquid in response to its container. The meniscus curve can be upward (concave), downward (convex), or flat, depending on the properties of the liquid and the container. When measuring the volume of a liquid, make sure that the line you are reading is even with the center of the meniscus.

Balances are used to measure the mass of an object. The mass is the amount of matter in an object. There are two types of balances used to measure mass: the triple-beam balance and electronic balance. The electronic balance is more common because it is easier to use.

CHOOSING AN APPROPRIATE SCALE

It is important to determine the most appropriate scaled unit to use when measuring items. Large items with a large mass would likely be measured using kilograms (kg). It is more efficient to say a person has a mass of 75 kg than to say a person has a mass of 75,000 grams. Measuring a few drops of water would make more sense in milliliters than liters. For length, small things like insects and fingernails should be measured in millimeters. Objects like the width of a piece of paper can be measured in centimeters, whereas the height of a door or a ceiling should be measured in meters. The distance between two towns can be measured in kilometers (km).

volumetric pipette. A device used for precise measurement of small amounts of liquid volume.
graduated cylinder. A narrow cylinder used to measure liquid volume.

Practice Problems

1. Which of the following values is appropriate for the height an adult human?

    A. 1.5 mm

    B. 1.5 cm

    C. 1.5 m

    D. 1.5 km

2. Which of the following is the meaning of the prefix "kilo"?

    A. 1,000

    B. 100

    C. 0.01

    D. 0.001

3. Which of the following tools could be used to measure the volume of a liquid sample?

    A. Triple-beam balance

    B. Flask

    C. Meterstick

    D. Ruler

4. A block of ice has a height of 10 cm, a width of 5 cm, and a length of 5 cm. What is the volume in cubic centimeters of the substance?

5. Two students measure the distance from one end of the school building to the other. One student measures a length of 2 km, and the other student measures a length of 200 cm. Which student most likely measured incorrectly? Why?

S.4.2 — Apply logic and evidence to a scientific explanation.

Scientific explanations of the world around us are based on evidence from observation and experimentation. Drawing meaningful conclusions from data is crucial in creating valid scientific explanations. It is also an important skill to be able to analyze scientific arguments for evidence. In this TEAS task, you will read scientific explanations, analyze the content, and evaluate the evidence provided.

DRAWING CONCLUSIONS

Empirical evidence, or evidence generated through experimentation, is a primary feature of science. Scientists collect data, analyze it, and then draw logical conclusions supported by the data. Conclusions in science are not drawn from just a few observations. Scientists study trends and patterns in large amounts of experimentally reproducible data. To have confidence in the data, scientists repeat experiments with the same **variables** and procedures. If repeated experiments have similar results, scientists can have confidence in the data and draw valid conclusions. TEAS tasks will ask you to draw conclusions based on data and other evidence. For example, consider a scientist is trying to determine how certain varieties of fertilizer affect the growth of grass. The TEAS task will present you with the scientist's experimental procedure and data. You will be asked to evaluate the scientist's procedure and data and draw a conclusion about the type of fertilizer that produces the most growth.

IDENTIFYING CAUSE-AND-EFFECT RELATIONSHIPS

Conclusions are often presented as cause–and–effect relationships. Although these relationships can be difficult to establish conclusively, scientists can use this simplified relationship to explain phenomena. Identifying cause and effect in a given scenario is necessary for completing TEAS tasks. For example, consider the scientist studying varieties of fertilizer. You may be asked to identify the effect of different fertilizers on grass growth.

Objectives
This objective includes, but is not limited to, the following examples of knowledge, skills, and abilities.
• Identify a logical conclusion based on the evidence provided in a chart, graph, or text.
• Identify the stated cause and effect in a scientific explanation.
• Use evidence to support a scientific explanation.

---

empirical evidence. Evidence generated through experimentation.

variables. The conditions in an experiment that may be changed or manipulated.

EVALUATING EVIDENCE

Conclusions rely on the evidence that supports them. Analyzing the reliability of evidence is important in evaluating the strength of a conclusion. Strong conclusions and theories are produced by reproducible and convincing data. The process of analyzing data includes evaluating the following factors: the presence of bias (either intentional or unintentional), controlled setting (changing only one variable at a time), accurate data collection, and replicable results. Bias sometimes occurs when experimenters influence results. For example, suppose the effectiveness of a new type of medicine is being tested. Experimenters or the people receiving the medicine may believe the medicine is effective, and this bias may influence their observations or conclusions unintentionally. To avoid this, some experiments use placebos to try and eliminate bias. A "*placebo*" is a substance with no medicinal effect that can be used as a control in an experiment. Common placebos are substances containing water and sugar. Experimenters and subjects do not know who is receiving the medicine and who is receiving the placebo. This helps to eliminate bias.

It is also important to analyze the experimental design when evaluating evidence. Larger sample sizes and repeated trials provide more confidence in the evidence collected. The design should also keep all conditions the same except for the variable being tested, which is called the "*independent variable*." The conditions being kept the same are called the "*controlled variables*." Keeping controlled variables the same provides further confidence that the results observed are caused by the variable under consideration. For example, consider the fertilizer experiment. Keeping all conditions such as temperature and amount of water provided the same for all the plants allows the experimenter to have more confidence that it is the fertilizer causing any changes or effects in plant growth.

---

placebo. A substance with no medicinal effect that can be used as a control in an experiment.

independent variable. The condition that is manipulated or changed in an experiment.

controlled variable. The condition that is kept the same in an experiment.

Practice Problems

Read the passage. Then answer the following questions.

A researcher collected data to measure the effectiveness of a new pain medication in treating chronic pain. Each patient was given a dose of medication every day at 8 a.m. and asked to rate their pain on a scale of 1-10. They were asked to rate their pain at 11 a.m. after the medicine had taken effect. Patient 1 received a placebo medicine containing a saline solution. Patients 2, 3, and 4 received the same doses of the new pain medication. The following table shows the results of the experiment.

Patient number	Pain rating (8 a.m.)	Pain rating (11 a.m.)
1	9	8
2	8	4
3	9	2
4	5	2

1. Which of the following conclusions can be drawn from the data?

    A. The pain medicine reduces patient pain after 3 hours.

    B. The pain medicine does not affect patient pain levels.

    C. In large doses, the pain medicine is effective.

    D. The correct time to take pain medicine is 9 a.m.

2. Which of the following describes what was done to try and avoid bias in this experiment?

    A. All patients were given the medicine when pain levels were highest.

    B. All patients had similar starting pain levels.

    C. A placebo was given to the patient who did not receive the medication.

    D. The experimenter followed the same directions each time when giving the medication.

3. The experimenter instructed patients to conduct similar activities during the 3 hours of testing. Which of the following is the name for this type of experimental factor?

    A. Data

    B. Independent variable

    C. Dependent variable

    D. Controlled variable

4. Which of the following experimental practices would strengthen the data supporting the conclusion?

    A. Testing multiple dosages of medicine

    B. Testing the medicine at different times of the day

    C. Testing more patients experiencing similar types of pain to see if the results are reproducible

    D. Removing the placebo group from further testing to prevent bias

5. Many trials of the experiment testing the new pain medication were conducted. Similar results were found among the placebo group and the group of patients who received the medicine. What conclusion would you make based on this data?

S.4.3 — Predict relationships among events, objects, and processes.

The natural world—including the human body—is constantly changing. Events such as hurricanes and drought affect many people, whereas specific ailments or diseases affect individuals. It is important to distinguish between the magnitude of large- and small-scale events, objects, and processes. This TEAS task focuses on the magnitude of events and processes. You will also be asked to determine causal relationships between events and the sequence of events and processes.

COMPARING MAGNITUDE

The human body has many cells, tissues, and organs. Each component of the body is a different size and is reported with a different scale. For example, the diameter of human hair can be measured in micrometers (millionths of a meter), and the height of a human would more commonly be measured in meters. The mass of atoms is measured using atomic mass units, whereas the mass of an elephant is measured in kilograms. Every measurement requires a unit, and the unit identifies the scale of the measurement, such as kilograms, grams, or milligrams. It is important to understand the concept of scale to compare the magnitude or size of objects and processes.

DETERMINING CAUSAL RELATIONSHIPS AND SEQUENCE

Causal relationships are difficult to determine with complete confidence. However, data can suggest a cause-and-effect relationship between two variables. Scientific studies can suggest causal relationships between variables. Examples of causal relationships include smoking and emphysema, high blood pressure and vascular disease, and alcohol consumption during pregnancy and fetal alcohol syndrome.

Determining a causal relationship can also involve determining the sequence of events that leads to a consequence. For example, if your body temperature increases above 37°C (98.6°F), your nerve cells send a signal to the brain. The brain then sends a signal to your sweat glands and you begin sweating. Another example is how the body maintains a proper level of blood glucose. As glucose rises, the pancreas releases insulin. Insulin allows the cells of the body to take in glucose. If blood glucose levels are too low, glucagon is released, causing the liver to break down glycogen into glucose. This TEAS task will ask you to determine causal relationships and sequence of events based on data provided.

Practice Problems

1. Which of the following units is most appropriate for measuring the height of a giraffe?

   A. Centimeters

   B. Meters

   C. Kilometers

   D. Millimeters

2. Which of the following units is most appropriate for measuring the mass of a coin?

   A. Grams

   B. Meters

   C. Kilograms

   D. Kilometers

3. Which of the following can lead to the breakdown of glycogen?

   A. High levels of insulin

   B. High levels of glucose

   C. Low levels of insulin

   D. Low levels of glucose

4. Researchers conducted an experiment on the effects of a new anti-mold product. Which of the following is the dependent variable that should be measured to establish an effect in this experiment?

   A. Amount of anti-mold product

   B. Amount of mold growth

   C. Humidity

   D. Temperature

5. Write three to five sentences describing the possible sequence of events of how the human body responds to high temperatures.

S.4.4 — Apply the scientific method to interpret a scientific investigation.

Science is propelled by investigation. Scientists determine hypotheses based on known evidence and then create investigations to test the hypotheses. For information to be validated, scientists submit their ideas for scrutiny by other scientists. This process of investigation is important to society's understanding of the world. This TEAS task will focus on **hypothesis** and investigations.

IDENTIFY A RELEVANT HYPOTHESIS BASED ON A GIVEN INVESTIGATION

Hypotheses are informed guesses about causal relationships that are generated by observation and initial data collection. A valid hypothesis is testable and has the potential for being proven wrong. Scientists develop hypotheses only after they begin to have ideas about relationships. This could be from observations or background research on a topic. The hypothesis is a guiding idea to develop a strong investigation or experiment. During the investigation, the hypothesis will

> ### Objectives
>
> This objective includes, but is not limited to, the following examples of knowledge, skills, and abilities.
>
> - Identify a relevant hypothesis based on a given investigation.
> - Describe a simple experimental design to test a hypothesis.
> - Identify dependent variables, independent variables, and experimental controls.
> - Determine whether experimental results or models support or contradict a hypothesis, prediction, or conclusion.

be accepted or rejected based on evidence collected from the investigation. Suppose a scientist wanted to determine the best conditions for germinating seeds. He or she may hypothesize that the seeds need to be in moist soil to germinate. Based on their investigation, the hypothesis will be supported or rejected based on data. An invalid hypothesis is either modified or replaced. The revised or alternative hypothesis is then tested by further experimentation.

DESCRIBE A SIMPLE EXPERIMENTAL DESIGN TO TEST A HYPOTHESIS

Scientific investigations collect experimental data to support or reject hypotheses. A **scientific hypothesis** is a prediction of what will occur in an experiment based on previous research. To test a hypothesis, an experiment must be set up in such a way that the data is accurate and valid. Consider the following experimental design.

Scientists are investigating the effect of water on germinating seeds. Their hypothesis is that water is necessary for seed germination. They have 100 seeds. Fifty seeds receive 25 mL of water each day, and 50 seeds receive no water. All other conditions such as amount of sunlight, temperature, soil conditions, and plant type are kept the same for every seed in the experiment. It is important to review the methodology of any investigation to determine if it is valid. This experiment only manipulates the water added to the seeds. Water is the independent variable. The observations of whether seeds germinate is the dependent variable. All other aspects that might affect the experiment are kept constant. These are the controlled variables.

---

hypothesis. An informed guess about a causal relationship that is generated by observation and initial data collection.

scientific hypothesis. A prediction of what will occur in an experiment based on previous research.

Another important aspect of an experimental design is sample size and the use of multiple trials. In this experiment, the sample size of each experimental group includes 50 seeds. Imagine if this experiment was only done with 1 seed in each group. What if the seed did not grow because it was defective? Testing on many seeds provides the scientist more data to analyze. The scientist should then repeat the experiment multiple times to make sure they obtain similar results.

IDENTIFY DEPENDENT VARIABLES, INDEPENDENT VARIABLES, AND EXPERIMENTAL CONTROLS

Scientists must develop strategies to controlled variables in an investigation. Variables are the parts of the experiment that could be changed or manipulated during the experiment. As you saw in the experiment on seed germination, there are three types of variables: independent, dependent, and control. Each experiment should manipulate only one variable: the independent variable. Examples of independent variables include type or concentration of a medicine. The independent variable is plotted on the x-axis of a graph. The dependent variable is what is measured after the independent variable is changed. It is the observed condition that responds to the manipulation of the independent variable. Examples of dependent variables include growth or response. The dependent variable is plotted on the y-axis of a graph. All other variables should be kept the same in an investigation. These are called "controlled variables," such as temperature and humidity. Controlling all other variables helps to establish a causal relationship between the independent and dependent variables.

The independent variable is the water, and the dependent variable is observing the germination of the seeds. All other variables, such as amount of sunlight, temperature, soil conditions, and type of plant, should be the same or controlled for all seeds in the experiment.

DETERMINE WHETHER EXPERIMENTAL RESULTS OR MODELS SUPPORT OR CONTRADICT A HYPOTHESIS, PREDICTION, OR CONCLUSION

After conducting investigations, scientists analyze their data to determine possible conclusions. Scientists accept or reject their hypothesis or prediction based on the data to form a conclusion. Conclusions are thus based on evidence and then subjected to scrutiny by other scientists. Scientists can submit their evidence to professional journals, where the investigation and data are reviewed. Only the most reliable experiments and data will pass the review process and be published. This process is called "peer review." Consider the following data to draw conclusions based on evidence.

Group	Number of Seeds Germinated
No water added	5 seeds
25 mL of water added	27 seeds

One conclusion that can be drawn from this data is that the evidence supports the hypothesis that seeds need water to germinate. This is because more seeds germinated (27 seeds) when water was added than without water (5 seeds germinated). In this TEAS task, be ready to determine if the data presented in a question provides evidence for a given hypothesis.

Practice Problems

Read the passage. Then answer the following questions.

Based on previous research, a group of scientists believe that fruit flies are attracted to rotting fruit. They design an experiment to test this hypothesis. The scientists place 20 fruit flies in a chamber. On one side of the chamber, they place an unripe banana. On the other side of the chamber, they place a rotten banana. After 5 minutes, they count how many fruit flies are on each side of the chamber.

1. Which of the following is the dependent variable in the experiment?

    A. Ripeness of the banana

    B. Size of the chamber

    C. Number of fruit flies placed in the chamber

    D. Number of fruit flies on each side of the chamber

2. Which of the following statements is the hypothesis in the experiment?

    A. Fruit flies are attracted to any type of fruit.

    B. If presented with a rotten banana, fruit flies will be attracted to it.

    C. Fruit flies live longer when exposed to unripe fruit.

    D. Fruit flies ripen fruit faster than when there are no fruit flies.

Read the passage. Then answer the following questions.

Juan Carlos hypothesizes that changing the color of light given to plants will affect their growth. He decides to test his prediction in an experiment. He sets up four groups of plants, giving each a different color of light. Each group has 10 radish plants all about 10 cm tall. He keeps all of them in the same temperature and gives them with the same amount of water each day. After 10 days, he records these results:

Light	Average Starting Height (cm)	Average Height after 10 days (cm)
Blue	10	17
Red	10	16
Green	10	11
Yellow	10	12

3. Which of the following is the independent variable in this experiment?

    A. Color of light

    B. Growth of the plant

    C. Number of plants

    D. Mass of the plants

4. Which of the following should be controlled in this experiment? (Select all that apply.)

    A. Color of light

    B. Growth of the plant

    C. Soil conditions

    D. Amount of water

5. Reread the experimental design regarding the effect of light color on plant growth. Which of the following is a hypothesis that would be supported by the data collected by Juan Carlos?

    A. Plant growth is unaffected by light color.

    B. If plants are grown in blue or red light, they will grow at faster rates than those grown in green or yellow light.

    C. If plants are grown in green or yellow light, they will grow at faster rates than those grown in blue or red light.

    D. Green or yellow light inhibits plant growth.

Science Key Terms

acid. A substance with a pH less than 7.

activation energy. The minimum energy needed to initiate a chemical reaction.

active immunity. Protection against a specific pathogen resulting from the production of antibodies in response to the presence of specific antigens.

active transport. Movement across a cell membrane that travels against the concentration gradient and thus requires energy.

adaptive defense. A specific response by the immune system to a given pathogen.

adaptive immune system. A kind of passive or active immunity in which antibodies to a particular antigen are present in the body.

adhesiveness. A measure of how well dissimilar particles or surfaces cling to one another.

adrenal. A gland above the kidney that produces hormones to regulate heart rate, blood pressure, and other functions.

aldosterone. A hormone secreted by the adrenal gland that increases reabsorption of sodium ions.

allele. A specific copy of a gene.

allergies. An immune response to a foreign agent that is not a pathogen.

alveoli. Tiny air sacs in the lungs where exchange of oxygen and carbon dioxide takes place.

amino acids. The monomers that make up proteins.

anaphase. The stage in mitosis in which the chromosomes are pulled apart to the poles and cell division begins.

anaphase I. The stage in meiosis I in which homologous chromosomes move to opposite ends of the cell.

anaphase II. The stage in meiosis II in which sister chromatids separate and move to opposite ends of the cell.

anatomical position. Standard positioning of the body as standing; feet together; arms to the side; with head, eyes, and palms of hands forward.

angiotensin II. A secretion that acts to restore blood volume and blood pressure by constricting blood vessels, stimulating thirst, and stimulating production of aldosterone and antidiuretic hormone.

anion. A negatively charged ion.

antagonist. The relaxed muscle in the pair of muscles that is involved in a given movement.

antibody-mediated immunity. A defense that employs B cells to create antibodies that tag pathogens for later destruction. Also known as humoral immunity.

antibody. A blood protein that counteracts a specific antigen.

antidiuretic hormone. A secretion from the pituitary gland that increases the amount of water able to be reabsorbed from a collecting duct.

antigen-presenting cell. A cell that displays foreign antigens with major histocompatibility complexes on their surfaces.

antigens. Substances on the surfaces of agents that act to identify them, to the body, as being native or foreign.

antimicrobial. A substance that kills or inhibits growth of microorganisms with minimal damage to the host.

anus. The opening of the rectum from which solid waste is expelled.

apocrine sweat gland. Accessory structures of the dermis that are in physical association with hair follicles, producing a secretion with an odor (possibly a sex pheromone to humans).

appendicular skeleton. The portion of the skeleton made up of our appendages—the bones of our arms, legs, hands, and feet.

arteries. Vessels that carry blood away from the heart toward other body parts.

asthma. A lung disease characterized by inflamed, narrowed airways and difficulty breathing.

atom. The fundamental constituent of matter that retains the properties of an element. It is the smallest unit that has a unique identity.

atomic mass. The sum of the masses of protons and neutrons in one atom of an element.

atomic number. The number of protons in the nucleus of an atom.

autoimmune disease. A pathology that results from the immune system mistaking part of the body as a pathogen.

autonomic nervous system. The part of the peripheral nervous system that regulates unconscious body functions such as breathing and heart rate.

axial skeleton. The portion of the skeleton consisting of the skull, ribs, sternum, and spinal column.

axon. A nerve fiber that carries a nerve impulse away from the neuron cell body.

bacteria. Unicellular organisms that are capable of causing disease.

B cells. Lymphocytes that mature in bone marrow and make antibodies in response to antigens.

ball and socket joints. Point of articulation that allows for abduction, adduction, circumduction, and rotation. The hip socket is one example of a ball and socket joint.

base. A substance with a pH greater than 7.

bolus. A mass of food that has been chewed and swallowed.

bone marrow. A soft material within spongey bone and medullary cavity of long bones.

bone. Hard, calcified material that makes up the skeleton.

Bowman's capsule. A cup-like structure that surrounds and collects filtrate from the glomerulus.

brittle bone disease. A group of diseases that affect collagen and result in fragile bones.

bronchi. The main passageways directly attached to the lungs.

bronchioles. Small passages in the lungs that connect bronchi to alveoli.

buffer. A solution of a weak acid and its conjugate base or a weak base and its conjugate acid. Buffers maintain the proper pH of the body.

canaliculi. Microscopic canals in ossified bone.

capillaries. Small vessels that connect smaller arteries, called arterioles, to smaller veins, called venules, and carry out gas exchange.

carbohydrates. Sugars and starches, which the body breaks down into glucose.

cardiac muscle. Involuntary muscle found in the heart.

cardiovascular system. The system comprised of the heart and blood vessels.

cartilage. Tough, flexible connective tissue found in parts of the body such as the ear.

catalyst. A substance that increases the rate of a chemical reaction without undergoing permanent chemical change by lowering the activation energy required for the reaction to occur.

cation. A positively charged ion.

cell-mediated immunity. A type of adaptive immunity in which T lymphocytes attack parasitic worms, cancer cells, transplanted tissues, or cells that contain pathogens.

cell (plasma) membrane. A cell organelle that maintains its environment through the property of selective permeability.

cells. The basic structural unit of an organism from which living things are created.

cellular functions. Processes that include growth, metabolism, replication, protein synthesis, and movement.

central nervous system. The part of the nervous system that consists of the brain and the spinal cord and acts as the command center for all communication and actions of the body.

ceruminous glands. Accessory structures that produce ear wax. They are found only in the dermis of the ear canal.

cervix. The passage that forms the lower part of the uterus.

chemical equation. Mathematical representation of a chemical reaction.

chromatid. One of the two duplicates of a chromosome formed during the cell cycle.

chromosome. A structure made of protein and one molecule of DNA that contains genetic information.

chyme. The semifluid mass of partly digested food that moves from the stomach to the small intestine.

codons. Triplets of nucleotides that code for amino acids.

cohesion. The tendency of similar molecules to stick to each other or group together.

collagen. The primary structural protein of connective tissue.

commensal microorganisms. Microscopic organisms that live in or on the human body without causing it harm.

compact (dense) bone. Bone containing densely packed osteons that make up the peripheral layer of bone.

complementary strand. A molecule of RNA (or a strand of DNA) synthesized from a complementary template strand.

compound. A substance made of two or more elements.

concentration of a solution. The quantity of solute in a given quantity of solution.

contraction. The process leading to shortening and/or development of tension in a muscle.

controlled variable. The condition that is kept the same in an experiment.

covalent bond. A chemical bond in which electron pairs are shared between atoms.

cutaneous vasoconstriction. A decrease in the diameter of blood vessels in the dermis that reduces blood flow through the skin.

cutaneous vasodilation. An increase in the diameter of blood vessels in the dermis that reduces blood flow through the skin.

cystic fibrosis. A genetic disorder that affects the lungs and other organs, characterized by difficulty breathing, coughing up sputum, and lung infections.

cytokines. Cell signaling molecules released primarily by helper T-cells and macrophages. Certain cytokines activate cytotoxic T-cells.

cytoplasm. The material within a eukaryotic cell that supports and suspends structures inside the cell membrane and transfers materials required for cellular processes.

cytotoxic T cells. The category of lymphocyte that attacks foreign cells.

dehydration reaction. A chemical reaction between two molecules in which a water molecule is released and a covalent bond forms; often requires an input of energy; polymers are built as a result of this reaction.

dendrite. A nerve fiber that carries a nerve impulse towards the neuron cell body.

dendritic cells. Antigen-presenting cells that process antigen material and present it to T cells.

density. The ratio of mass to volume.

deoxyribonucleic acid (DNA). The material that contains genetic information and is responsible for directing protein synthesis in living organisms.

deoxyribose sugar. The sugar portion of a deoxyribose nucleotide.

dermis. The middle layer of skin.

diabetes. Pathologically high blood sugar levels that result from a pancreatic hormone regulation malfunction.

diastole. The portion of the cardiac cycle in which the heart refills with blood.

diffusion. The passive movement of a substance from an area of high concentration to an area of low concentration.

dihybrid cross. A cross between parents heterozygous at two specific genes.

dilution. The addition of solvent to decrease the concentration of solute in a solution.

directional terminology. Words used to explain relationships of locations of anatomical elements (distal, posterior, medial, etc.).

disease. A condition that deteriorates the normal functioning of the cells, tissues, and/or organs.

diuretic. Any substance that causes water to be lost from the body through urination.

dominant. Refers to the most powerful trait or the allele for that trait.

eccrine sweat glands. Accessory structures originating throughout the dermis of the human body that secrete sweat, used primarily for regulation of body temperature.

electron. A negatively charged atomic particle.

electron microscope. A magnification instrument that forms an image using a beam of electrons that travel at high speeds and form a wavelike pattern.

element. Pure substances that cannot be broken into simpler substances.

empirical evidence. Evidence generated through experimentation.

endocrine gland. A gland that secretes hormones. A duct-less gland.

endothermic. Involving absorption of heat.

enzymatic digestion. The breakdown of food by enzymes for absorption.

enzyme. A substance produced by a living thing that acts as a catalyst. A catalyst that speeds up a chemical reaction by lowering the activation energy; in cells, most enzymes are proteins.

epidermis. The outer layer of the skin.

epinephrine. A polar, water-soluble hormone released by the adrenals in response to stress. Also known as adrenaline.

epiphyseal plate. Hyaline cartilage in long bones where bone elongation happens. Also known as the growth plate.

equilibrium. The stage of a chemical reaction in which both reactants and products are present and their concentrations no longer change.

estrogen. A female sex hormone released by the ovaries.

excretion. Elimination of metabolic waste from the body.

exocrine gland. A gland that produces secretions having an extracellular effect, such as chemical digestion. These secretions leave the gland by way of a duct.

exothermic. Involving release of heat.

fallopian tubes. Tubes that carry eggs from the ovaries to the uterus.

fatty acid. A molecule composed of a long hydrocarbon chain with a carboxylic acid group on one end.

fertilization (or conception). The fusion of the egg and sperm.

filtrate. Materials, including water, that leave the blood through the walls of the glomerular capillaries to enter the Bowman's capsule.

flat bones. Thin bones that have a plate-like shape, such as bones of the cranium.

follicle-stimulating hormone. A hormone secreted by the anterior pituitary that stimulates development of eggs in ovaries and sperm in testes.

follicle. Saclike structure that contains and allows for maturation of the female ovum (egg) within the ovary.

fungi. Eukaryotic organisms that obtain nutrients by absorbing organic material from their environment (decomposers) through symbiotic relationships with plants or harmful relationships with a host.

gall bladder. The organ that stores bile.

gamete. Sex cell; in males the sperm, in females the eggs (ova).

gene. A sequence of DNA that is the basic unit of heredity.

genetic code. The set of 64 codons that specify the 20 amino acids.

genome. The complete set of genetic information in a cell.

genotype. The genetic makeup of an individual.

gigantism. Excessive growth resulting from overproduction of growth hormone.

gland. An organ that secretes a substance.

glomerulus. A network of capillaries from which blood pressure pushes water, salt, glucose, amino acids, and urea from the blood.

glucagon. A hormone secreted by the pancreas that stimulates its target cells in the liver to convert hepatic glycogen stores into glucose and release that glucose into the blood.

glycerol. A sugar compound that serves as the backbone for triglycerides and phospholipids.

Golgi apparatus. A cell organelle that processes proteins and lipid molecules.

gonad. Reproductive organ that produces gametes; in males the testes, in females the ovaries.

graduated cylinder. A narrow cylinder used to measure liquid volume.

gram. Metric unit of mass.

group. A column of elements in the periodic table.

growth hormone. A secretion of the anterior pituitary that stimulates tissue growth. Also known as somatotropin.

hair follicles. Tubes arising from the dermis surrounded by invaginations of epithelial tissue, from which hair growth occurs.

Haversian canal. Channels in bone that contain blood vessels and nerves. Also called the central canal.

heart. Muscular organ that pumps blood throughout the body.

helper T cell. A type of lymphocyte that secretes interleukins, a protein that triggers the action of other cells, including the attack of foreign cells by the cytotoxic T cell.

hemoglobin. Protein in red blood cells that carries oxygen from the lungs to the rest of the body.

heterozygous. The state of carrying different alleles of a gene; e.g., Aa.

hinge joint. A joint that allows for flexion and extension of the more distal bone along only one plane.

histamine. A white blood cell secretion that triggers capillary permeability and vasodilatation.

homeostasis. The maintenance of a constant internal environment.

homozygous. The state of carrying a pair of identical alleles of a gene; e.g., AA or aa.

hormone. A chemical messenger produced by a gland and transported by the bloodstream that regulates specific processes in the body.

host. A larger organism on/in whose body a parasite lives.

hyaline cartilage. The kind of connective tissue that protects bone in articulating joints.

hydrogen bond. A type of non-covalent bond; a weak attraction between a hydrogen atom bound to an electronegative atom and a second highly electronegative atom.

hydrolysis reaction. A chemical reaction in which a water molecule cleaves a covalent bond to form two products; monomeric subunits of polymers are cleaved from a polymer by this reaction.

hydrophilic. Water loving.

hydrophobic. Water fearing.

hyperthyroidism. A malfunction of regulatory feedback loops leading to the overproduction of thyroid hormone.

hypodermis. The deepest layer of the skin.

hypothalamus. A location in the brain that integrates the endocrine and nervous systems.

hypothesis. An informed guess about a causal relationship that is generated by observation and initial data collection.

immune system. A system that protects the body from disease-causing agents known as pathogens by responding to substances on the surfaces of agents that the body perceives as foreign.

immunoglobulin. An antibody.

independent variable. The condition that is manipulated or changed in an experiment.

infectious/communicable diseases. Diseases that spread from one person to another.

inflammation. The resulting redness, swelling, heat, and pain in an area of defense by innate immunity.

inheritance. Transmission of characteristics to offspring.

inhibiting hormones. Chemical messengers that restrict the production of certain hormones.

innate defense. A nonspecific response to pathogens by the immune system

innate immune system. A collection of nonspecific barriers and cellular responses that serve as an inborn first and second line of defense against pathogens.

insulin. A hormone that triggers the influx of glucose into cells, thus lowering blood glucose levels.

integumentary system. An organ system comprised of skin and its associated organs.

interferons. Proteins secreted by leukocytes when they are infected with viruses.

interphase. The stage in mitosis or meiosis in which DNA replicates.

involuntary. Without intentional control.

ion. A positively or negatively charged atom or molecule.

ionic bond. The bond between two oppositely charged ions.

irregular bones. Bones that do not fit into the three bone shape categories: flat bone, long bone, short bone.

isotopes. Atoms of the same element that have different numbers of neutrons but the same numbers of protons and electrons.

joints. Places in the skeletal system where bones meet other bones. Some joints are movable, and some are immovable because the bones are fused together.

keratin. A tough protein made by epithelial keratinocytes.

kidneys. The pair of organs that regulate fluid balance and filter waste from the blood.

kinetic molecular theory. A theory stating that the molecules that make up all matter are in constant motion, and the temperature of a substance is directly proportional to the average kinetic energy of its molecules.

lacunae. Microscopic pits in bones that contain osteocytes and connect to each other within an osteon by way of canaliculi.

lamellae. Layers of bone, tissue, or cells walls.

large intestine. Comprised of the cecum, colon, rectum, and anal canal, it is where vitamins and water are absorbed before feces is stored prior to elimination.

le Chatelier's principle. A principle stating that when a chemical reaction at equilibrium is perturbed, it responds by proceeding in a direction that will restore the equilibrium.

length. Measurement of distance from end to end.

leukocyte. White blood cells, which protect the body against disease.

ligaments. A tough connective tissue that attaches bone to bone.

lipase. Pancreatic enzyme that breaks down fat.

lipids. Fatty acids and their derivatives that are insoluble in water.

liter. Measurement of liquid volume.

liver. The organ that produces bile, regulates glycogen storage, and performs other bodily functions.

long bones. Bones that have a pronounced longitudinal axis.

luteinizing hormone. A hormone secreted by the anterior pituitary that is responsible for triggering ovulation in ovaries and the production of testosterone by testes.

lymph. Clear fluid that moves throughout the lymphatic system to fight disease.

lymphocyte. A category of white blood cells that includes natural killer cells, B-cells, helper T-cells, and cytotoxic T-cells.

lysosome. A cell organelle that aids in digestion and the recycling of old cell materials.

macromolecules. Very large molecules, four major types of which are important to living things: carbohydrates, proteins, lipids, and nucleic acids.

macrophage. A large white blood cell that ingests foreign material.

mass. A measurement of inertia, commonly considered the amount of material contained by an object and causing it to have weight in a gravitational field.

mediastinum. The area between the two lungs.

meiosis. Specialized cell division used to create haploid gametes in diploid organisms.

memory cell. A lymphocyte that responds to an antigen upon reintroduction.

Mendelian inheritance. Inheritance of traits that follow Gregor Mendel's two laws and the principle of dominance.

metal. A substance that is a good conductor of electricity and heat, forms cations by loss of electrons, and yields basic oxides and hydroxides.

metaphase. The stage in mitosis in which chromosomes align.

metaphase I. The stage in meiosis I in which pairs of homologous chromosomes align.

metaphase II. The stage in meiosis II in which individual chromosomes align.

microbes/microorganisms. Organisms that cannot be seen with the naked eye and may be classified as bacteria, viruses, fungi, protozoa (including algae), or animals.

mineral resorption. The osteoclasts' removal of calcium from bone so it can enter the bloodstream.

mineralization. Deposition of hydroxyapatite onto the highly organized collagen matrix in bone.

mitochondrion. The site of energy production in a cell.

mitosis. Cell division in eukaryotes that produces two daughter cells, each with the same chromosome number as the parent cell.

mole. A unit of a substance that is equal to exactly $6.02214076 \times 10^{23}$ particles of that substance.

molecule. An arrangement of two or more atoms bonded together.

monohybrid cross. A cross between parents heterozygous at one specific gene.

monomers. Molecules that can bond to similar or identical molecules to form a polymer.

mouth. The oral cavity at the entry to the alimentary canal.

muscle. Fibrous tissue that produces force and motion to move the body or produce movement in parts of the body.

muscular system. An integrated system in the body that is vital for controlling involuntary and voluntary movement.

mutation. A permanent change in the nucleotide sequence of DNA that may arise during replication.

negative feedback. A mechanism that includes the monitoring for specific homeostatic levels and a signal to a gland. This signal stimulates or inhibits the gland's secretion in order to maintain homeostasis or cause compensations that returns the level to homeostasis.

nephron. A system of microscopic tubes in the kidneys that use various pressure levels to remove wastes and reabsorb important molecules and water.

nerve. A long bundle of neuronal axons that transmits signals to and from the central nervous system.

nervous system. A complex system that controls and affects every part of the body in daily life functions and in the constant drive to maintain homeostasis. neuron. Cell of the nervous system that conducts the electrical nerve impulse.

neutralization reaction. A chemical reaction in which mixing an acid with a base causes the H⁺ from the acid to combine with the OH⁻ from the base, forming water.

neutron. An atomic particle with no electric charge.

non-Mendelian inheritance. Inheritance of traits that do not follow Mendelian patterns of inheritance.

noncovalent bond. A relatively weak bond, like a hydrogen bond or an ionic bond; in macromolecules, many noncovalent bonds work together to give the macromolecule its functional three-dimensional shape.

noninfectious diseases. Diseases that cannot be transmitted directly from one person to another.

nonmetal. Any element or substance that is not a metal.

nucleic acids. Long molecules made of nucleotides; DNA and RNA.

nucleotides. The monomers used to build DNA and RNA.

nucleus. A large organelle within a cell that houses the chromosomes and regulates the activities of the cell.

nucleus (atom). The central part of an atom that contains the protons and neutrons.

orbital. An area around the nucleus where an electron can be found.

organ. A structure formed from various tissues that performs a specific function in an organism.

organ systems. Functional groups of organs that work together within the body: circulatory, integumentary, skeletal, reproductive digestive, urinary, respiratory, endocrine, lymphatic muscular, nervous.

organelle. A specialized part of a cell that has a specific function and is found in the cell's cytoplasm.

organic molecule. A molecule found in a living thing that contains carbon.

osmosis. A specific type of diffusion in which water moves across a semipermeable membrane from an area of high concentration to an area of low concentration.

osteoarthritis. Degenerative joint disease.

osteoblasts. Osteocytes are star-shaped cells that maintain bone and are able to sense physical stresses. Their long projections connect to each other through the canaliculi of bones.

osteoclasts. Cells that remove bone.

osteocytes. Osteocytes are star-shaped cells that maintain bone and are able to sense physical stresses.

osteogenesis imperfecta. Brittle bone disease.

osteons. Tubular structures that make up compact bone.

osteoporosis. A disease that causes brittle, fragile bones.

ova (eggs). Female gametes.

ovaries. The female gonads. Organs in which eggs are produced for reproduction.

oxytocin. A hormone made by the hypothalamus and stored in the posterior pituitary. One of its functions is to stimulate uterine contractions during childbirth.

pancreas. The gland of the digestive and endocrine systems that produces insulin and secretes pancreatic juices.

parasites. Microbes that are not free-living and must find a host from which to gain nutrients.

parathyroid. An endocrine gland in the neck that produces parathyroid hormone.

passive immunity. Temporary immunity gained by a body that has acquired antibodies from an outside source.

passive transport. Movement across a cell membrane that does not require energy input.

pathogen. An infectious agent.

pepsin. A stomach enzyme that breaks down proteins.

peptide bond. The link between amino acids in a protein.

penis. Organ for elimination of urine and sperm from the male body.

perfusion. The passage of fluid to an organ or a tissue.

period. One of seven horizontal rows in the periodic tables.

periodic table. The table of elements expressed as columns and rows.

periosteum. A thin layer that surrounds bone and is the surface for attachment of tendons and ligaments.

peripheral nervous system. The part of the nervous system that consists of all the nerves and ganglia that branch out from the brain and spinal cord to the rest of the body, allowing signals sent by the brain to reach their target destinations.

peristalsis. A series of muscle contractions that move food through the digestive tract.

pH. A logarithmic scale based on the amount or concentration of hydrogen ions (H^+) in a solution, calculated as $pH = -\log[H^+]$ and used to express acidity or basicity.

phagocytosis. Ingestion of particles by a cell or phagocyte.

phenotype. Physical appearance of a trait formed by genetics and environment.

phosphate group. A phosphorus atom bound to four oxygen atoms.

phosphodiester bond. A covalent bond that links two nucleotides together in a nucleic acid molecule.

pineal gland. A small gland near the center of the brain that secretes melatonin.

pituitary gland. The endocrine gland at the base of the brain that controls growth and development.

placebo. A substance with no medicinal effect that can be used as a control in an experiment.

plasma. Clear pale yellow component of blood that carries red blood cells, white blood cells, and platelets throughout the body.

pleura. A membrane around the lungs and inside the chest cavity.

polymer. A substance composed of similar units bonded together.

polysaccharides. Carbohydrate polymers made of many sugar molecules.

positive feedback. A mechanism that stimulates glandular secretions to continue to increase, temporarily pushing levels further out of homeostasis, until a particular biological effect is reached (e.g., expulsion of the fetus during childbirth).

prime mover. The contracting muscle in the pair of muscles that is involved in a given movement; also called the agonist.

products. In a chemical equation, the substances on the right side of the equation; the substances that are formed in a chemical reaction.

prophase. The stage in mitosis in which chromosomes condense in preparation for being pulled apart.

prophase I. The stage in meiosis I in which chromosomes condense and form homologous pairs.

prophase II. The stage in meiosis II in which chromosomes in the haploid daughter cells condense.

prostate. The gland in males that controls the release of urine and secretes a portion of semen that enhances motility and fertility of sperm.

proteins. Molecules composed of amino acids joined by peptide bonds.

proton. A positively charged atomic particle.

protozoans/protists. Unicellular aerobic eukaryotes. They are the largest group of organisms in the world in terms of numbers, biomass, and diversity.

proximal tubule. The first location where glucose and other useful solutes are reabsorbed back into the blood through the walls of surrounding capillaries. It connects the Bowman's capsule to the Loop of Henle.

puberty. A physiological period in which changes in hormone levels cause a general "growth spurt" and development of secondary sex characteristics.

Punnett square. A square diagram used to determine the various genotype combinations that may be passed from parent to offspring and their likelihood of occurring.

reactants. In a chemical equation, the substances on the left side of the equation; the starting materials in a chemical reaction.

recessive. Refers to traits that are masked if dominant alleles are also present; also refers to the allele for that trait.

rectum. The last section of the large intestine, ending with the anus.

reference planes. Planes dividing the body to describe locations: sagittal, coronal, and transverse.

reflex. An involuntary action to a stimulus.

relaxation. Release of tension in a muscle.

releasing hormones. Chemical messengers that stimulate the production of certain hormones.

renal arteries. The two branches of the abdominal aorta that supply the kidneys.

renal cortex. The outer layer of the kidney.

renal medulla. The innermost part of the kidney.

renal pelvis. The center of the kidney where urine collects before moving to the ureter.

renal vein. A vein carrying blood from a kidney to the inferior vena cava.

renin. An enzyme released by the kidney when reduced blood pressure is detected by baroreceptors in aorta and carotid arteries.

rheumatoid arthritis. A progressive autoimmune disease that causes joint inflammation and pain.

ribonucleic acid (RNA). An important biological macromolecule that is present in all cells and controls the intermediate steps involved in protein synthesis.

ribosome. A protein-RNA complex that is the site of protein synthesis.

rough endoplasmic reticulum. A cell organelle containing ribosomes that synthesizes and processes proteins in the cell.

saliva. The clear liquid found in the mouth, also known as spit.

salt. A chemical compound formed from the reaction of an acid with a base, with at least part of the hydrogen of the acid replaced by a cation.

saturated solution. A solution containing the maximum possible amount of solute.

sarcomere. Contracting unit of a muscle.

scientific hypothesis. A prediction of what will occur in an experiment based on previous research.

scrotum. The pouch of skin that contains the testicles.

sebaceous glands. Accessory structures originating in the dermis that secrete sebum onto hair emerging from the hair follicle.

short bones. Bones that are similar in both length and width, such as those found in the wrist. They have limited articulation with each other as gliding joints.

SI units (Système Internationale). International System of Units based on meters, kilograms, seconds, amperes, Kelvin, candela, and mole. Commonly known as the metric system.

skeletal muscles. Muscles that attach to bones and are connected to and communicate with the central nervous system.

skeletal system. The system of bones in the body that provides protection for delicate organs and serves as the scaffold against which muscles pull for movement. It has three main functions: movement, protection, and storage of minerals and fat.

skin. The thin layer of tissue that covers the body.

small intestine. The part of the GI tract between the stomach and large intestine that includes the duodenum, jejunum, and ileum, where digestion and absorption of food occurs.

smooth endoplasmic reticulum. A cell organelle that synthesizes and concentrates lipids in the cell; does not contain ribosomes.

smooth muscle. Muscle that can be found in the walls of hollow organs, such as the stomach and intestines.

solute. The substance that dissolves in a solvent to form a solution.

solution. A homogeneous mixture of two or more substances whose components are uniformly distributed on a microscopic scale.

solvent. The substance in which a solute is dissolved to form a solution.

somatic nervous system. The part of the peripheral nervous system that controls conscious skeletal muscle function.

sperm. Male gametes.

spongy bone. A type of bone having fewer osteons, and therefore, lighter than compact (dense) bone.

steroid hormones. Hormones made from cholesterol.

stomach. The organ between the esophagus and small intestine in which the major portion of digestion occurs.

subcutaneous. Under the dermis.

sublimation. The transition of a substance from solid to gas without passing through the liquid state.

sugars. The monomers used to build polysaccharides; also molecules made of two or a few monosaccharide units that are used for fuel in the body.

supersaturated solution. A solution that has been raised to a higher temperature in order to dissolve more solute than would be possible at room temperature.

surfactant. A lipoprotein secreted by alveoli and found in the lungs that facilitates breathing by reducing surface tension.

sutures. Joints, such as those between the plates of the skull, that do not allow motion.

sweat. Perspiration excreted by sweat glands through the skin.

synapse. The structure that allows neurons to pass signals to other neurons, muscles, or glands.

systole. The portion of the cardiac cycle in which the heart expels blood.

T cells. White blood cells that mature in the thymus and participate in an immune response.

target site. A particular cell type or organ on which a specific hormone can have an effect.

telophase. The stage in mitosis in which two nuclei form and the daughter cells separate.

telophase I. The stage in meiosis I in which nuclear membranes form as the cell separates into two haploid daughter cells with chromosomes consisting of two sister chromatids.

telophase II. The stage in meiosis II in which nuclear membranes form as the two daughter cells from meiosis I separate into four haploid daughter cells with chromosomes consisting of a single chromatid each.

template strand. A sequence of bases on a strand of DNA that is used to form a complementary mRNA molecule.

tendons. Tough connective tissue that attaches muscle to bone.

testes (testicles). The male gonads. The organs that produce sperm.

testosterone. The hormone that stimulates male secondary sexual characteristics.

thymus. The lymphoid organ that produces T-cells.

thyroid gland. The gland in the neck that secretes hormones that regulate growth, development, and metabolic rate.

tidal volume. The amount of air breathed in a normal inhalation or exhalation.

tissue. A group of cells with similar structure that function together as a unit, but at a lower level than organs.

trachea. The windpipe, which connects the larynx to the lungs.

transcription. The synthesis of RNA from a DNA template.

translation. Protein synthesis that takes place after mRNA exits the nucleus and binds to a ribosome.

trypsin. Pancreatic enzyme that breaks down protein

tubular reabsorption. Movement of useful material from filtrate back into the bloodstream.

unsaturated solution. A solution containing less than the maximum possible amount of solute.

urea. The main nitrogenous part of urine.

ureter. The duct that delivers urine from the kidney to the bladder.

urethra. The duct that delivers urine from the urinary bladder to the outside of the body.

urinary bladder. The structure that stores urine in the body until elimination.

urinary system. Is composed of the kidneys, ureters, urinary bladder, and urethra and function in the excretory process

urine. Liquid waste excreted by the kidneys.

uterus. The womb.

vaccination. The process of introducing weakened or killed antigens to a body in order to elicit an immune response.

vaccine. A solution of dead or weakened pathogen introduced to the body for the purpose of stimulating antibody production for that pathogen.

vacuole. A cell organelle that serves as storage for a variety of substances, including water, toxins, and carbohydrates.

vagina. The canal that connects the external genitals to the cervix in the female.

valence electron. An electron in an outer orbital that can form bonds with other atoms.

variables. The conditions in an experiment that may be changed or manipulated.

vas deferens. The duct in which sperm moves from a testicle to the urethra.

veins. Vessels that carry blood toward the heart from other body parts.

ventilation. The exchange of oxygen with carbon dioxide in the lungs. .

virus. A noncellular entity that consists of a nucleic acid core (DNA or RNA) surrounded by a protein coat.

viscera. The internal organs in the main cavities of the body.

vitamin D. A vitamin made by the skin that helps the intestine absorb dietary calcium.

Volkmann canal. Channels in bone that transmit blood vessels and communicate with Haversian canals. Also called perforating canals.

volume. The amount of space something takes up.

volumetric pipette. A device used for precise measurement of small amounts of liquid volume.

voluntary. With intentional control.

zygote. Fertilized egg with full set of genetic material resulting from merging of egg and sperm nuclei.

Practice Problems Answer Key

S.1.1

1. Options B and E are correct. "Superior" refers to "above" on a human in anatomical position, which would make the trachea and brain superior to the lungs. The stomach is inferior to the lungs, the diaphragm is inferior to the lungs, and the heart is medial to the lungs.

2. Distal refers to "farthest away." The thumb is farthest away from the shoulder of the body.

3. Option C is correct. The coronal or frontal plane divides the body front and back; "anterior" references the front of the body and "posterior" references the back. "Superior" and "inferior" reference the transverse or cross-sectional plane, "distal" and "proximal" indicate relative distance, and "lateral" and "medial" indicate proximity to a medial line.

4. Option A is correct. "Dorsal" and "lumbar" both relate, either directionally or regionally, to the back. "Umbilical" refers to the navel, "crural" refers to the shin area, "orbital" refers to the region of the skull around the eye, and "patellar" refers to the front of the knee.

5. Options B and C are correct. The mouth, nose, cheek, and eye socket are all to the front of the skull, while the occipital region refers to back base of the skull. Digits or phalanges are fingers or toes, which do occur on hands and feet. However, the armpit is not above the head. And while the armpit, upper arm, elbow, and forearm are upper limb structures, the hollow behind the knee and calf are not.

S.1.2

1. Option D is correct. The diaphragm is a muscle that increases and decreases the volume in the lungs. The trachea and alveoli function in transporting air and gas exchange. The heart is part of the circulatory system.

2. Option B is correct. The thin walls decrease the distance between the air and bloodstream, increasing the rate of diffusion. Increasing the distance would decrease the rate of diffusion. Small and numerous alveoli increase the surface area, which increases the rate of diffusion.

3. Option C is correct. The respiratory system exchanges oxygen and carbon dioxide. Gas exchange affects the pH of blood, but that is not the primary role of the system. Transporting gases is a role of the circulatory system.

4. Option A is correct. The right lung has three lobes, the superior, middle and inferior. The left lung has two lobes, the superior and inferior. The right lung has more space because the heart is located toward the left side of the body.

5. Increasing the tidal volume will increase diffusion of carbon dioxide out of the bloodstream. Oxygen will increase in the bloodstream. Changing the tidal volume will not have a direct effect on heart rate or surfactant.

S.1.3

1. Option C is correct. The heart is made up of four chambers, two atria and two ventricles. Blood cells travel through the heart chambers.

2. Option A is correct. Red blood cells contain hemoglobin, which transports oxygen.
   - Plasma helps control body temperature and transport substances.
   - Dissolved gases can be found in the blood but do not transport substances.
   - Leukocytes are white blood cells that help guard against infection.

3. Option D is correct. The right ventricle pumps blood toward the lungs.
   - The left atrium accepts blood from the lungs.
   - The right atrium accepts blood from the body.
   - The left ventricle pumps blood to the body.

4. Option C is correct. Veins transport blood from the lungs or the body to the heart. Veins can carry oxygenated or deoxygenated blood.

5. The right and left ventricles have thicker walls than the two atria. Thicker muscular walls are needed to generate the pressure to pump blood out of the heart to the pulmonary and systemic circuits.

S.1.4

1. Option A is correct. Digestion begins in the mouth with mechanical and chemical digestion. The other organs play a role but do not start digestion.

2. Option B is correct. With the help of pepsin, protein starts to break down in the stomach. The small intestine also breaks down proteins with the secretion of trypsin from the pancreas, but this is after the food passes through the stomach.

3. Option B is correct. Microvilli absorb nutrients in the small intestine. Enzymes and hormones aid in digestion, but they do not absorb.

4. Option C is correct. Peristalsis refers to the muscle contractions that move food through the digestive tract.

5. Starch begins to breakdown in the mouth. Chewing breaks the food fragments into smaller pieces. Amylase chemically speeds up the process of starches breaking down into smaller molecules. Muscle contractions in the stomach break down food particles into chyme. Then, in the small intestines, more enzymes released by the pancreas break down the starches into simple sugars.

S.1.5

1. Options A and C are correct. Walking and talking controlled by voluntary nerve signals. Breathing, digestion, and heartbeats are controlled by the autonomic nervous system.

2. Option C is correct. Synapses allow for the passing of signals to another nerve cell or a muscle cell.

   • Axons are structures that carry nerve impulses away from nerve body.

   • Synapses are junctions between a nerve axon terminal and another cell.

3. Option C is correct. The central nervous system acts as the central command for all communication and actions of the body.

   The peripheral nervous system is responsible for transmitting the electrical signals from the brain to the rest of the body and back again.

4. Option C is correct. Sensory nerves send messages to the brain.

   • Skeletal and smooth refer to types of muscles and not nerves.

   • Motor nerves send messages from the brain to the muscles

5. The central nervous system is comprised of the brain and spinal cord. It controls the regulation of body systems. The peripheral nervous system is made up of all of the neurons that connect the central nervous system to the rest of the body. It is responsible for sending the messages to the brain or from the brain to designated targets.

S.1.6

1. Option B is correct. Muscles contain long myofibrils made of sarcomere units, each consisting of actin (thin filaments) and myosin (thick filaments).

2. Option A is correct. Tendons attach muscle to bone.

   • Ligaments and cartilage connect bone to bone and help stabilize joints.

3. Option A is correct. Skeletal muscles are voluntary.

   Smooth and cardiac muscles are often involuntary and control things like heartbeats, breathing, and digestion.

4. Option A is correct. The deltoids are the shoulder muscles.

   The pectoral muscles are in the chest, the trapezius muscles are in the upper back, and the abdominal muscles are in the abdominal area of the body.

5. Muscles are connected to nerve fibers. The hot stove is felt, and a message is sent to the brain. The nervous system sends a signal back to the muscles. The receptors in the muscles of the hand and arm receive the signal and respond. This causes the muscles to contract and move the hand away.

   Afferent nerves carry the hot sensation to the brain. Efferent nerves carry neurotransmitters which synapse with muscles of the hand which cause them to contract, removing the hand."

S.1.7

1. Option A is correct. Ovaries produce the female gamete (eggs).
   - Testes produce male gametes (sperm).

2. Option D is correct. Sperm is released into the vagina and travels into the uterus and fallopian tubes. If an egg is present, there is a good chance it will be fertilized by a sperm cell.
   - The vagina is where sperm are released by the penis during sexual intercourse, but it then travels to the uterus and fallopian tubes.
   - Vas deferens are found only in the male reproductive system.

3. Option B is correct. Estrogen is a hormone that plays a role in egg maturation.
   - Estrogen does not play a role in the male production of sperm cells.
   - Implantation is the process by which a blastocyst implants into the endometrium of the uterus, and estrogen does not play a role in that process.
   - Fertilization is the fusion of an egg and a sperm cell.

4. Options B, C, and D are correct. Hormones released during puberty do not lead to heart growth.
   - Hormones released during puberty lead to egg production in females and sperm production in males.
   - Puberty hormones lead to secondary sexual characteristics such as facial hair in men.

5. Male gametes, or sperm, are produced by the testes, whereas female gametes, or eggs, are produced by the ovaries. Sperm are constantly produced, but eggs are developed and matured cyclically. Eggs are typically released one at a time, but many sperm can be released at once during ejaculation.

S.1.8

1. Option D is correct. The epidermis is the outermost layer that forms a barrier of protection.
   - The dermis is the middle layer of the skin.
   - Sebaceous and sudoriferous refer to glands found in the skin.

2. Option B is correct. Melanocytes produce melanin that protect the body from ultraviolet radiation.
   - Secretion occurs in the glands of the skin.
   - The skin produces vitamin D by absorbing ultraviolet radiation, but melanocytes are not responsible for its production.
   - Nerve endings are responsible for sensing the environment.

3. Option A is correct. Hair follicles are found in the middle layer of skin, the dermis.
   - Sebaceous and sudoriferous glands are also found in the dermis but are not layers of skin.
   - The epidermis is above the dermis and does not contain hair follicles.

4. Option D is correct. The epidermis has an outer layer of dead cells.
   - The dermis and hypodermis are layers of skin, but they do not form layers of dead cells like the epidermis.
   - Blood vessels are found in skin but do not make up layers of the skin.

5. If the body gets too hot, the integumentary system uses homeostatic strategies to cool it off. Sweat is secreted by the sweat glands. As the water in sweat evaporates, the skin is cooled. Blood vessels also dilate and move closer to the skin surface to try and cool it.

S.1.9

1. Option B is correct. Chemical signals travel through the bloodstream. Electrical signals are part of the nervous system. Physical, audio, and visual signals are received by the nervous system.

2. Option A is correct. The hypothalamus integrates the endocrine and nervous system. It secretes both releasing and inhibiting hormones, which are sent to the pituitary gland. The pituitary secretes a number of hormones sent to other cells. The pancreas secretes hormones to control glucose levels. The liver is not an endocrine gland and is an accessory organ of the digestive system.

3. Option B is correct. The pineal gland secretes melatonin, which helps regulate the body's sleep cycle.

   - Growth hormone is secreted by the pituitary gland. Insulin and glucagon are secreted by the pancreas. Luteinizing hormone is released by the pituitary gland.

4. Option B is correct. The adrenal glands release epinephrine. Although the other glands listed release hormones, only the adrenal gland secretes epinephrine.

5. After eating food, blood glucose levels rise. The pancreas responds by releasing insulin, which promotes glucose being taken up by cells. This leads to a decrease in blood glucose level because glucose leaves the bloodstream.

S.1.10

1. Option B is correct. The urethra is a tube that empties the bladder. It also transports sperm in males.

   - The ureter is the connecting tubule from the kidney to the bladder.
   - The uterus is a female reproductive structure.
   - The urinary bladder stores urine before it is excreted.

2. Option A is correct. Nitrogen in the form of urea in the urine results from the metabolism of proteins.

   - Sodium chloride levels are regulated, but they do not result from digestion.
   - Protein is not a waste product.
   - Carbon is not a waste product.

3. Option B is correct. Without kidneys that function properly, the human body would not be able to filter out waste in the blood.

   - The capillaries in the lungs, and not in the kidneys, remove carbon dioxide from the blood.
   - Kidneys do not fill with urine. Waste is transported from the kidneys to the bladder.
   - Without functional kidneys, urea would not be produced. Therefore, urine production would not increase.

4. Option C is correct. The nephron is the microscopic tubule system that filters and reabsorbs.

   - Renal capillaries absorb and reabsorb molecules but are not the functional unit.
   - The glomerulus is a part of the nephron.
   - The cortex is the layer where part of the nephron is located.

5. The pressure of the blood helps the glomerulus filter out wastes and return vital nutrients through the renal vein to the blood. Renin is a hormone that is released by the kidneys and helps to regulate blood pressure by retaining or removing water and salt.

S.1.11

1. Option B is correct. Mucus can trap pathogens entering an opening in the body such as in the nasal cavity.

   - Histamines, T cells, and macrophages play roles in the immune response once pathogens have invaded the body.

2. Option B is correct. Histamines are released to stimulate blood flow to the area of the cut, allowing white blood cells to infiltrate the area.

   - Although vaccination, antigens, and T cells are important parts of the immune system, they are not the response to a cut.

3. Option B is correct. Plasma cells produce and release antibodies.

   - T cells, memory cells, and macrophages are all types of white blood cells. Their function is not to produce and release antibodies.

4. Option C is correct. Vaccinations allow the body to recognize and produce antibodies to use in the case of future infection by that pathogen. Vaccinations are not administered to produce an inflammatory response. Vaccinations are active, and not passive, immunity. Vaccinations do not increase macrophage production.

5. Allergies are caused by a substance that enters the body and triggers an immune response even when there is not an invading pathogen. The substance causing the allergy triggers histamine to be released, which can cause sneezing and mucus secretion.

S.1.12

1. Option A is correct. Osteoclasts break down bone material. Osteoblasts build up bone material, canaliculi are channels in the matrix, and osteocytes are mature bone cells.

2. Option C is correct. Carpals and tarsals are examples of short bones. They have the same length and width. Skull bones are either irregular or flat bones. The humerus, radius, and ulna are long bones, and the scapula is a flat bone.

3. Option D is correct. The covering at the end of long bones, where joints form, needs hyaline cartilage to reduce the friction of movement. The matrix forms from osteoblasts. Cartilage does not become bone, although it is important in the formation of such, and collagen strengthens the skeletal system.

4. Option C is correct. More bone is being broken down than is being built up, causing bones to weaken and become brittle. Osteoclasts break down bone faster than osteoblasts deposit minerals, and osteoporosis is not caused by pathogens or ligament degradation.

5. The bones of the skeleton connect to the skeletal muscles with a connective tissue known as a "tendon." When the brain sends a message for movement to occur, the intended muscle will contract. When the muscle contracts, it shortens, pulling the bone it is connected to, creating movement.

S.2.1

1. Chemicals, cells, tissues, organs, organ systems, organism

2. Option A is correct. The ribosomes synthesize proteins in a cell. Mitochondria are responsible for energy production; cilia are responsible for movement; and vesicles store molecules.

3. Option B is correct. Mitochondria are involved in energy production. Ribosomes make proteins, the cytoskeleton gives form to a cell, and the cell membrane maintains what enters and leaves a cell.

4. Option A is correct. The nucleus is responsible for housing DNA, which stores genetic information. Ribosomes are involved in making proteins, the cell membrane surrounds and protects the cell, and lysosomes are involved in the digestion and recycling of molecules.

5. In mitosis, cells duplicate for tissue growth and repair. One cell divides into two genetically identical daughter cells. In meiosis, the nucleus of a germ cell splits through two fissions into four sex cells, each with half the genetic material of the original cell.

S.2.2

1. Option D is correct. Adenine pairs with thymine.
    - Cytosine pairs with guanine.
    - Adenine does not pair with itself.

2. Option C is correct. Humans have 23 pairs of chromosomes.

3. Option C is correct. Nucleotides form strings of DNA that make up genes. Genes make up chromosomes.
    - Nucleotides are the smallest unit.
    - Chromosomes are made up of many genes.

4. Option B is correct. A gene codes for a protein.

5. Genes are segments of DNA that can code for specific proteins. RNA controls the steps involved in protein synthesis. Genes made of DNA are located on larger structures called "chromosomes."

S.2.3

1. Option A is correct. Capital letters are used for dominant alleles. Homozygous genotypes have two of the same alleles.
    - Ww is heterozygous.
    - ww is homozygous recessive.
    - WX is not a Mendelian configuration.

2. The correct answer is 75%.
    - Performing a Punnett square will reveal that three out of four genotypes will result in green seed phenotypes.

3. Option C is correct. Phenotypes are the expressed traits of genotypes.

   - Heritable is used to describe traits that are passed down from one generation to the next.
   - Genotypes are the two alleles an individual has for a particular trait.
   - P generation is used to define the parent generation in a Mendelian cross.

4. Option A is correct. Non-Mendelian traits are due to the presence of more than simple dominance or recessiveness.

   - Traits must be inheritable and follow the Law of Independent Assortment, which states that traits are inherited randomly.
   - Each trait has one dominant and one recessive allele. If this is not the case, the traits follow non-Mendelian inheritance patterns.

5. Heterozygous crosses result in a 3:1 phenotypic ratio.

S.2.4

1. Option A is correct. Glucose is a carbohydrate monomer.

   - Lipids like fats and oils are made up of fatty acids, and a carbohydrate can be made up of fatty acids.
   - Proteins are made up of monomers called "amino acids."
   - Nucleic acids are made up of monomers known as "nucleotides."

2. Option D is correct. Deoxyribonucleic acid, or DNA, stores copies of genetic information.

   - Carbohydrates perform many functions such as storing sugar (starch) and providing structural support (cellulose).
   - Lipids store energy and can serve as chemical messengers.
   - Proteins have many functions, including controlling the rate of reactions (enzymes), regulating cell processes, and building important cell structures.

3. Option B is correct. Enzymes are proteins, so they are made up of amino acids.

   - Glucose and fructose are carbohydrate monomers.
   - Nucleotides are nucleic acid monomers.
   - Fatty acids are found in lipids.

4. Option B is correct. Oil is made up of lipids.

   - Potatoes are full of starch, which is a carbohydrate.
   - Chicken contains protein.
   - Lettuce is mostly a carbohydrate known as "cellulose."

5. Briefly describe a function of each macromolecule.

   - Macromolecules perform different functions for living things.
   - Carbohydrates are used as a source of energy and for structural purposes.
   - Lipids can form membranes and store energy. They are used as chemical messengers.
   - Nucleic acids store genetic information and help transmit information needed to make proteins.
   - Proteins form many body structures, form enzymes used in metabolism, provide immunity, form cell membrane transport channels, and can even be used as an energy source.

S.2.5

1. Option C is correct. Pathogens are disease-causing micro-organisms. Decomposers are organisms that decompose organic material. Prokaryotes are a distinction of cells that lack a nucleus. Eukaryotes are a type of cell that have a nucleus.

2. Option A is correct. Every virus's core contains either DNA or RNA as its genetic material. Enzymes are protein catalysts, not viruses. Viruses contain either RNA or DNA, never both.

3. Option D is correct. The electron microscope is able to achieve magnification of specimens that far exceeds that of any light microscope and with greater resolution. Bright-field, dark-field and fluorescence microscopes are a type of light microscopes.

4. Options B, C, and D are correct. A mosquito is not considered a microorganism. It is a parasite that can be seen with the naked eye. Protozoa, bacteria, and fungi are all considered microorganisms.

5. Infectious diseases are diseases that spread from one person to another and are commonly called communicable diseases. They are caused by microorganisms called pathogens such as bacteria, protozoans, virus and other such microbes. Non-infectious diseases do not spread to others and they remain within a person who has contracted them. These diseases are not caused by pathogens, but by other factors such as age, nutritional deficiency, gender heredity, and lifestyle.

S.3.1

1. Option A is correct. To determine the type of atom, use the number of protons to determine the atomic number and then find it on the periodic table.
   - Sodium has an atomic number of 11, but that is the number of neutrons in this atom.
   - Calcium has protons.
   - Boron has 5 protons.

2. Option C is correct. The atomic mass is determined by adding the protons and neutrons. Because all carbon atoms have six protons, the number of neutrons must have changed.
   B. The charge of an atom will help determine the number of electrons.
   C. If the number of protons increased or decreased, the atom would no longer be carbon.

3. Option A is correct. Calcium will give away the two electrons to have a full valence shell.
   - Gaining two electrons will give calcium a valence shell of four. It needs eight to fill it.
   - Changing the protons will not affect the valence shell but would turn calcium into another element.
   - Although gaining six electrons would fill the valence shell, it is easier for calcium to lose two than gain six electrons.

4. Option A is correct. This ion of oxygen has 8 protons and electrons, giving it a charge of −2.
   B. Negatively charged ions are called anions.
   C. Use oxygen's atomic number to determine the number of protons.

5. Solution as follows.

Element name	Element symbol	Proton number	Neutron number	Electron number	Atomic number	Atomic mass (amu)
Hydrogen	H	1	0 to 2	1	1	1
Nitrogen	N	7	7	7	7	14
Platinum	Pt	78	117	78	78	195
Chlorine	Cl	17	18	17	17	35
Potassium	K	19	20	19	19	39
Helium	He	2	2	2	2	4

S.3.2

1. Option C is correct. Freezing is a phase change from liquid to solid as a result of the loss of heat.
   - Melting is a phase change from solid to liquid that requires heat.
   - Evaporation is a phase change from liquid to gas that requires heat.
   - Sublimation is a phase change from solid to gas that requires heat.

2. Option B is correct. Liquids have no definite shape but definite volume.
   - Solids have a definite shape and volume.
   - Gases have no definite shape or volume.
   - No state of matter has a definite shape and no definite volume.

3. The correct answer is 4 g/cm^3 or 4 g/mL. This is the correct ratio of mass to volume: 22.5 divided by 5. The reason the answer is 4 rather than 4.5 is the presence of only one significant figure in the volume quantity.

4. Option B is correct. If the temperature is raised above the triple point, the substance can only exist as a liquid and gas.

5. The solid pieces of ice will absorb energy from the hot environment. As heat is added, the forces holding the water molecules together will break, and the water molecules will separate from one another.
   - As this happens, the solid ice will lose its shape and turn into water as the molecules move away from one another. As more heat is absorbed, the water molecules will move even more rapidly and spread further apart as the water evaporates into gas.

S.3.3

1. Option A is correct. Elements in the same group have similar properties and the same number of valence electrons.

    - The elements in the other options (rubidium [1], oxygen [6], neon [8]) do not have the same number of valence electrons as strontium (2).

2. Options D and E are correct. K (potassium) and sodium (Na) are metals, and Cl (chlorine) is a nonmetal.

    - In the other options, both elements in each compound are nonmetals, and the bonds between them are covalent.

3. Option A is correct. It works out to a total of (nitrogens) and (hydrogens) on each side of the reaction.

    - The other options do not give the same number of atoms on the reactant and product sides.

4. Option C is correct. There are $25O_2$ ($\times 2 = 50$ on the left and $16CO_2$ plus $18H(\times 2 + \times 1 = 50$ on the right.

    - None of the other options calculate the numbers correctly.

5. 4 moles. From the balanced reaction, the ratio of moles of AgCl to moles of Ag is equal.

S.3.4

1. Option A is correct. Adding a product perturbs the equilibrium, and it is reestablished by forming more reactants. Decreasing the temperature of an exothermic reaction drives it to the right. Adding a reactant drives the reaction to the right. Removing a product pulls the reaction to the right.

2. Option A is correct. Adding a reactant increases the likelihood of collisions forming products.

    - Increasing the temperature increases the rate of endothermic reaction, not exothermic.
    - Adding a product decreases the rate.
    - Increasing the pressure increases temperature, and drives this exothermic reaction to the left, slowing down the forward reaction.

3. Option C is correct. Catalysts lower the activation energy.

    - Reactants are converted to products more readily with a catalyst because the catalyst lowers the energy barrier.
    - Adding product would slow the reaction and has no effect on the activation energy. .
    - Time does not have an effect on activation energy.

4. Options C and D are correct.

    - Decreasing the pressure would decrease the rate of collisions between substances, decreasing the rate of reaction.
    - Decreasing the concentration of the reactants would slow down the reaction. Fewer collisions would happen between reactants if they were less concentrated.
    - Adding temperature to an endothermic reaction or enzymes would increase the reaction rate.

5. Option C is correct. Enzymes lower the activation energy, which increases the rate of both the forward and reverse reactions.

    - Enzymes do not affect equilibrium; therefore, they would not shift the direction of the reaction or cause it to go to completion.

S.3.5

1. ppm. Ppm is milligrams of solute per kilogram of solution.

    0.05 kg = 0.05 × 10,000 = 50,000 mg = 50,000 ppm

2. Option B is correct. The solubility of most solid and liquid solutes increases with increase in temperature.

    - The solvent constitutes a greater proportion in a solution.
    - Vitamins with hydrophilic structures are water-soluble.
    - The solubility of gas decreases with increase in temperature.

3. Option B is correct. Diffusion is the movement of molecules from a region of high concentration to a region of low concentration.

    - Diffusion does not change the state of matter.
    - Diffusion takes place passively.
    - Diffusion is not specific to water; osmosis is specific to the movement of water.

4. Option C is correct. During osmosis, water moves from areas of high concentration to low concentration. Because there are large concentrations of sodium dissolved in water inside the cell, the concentration of water would be lower inside the cell.

5. The polarity of water allows it to form hydrogen bonds and demonstrate both cohesive and adhesive properties. Breaking up the multitude of hydrogen bonds between water requires a lot of energy. So, water has high specific heat and high heat of vaporization.

S.3.6

1. Option A is correct. HI is hydroiodic acid, and in water it dissociates, forming H^+ and I^-.

    - CO_2 does not produce or donate H^+ in water; if anything, it can be seen to accept H^+. NH_3 is a base, and KCl is an ionic compound.

2. Options A, C, and E are correct. KOH, NH, and NaOH can produce OH^- in water.

    - HCl and HI are both acids.

3. Option B is correct. Acids have a pH lower than 7.

    - Although substances with a pH lower than 2 are all acids, not all of these substances are that strong of an acid.
    - Substances with a pH of 7 are neutral.
    - Substances with a pH above 7 are bases.

4. Option D is correct. In a neutralization reaction, water and salt are formed.

    - A. The reaction is reversible, as indicated by the double arrow.
    - H2PO is acting as an acid because it is dissociating to release a hydrogen ion.
    - H_2PO and HPO_4 could be used to make a buffer because they represent a conjugate acid ($H_2PO_4^-$) and a conjugate base (HPO_4^{2-}).

5. $H_2SO_4 + Ca(OH)_2 \rightarrow 2H_2O + CaSO_4$

S.4.1

1. Option C is correct. 1.5 meters would be the correct height for an adult human.

    - The width of a fingernail is 1.5 mm, which is quite small.
    - The width of a small insect is 1.5 cm, which is also quite small.
    - A measurement of 1.5 km is quite large; 1.5 kilometers is 4921.26 feet.

2. Option A is correct. Kilo- means 1,000.

    - 100 is hecta.
    - 0.01 is centi.
    - 0.001 is milli.

3. Option B is correct. A flask would be used to measure the volume of a liquid.

    - Triple-beam balances measure mass.
    - Graduated cylinders measure volume.
    - Rulers measure length.

4. The correct answer is 250 cm³. To find the mass, you would multiple the length, width, and height.

5. The student who measured 200 cm is incorrect. A measurement of 2 m is about the height of a door, which would be way too small for the width of an entire building.

S.4.2

1. Option A is Correct. All three patients reduced their pain levels after taking the medication.

    - Because patients reported a decrease in pain levels, there is no evidence that the pain medicine does not affect pain levels.
    - The size of the dose was not tested in this experiment.
    - The time the medicine was given was not being tested in this experiment.

2. Option C is correct. The clients who did not receive the medication received a placebo instead.

    - There is no indication pain levels were highest at 8 am.
    - Client 4 had a lower starting pain level than clients 1, 2, and 3.
    - Always following the same procedure would increase the data's reliability, but not necessarily by eliminating bias.

3. Option D is correct. Keeping conditions the same is a control variable.

    - The independent variable is the medication.
    - The dependent variable is the pain rating.
    - The data in the experiment is provided in the table.

4. Option C is correct. Increasing the sample size would strengthen the data set.

    - Option A and Option B are ways to test other variables.
    - Option D would weaken the data because there would not be a group to compare with.

5. If the placebo group rated similar losses of pain as those who received the medicine, it would support the conclusion that the medicine does not have an effect on pain levels.

S.4.3

1. Option B is correct. Meters is the most appropriate unit for measuring the height of a giraffe.

   - Centimeters and millimeters are too small to measure the giraffe.
   - Kilometers is too big of a unit to measure the height of a giraffe.

2. Option A is correct. Grams is the most appropriate unit for measuring the mass of a coin.

   - Meters and kilometers measure length.
   - Kilograms is too large of a unit to measure the mass of a coin.

3. Option D is correct. Low levels of glucose lead to the release of glucagon, which breaks down glycogen.

   - High levels of insulin lead to glucose being absorbed by cells.
   - High levels of glucose lead to the release of insulin.

4. Option B is correct. The amount of mold growth is the dependent variable. This variable should be measured to determine the effect of the new anti-mold product.

   - The amount of anti-mold product is the independent variable. This is the variable being changed to determine whether it has an effect on mold growth.
   - Humidity and temperature are control variables. These should be kept the same so that the independent variable is the only aspect being changed.

5. When your body temperature increases above 37°C (98.6°F), nerve cells send a signal to the brain. The brain then sends a signal to your sweat glands and you begin sweating. The perspiration helps to cool the skin, resulting in lowered body temperatures.

S.4.4

1. Option D is correct.

   - The ripeness is the independent variable.
   - Options B and C are variables, but they are controlled in the experiment.

2. Option B is correct.

   - Options A, C, and D will not be supported or refuted by this experiment.

3. Option A is correct. The light is what the experimenter is manipulating.

   - This is the dependent variable.
   - This is a controlled variable.
   - This is not part of the experiment.

4. Option C and D are correct. Soil conditions and amount of water may affect the outcome; therefore, they should be controlled.

   - Option A is the independent variable.
   - Options B is the dependent variable.

5. Option B is correct.

   - Options A, C, and D will not be supported or refuted by this experiment.

Science Unit Quiz

1. Which of the following terms is used to describe the amount of air in a normal inhalation or exhalation?

   A. Perfusion

   B. Tidal volume

   C. Ventilation

   D. Residual volume

2. Which of the following blood vessels carries deoxygenated blood from the heart to the lungs?

   A. Pulmonary vein

   B. Pulmonary artery

   C. Aorta

   D. Vena cava

3. In which of the following actions is the autonomic nervous system engaged?

   A. Lifting weights

   B. Holding your breath

   C. Walking

   D. Digestion

4. During inhalation, where would you expect to find a higher concentration of oxygen?

   A. In the capillaries

   B. In the alveolar air space

   C. In the pulmonary artery

   D. In the heart

5. Where does blood flow next after being oxygenated in the lungs?

   A. Pulmonary artery

   B. Pulmonary vein

   C. Inferior vena cava

   D. Aorta

6. Which of the following is the name of the structure that releases an enzyme that breaks down starch in the mouth?

   A. Salivary gland

   B. Pancreas

   C. Liver

   D. Gallbladder

7. Which type of tissue would you find in the heart?

   A. Skeletal muscles

   B. Non-striated muscle

   C. Smooth muscles

   D. Cardiac muscles

Use the graph below to answer the question.

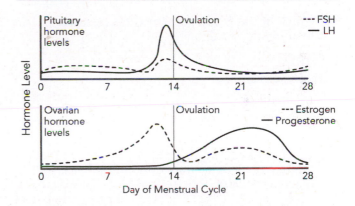

8. According to the graph, which of the following identifies when fertilization is most likely?

   A. Between day 0 and 7

   B. After luteinizing hormone (LH) levels peak and begin to decline

   C. Before ovulation

   D. When estrogen levels are highest

9. What is the name for the hormone responsible for male secondary sex characteristics?

   A. Luteinizing hormone

   B. Estrogen

   C. Testosterone

   D. Follicle-stimulating hormone

10. Which of the following would result from a decrease in body temperature?

    A. Blood vessels near the surface of the body would dilate.

    B. Blood vessels near the surface of the body would constrict.

    C. Sweat glands would excrete sweat.

    D. Cheeks would become more flushed.

11. Which of the following is where melanocytes are found?

    A. Epidermis

    B. Dermis

    C. Hypodermis

    D. Sebaceous glands

12. Which of the following is an immediate result of the adrenal gland releasing epinephrine into the blood?

    A. Weight gain

    B. Increased muscle growth

    C. Breakdown of glycogen

    D. Increase in heart rate

13. Which of the following structures releases insulin and glucagon?

    A. Adrenal

    B. Hypothalamus

    C. Pancreas

    D. Pituitary

14. Which of the following substances is the fluid that contains urea, water, and salts that is released through the urethra?

    A. Urine

    B. Filtrate

    C. Blood

    D. Nephron

15. Which of the following is a nonspecific barrier of the immune system?

    A. Mucus

    B. Antibodies

    C. Interferons

    D. B cells

16. Which of the following diseases is caused by a virus that infects T cells?

    A. Allergies

    B. Asthma

    C. Autoimmune

    D. Acquired immune deficiency syndrome (AIDS)

17. Which of the following functions is an example of how the skeletal and neuromuscular system work together?

    A. Body movement

    B. Organ protection

    C. Heat production

    D. Calcium storage

18. Rearrange the terms below in the order of the anatomical subregions.

    A. Antebrachium

    B. Phalanges

    C. Antecubital

    D. Brachium

    E. Carpal

19. Which of the following is classified as a carbohydrate?

    A. DNA

    B. Endorphin

    C. Glycogen

    D. Amylase

20. Which of the following best describes the relationship between a chromosome and a gene?

    A. Each gene forms its own chromosome.

    B. Each chromosome contains a single gene.

    C. Each gene contains a specific number of chromosomes.

    D. Each chromosome contains a specific number of genes.

21. A purple-flowered pea plant and a white-flowered pea plant were crossed. The allele for purple flowers is dominant, and the allele for white flowers is recessive. Of 1,000 offspring, 498 were purple-flowered pea plants, and 502 were white-flowered peas plants. Based on these results, which of the following can be concluded about the parent plants?

    A. The white-flowered pea plant is homozygous dominant.

    B. The white-flowered pea plant is heterozygous.

    C. The purple-flowered pea plant is heterozygous.

    D. The purple-flowered pea plant is homozygous dominant.

22. Which of the following cell structures contain cristae?

A. DNA

B. Smooth endoplasmic reticulum

C. Mitochondria

D. Peroxisomes

23. Which of the following describes the function of the plasma membrane?

A. It provides energy to the cell.

B. It helps to synthesize proteins.

C. It maintains the cell's internal environment.

D. It produces adenosine triphosphate (ATP) for cells.

24. Thymine is replaced by which of the following nitrogen bases in RNA?

A. Ribose

B. Uracil

C. Guanine

D. Cytosine

25. Which of the following are possible allele combinations for a child's blood type, if both parents have type A blood? (Select all that apply.)

A. IA, IA

B. IA, i

C. IB, IB

D. IA, IB

E. i, i

26. Which of the following types of microscopes uses something other than light to form a specimen image?

A. Bright-field

B. Dark-field

C. Fluorescence

D. Electron

27. Which of the following microscopic organisms are decomposers and the cause of many skin diseases?

A. Protozoans

B. Algae

C. Fungi

D. Viruses

28. Which of the following statements describes the subatomic particles that make up an atom?

A. Protons and electrons are about the same size and are found in the nucleus.

B. Protons and neutrons have about the same mass and can be found in the nucleus.

C. Electrons are found in the nucleus and make up most of the mass of an atom.

D. Protons are the only particles with mass and can be found in the nucleus.

Use the graph below to answer the question.

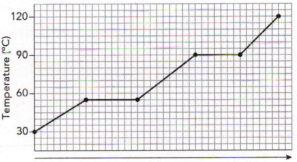

29. A substance in a solid state is put on a hot plate with a thermometer. Every minute, the temperature of the substance is recorded. According the graph, what is happening to the substance?

A. As heat is added, the substance is becoming more and more dense.

B. As heat is added, the particles holding the substance together are becoming stronger.

C. As heat is added, the substance absorbs energy, and its temperature increases.

D. As heat is added, the substance is maintaining room temperature by absorbing the energy.

30. Which of the following is an example of an ionic compound?

A. NaCl

B. CO

C. $C_6H_{12}O_6$

D. H_2O

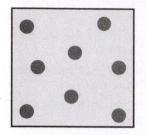
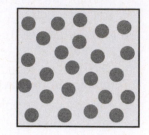

31. The diagram shows two substances contained in equal size containers. Which of the following statements best explains the density of the substances?

    A. Both substances have equal densities because they have equal volumes.

    B. The first substance is less dense because it has more volume and less mass.

    C. The first substance is less dense because it has less mass in the same amount of volume.

    D. The first substance is denser because it has less mass in the same amount of space.

$$3CaCl_2 + 2Na_3PO_4 \rightarrow Ca_3(PO_4)_2 + 6NaCl$$

32. The coefficients in the chemical reaction equation above show the quantities of the substances in the reaction. Which of the following units are assumed to represent the quantities?

    A. Moles

    B. Grams

    C. Atoms

    D. Molecules

33. A cup of tea with a volume of 200 mL contains 0.02 mol sucrose. What is the molar concentration of sucrose? (Round the answer to the nearest tenth. Use a leading zero if it applies. Do not use a trailing zero.)

$$N_2 + 3H_2 \rightarrow 2NH_3$$

34. Which of the following will increase the rate of the exothermic reaction shown above?

    A. Decreasing the pressure

    B. Increasing the temperature

    C. Adding a catalyst

    D. Adding ammonia (NH_3)

$$CH_3COOH + H_2O \rightleftharpoons$$
$$CH_3COO^- + H_3O^+$$

35. Which of the following is true about the above reaction of acetic acid (CH_3COOH) and water?

    A. This is a strong acid dissociation.

    B. The reaction is an acid–base neutralization reaction.

    C. H_2O is acting as Bronsted–Lowry acid.

    D. H_2O is acting as Bronsted–Lowry base.

36. Which of the following is the purpose of using control groups in an investigation?

    A. To establish a standard for data comparison

    B. To provide the correct answer to an investigation

    C. To determine the dependent variables

    D. To function as a third variable group

37. Which of the following instruments would most accurately measure 0.1 mL of a liquid?

    A. A 50-mL beaker

    B. A micropipette

    C. A graduated cylinder

    D. An Erlenmeyer flask

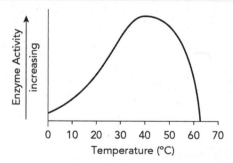

38. Joseph and Demarius conducted an experiment on the activity of an enzyme. They tested whether the enzyme activity changed at different temperatures from 10° to 60° C. Based on the graph, which of the following best describes the relationship between enzyme activity and temperature?

    A. Enzyme activity is greatest at temperatures below 30° C.

    B. Enzyme activity decreases between 20° and 30° C.

    C. Enzyme activity is unaffected by temperature changes.

    D. Enzyme activity is greatest at 40° C.

39. What tool and unit would be used to find the volume of a brick?

A. Ruler and cm³

B. Ruler and m³

C. Balance and g

D. Graduated cylinder and mL

An experiment is conducted to test the effects of caffeine on heart rate. Four trials are set up. In each trial, a daphnia, a small water organism, is given different amounts of caffeine. After 5 minutes, the number of heart beats are counted for 1 minute. The results are shown in the table.

Amount of caffeine	Heartbeats/minute
0 mg	180
0.5 mg	195
1 mg	207
1.5 mg	217
2 mg	0

40. Which of the following explanations states a logical cause and effect of caffeine on the heart beats of daphnia?

A. Daphnia need caffeine to pump blood throughout their body.

B. Caffeine causes daphnia to lower their heart rates over time.

C. Caffeine does not affect daphnia's heart rate.

D. Daphnia given too much caffeine may die.

41. Which of the following experimental practices would strengthen the conclusion made about daphnia and caffeine?

A. The experimenter should test the experiment with other substances besides caffeine.

B. The experimenter should test the experiment using different organisms.

C. The experimenter should test each condition more than once.

D. The experimenter should collect data after 10 minutes instead of 5 minutes.

42. Which of the following is the dependent variable in this experiment?

A. Length of time measuring heart beats

B. Amount of caffeine

C. Number of heart beats

D. Type of organism

43. Which of the following hypotheses is supported by the data?

A. All organisms increase their heart beats when given caffeine.

B. Organisms decrease their heart beats when exposed to caffeine.

C. When given caffeine, daphnia increase their heart rate.

D. When given caffeine, daphnia decrease their heart rate.

---

44. Which of the following best explains the maintenance of a nearly constant average temperature on the surface of the Earth?

A. The amounts of solar energy absorbed and radiant energy emitted by the Earth exist in equilibrium.

B. Photosynthesis in plants and other organisms consumes the majority of incoming solar radiation.

C. Energy emitted by nuclear reactions in the Earth's crust exceeds energy loss by radiation from the Earth.

D. The Sun provides a continuous source of radiant energy entering the Earth's system at a constant rate.

Quiz Answers

1. A. Perfusion is the movement of fluid to a tissue.
   B. **CORRECT.** Tidal volume is the amount of air in a normal inhalation or exhalation.
   C. Ventilation is a synonym for breathing in any capacity.
   D. Residual volume is the amount of air that remains in the alveoli after exhalation.

2. A. The pulmonary vein brings oxygenated blood back to the left atrium from the lungs.
   B. **CORRECT.** The pulmonary artery is part of pulmonary circulation. The pulmonary artery carries deoxygenated blood from the right ventricle, divides into the right and left pulmonary arteries, and delivers deoxygenated blood to the right and left lung.
   C. The aorta is responsible for bringing oxygenated blood from the left ventricle to the rest of the body.
   D. The vena cava is responsible for bringing back deoxygenated blood to the right atrium.

3. A. Lifting weights is an example of a voluntary action, which is controlled by the somatic nervous system.
   B. Holding your breath is an example of a voluntary action, which is controlled by the somatic nervous system.
   C. Walking is an example of a voluntary action, which is controlled by the somatic nervous system.
   D. **CORRECT.** Digestion is an involuntary action that the autonomic nervous system controls.

4. A. During inhalation, the lungs fill with oxygenated air from the environment. The blood in the capillaries will have a low level of oxygen because it just returned from the body.
   B. **CORRECT.** During inhalation, the lungs fill with oxygenated air from the environment. Therefore, the alveolar air space will have a higher concentration of oxygen.
   C. The pulmonary artery is not directly affected by inhalation.
   D. The heart is not directly affected by inhalation.

5. A. The pulmonary artery carries blood to the lungs.
   B. **CORRECT.** The pulmonary vein carries blood back from the lungs. Because the blood recently visited the lungs, it is now oxygenated.
   C. The inferior vena cava carries blood back to the heart from the lower part of the body.
   D. The aorta carries oxygenated blood to the body after it returns to the heart.

6. A. **CORRECT.** The salivary glands secrete amylase, an enzyme that breaks down starch.
   B. The pancreas is related to digestion but releases enzymes that are used in the small intestine.
   C. The liver secretes bile, an emulsifier that breaks apart fat and lipid globules
   D. The gallbladder stores bile, which is used in the breakdown of fat and lipid globules.

7. A. Skeletal muscles generally attach to bones to allow voluntary body movements. See S.1.6 for related information.
   B. Non-striated muscle is the same as smooth muscle and is involved in the involuntary contraction of hollow internal organs, such as the bladder and intestines. See S.1.6 for related information.
   C. Smooth muscles are involved in the involuntary contractions of hollow internal organs, such as the bladder and intestines. See S.1.6 for related information.
   D. **CORRECT.** The term "cardiac" refers to the heart. The heart is made up of muscle and connective tissue. The muscle found in the heart is known as "cardiac muscle" and contracts involuntary. When it contracts, it pushes blood throughout the body. See S.1.6 for related information.

8. A. This is the time period before ovulation (days 0 to 14), so there will not be a mature egg in the Fallopian tubes to be fertilized.
   B. **CORRECT.** Luteinizing hormone (LH) levels peak right before ovulation, or the release of a mature egg. After ovulation, LH levels begin to decline. Because ovulation happens, an egg will be in the Fallopian tubes and able to be fertilized if sperm are present.
   C. Before ovulation there will not be a mature egg in the Fallopian tubes to be fertilized.
   D. Estrogen levels are highest before ovulation, so this answer is incorrect.

9. A. Although luteinizing hormones send important signals related to the reproductive system, they are not responsible for the development of these characteristics.

   B. Although estrogen sends important signals related to the reproductive system, it is not responsible for the development of these characteristics.

   C. **CORRECT.** Testosterone signals tissues in the body to develop secondary sex characteristics like facial hair and growth of muscles.

   D. Although follicle-stimulating hormone sends important signals related to the reproductive system, it is not responsible for the development of these characteristics.

10. A. Blood vessels dilate when the body temperature rises to allow blood to release heat through the skin.

    B. **CORRECT.** To prevent heat from leaving through the surface of the skin, blood vessels constrict so that less blood is carried to the surface of the skin to maintain core body temperature.

    C. Sweat glands excrete sweat when the body temperature rises. When the sweat evaporates, it has a cooling effect.

    D. Cheeks flush when the body temperature rises to allow blood to release heat through the skin.

11. A. **CORRECT.** Melanocytes are found in the upper layer of skin, the epidermis. These cells release melanin, which helps protect cells below.

    B. Melanocytes are not found in the lower dermis layer of skin.

    C. Melanocytes are not found in the lower hypodermis layer of skin.

    D. The sebaceous glands excrete waste and do not contain melanocyte cells.

12. A. Epinephrine is released by the adrenal gland during stress and causes an increase in weight gain. It is a long-term effect of epinephrine release into the blood.

    B. Epinephrine is released by the adrenal gland during stress and causes an increase in muscle strength. However, this is not an immediate effect of epinephrine release into the blood.

    C. Epinephrine is released by the adrenal gland during stress and causes an increase in the breakdown of glycogen into glucose. However, this is not an immediate effect of epinephrine release into the blood.

    D. **CORRECT.** Epinephrine is released by the adrenal gland during stress and immediately causes an increase in heart rate. This is a rapid response to perceive danger and is called the fight-or-flight response.

13. A. The adrenal medulla secretes epinephrine and norepinephrine. The adrenal cortex secretes glucocorticoids and mineralocorticoids.

    B. The hypothalamus secretes releasing and inhibiting hormones, not insulin and glucagon.

    C. **CORRECT.** The pancreas releases insulin and glucagon to regulate blood sugar levels.

    D. The anterior pituitary secretes various tropic hormones. The posterior pituitary secretes antidiuretic hormone and oxytocin.

14. A. **CORRECT.** Urine is the name for the fluid secreted by the urinary bladder through the urethra. It contains substances that the body needs to get rid of.

    B. Filtrate is a material filtered out of the blood through the nephrons of the kidney; it contains water and urea, but in different concentrations.

    C. Urea and other wastes are removed from the blood by filtration in the kidney to make urine. Urine is removed from the body through the urethra.

    D. Filtrate is a material filtered out of the blood through the nephrons of the kidney. While still in the nephron, water and other important molecules are filtered back through and reabsorbed by the body.

15. A. **CORRECT.** Mucus lines the openings in the body to try and prevent pathogens from entering. For example, mucus can be found in the lungs.

B. Antibodies are more specific responses to certain pathogens.

C. Interferons are more specific responses to certain pathogens. Interferons are used by the body to stop viruses.

D. B cells release antibodies for particular bacteria pathogens.

16. A. Allergies are not considered a virus.

B. Asthma is an illness that affects the bronchi of the lungs; it is not a virus.

C. Autoimmune disease is a condition that causes the immune system to mistakenly attack the body.

D. **CORRECT.** Acquired immune deficiency syndrome (AIDS) is caused by a virus, known as human immunodeficiency virus (HIV), that infects and kills T cells. Without T cells, the body is less competent at fighting other diseases.

17. A. **CORRECT.** Although these are all functions of the skeletal system, body movement is the function that needs both the skeletal and muscular systems.

B. Organ protection is a function of the skeletal system only.

C. Heat production is a function of the muscular system only.

D. Calcium is stored in bones, so it is a function of the skeletal system only.

18. Brachium is the first subregion. The upper limb starts from the shoulder joint. The brachium is the upper arm.

Antecubital region is the second subregion. The antecubital region is the front of elbow.

Antebrachium is the third subregion. The antebrachium is the forearm.

Carpal is the fourth subregion. The carpal is the wrist.

Phalanges is the fifth subregion. The phalanges are the fingers.

19. A. DNA is classified as a nucleic acid.

B. Endorphins are neurotransmitters secreted by neurons.

C. **CORRECT.** Glycogen is a storage form of carbohydrates in animals. Glycogen is found in the liver and in skeletal muscles of humans and is used for energy production.

D. Amylase is a protein enzyme which breaks down carbohydrates.

20. A. Chromosomes contain genes, not the other way around.

B. Chromosomes contain many genes.

C. Chromosomes contain genes.

D. **CORRECT.** An individual chromosome is where specific sequences of DNA called "genes" are found. DNA is the foundational material found in genes and, therefore, in chromosomes.

21. A. In Mendelian genetics, homozygous means two of the same allele, and heterozygous means different alleles. If the white-flowered plant had been homozygous dominant, the dominant allele would have been expressed in all the offspring, resulting in 1,000 white-flowered pea plants. See S.2.3 for related information.

B. In Mendelian genetics, homozygous means two of the same allele, and heterozygous means different alleles. In order for a recessive phenotype to be expressed, the genotype must be homozygous for the recessive allele. Since white flowers are recessive, the white-flowered plant must be homozygous. See S.2.3 for related information.

C. **CORRECT.** In Mendelian genetics, homozygous means two of the same allele, and heterozygous means different alleles. A dominant phenotype can be either homozygous or heterozygous. If the purple-flowered plant had been homozygous, the dominant allele would have been expressed in all the offspring, resulting in 1,000 purple-flowered pea plants. For there to be any homozygous recessive white-flowered pea plants, the purple-flowered plant had to contribute a recessive allele. See S.2.3 for related information.

D. In Mendelian genetics, homozygous means two of the same allele, and heterozygous means different alleles. A dominant phenotype can be either homozygous or heterozygous. If the purple-flowered plant had been homozygous, the dominant allele would have been expressed in all the offspring, resulting in 1,000 purple-flowered pea plants. Since there were homozygous recessive white-flowered pea plants, the purple-flowered plant had to contribute a recessive allele, so it could not be homozygous dominant. See S.2.3 for related information.

22. A. DNA is a molecule composed of two chains of nucleotides that coil around each other to form a double helix.

B. The smooth endoplasmic reticulum is a series of membranes used in processing cell products such as lipids.

C. **CORRECT.** Cristae are the internal, folded membranes of mitochondria where cellular respiration occurs.

D. Peroxisomes have a single membrane that surrounds the digestive enzymes, which detoxify harmful cell waste products.

23. A. Only mitochondria, not the plasma membrane, generate energy for the cell.

B. Ribosome, not the plasma membrane, helps in the synthesis of proteins.

C. **CORRECT.** The plasma membrane is a semi-permeable layer that allows only some substances to enter and exit the cell. In this role, it maintains the internal environment of the cell.

D. Only mitochondria, not the plasma membrane, generate chemical energy in the form of ATP molecules.

24. A. Ribose is a structural component of RNA, not a nitrogen base.

B. **CORRECT.** Uracil replaces thymine when DNA is copied to mRNA.

C. Guanine is a nitrogenous base that is found in DNA and RNA. It is not replaced by thymine.

D. Cytosine is a nitrogenous base that is found in DNA and RNA. It is not replaced by thymine.

25. A. **CORRECT.** Allele combinations for type A blood are IA, IA and IA, i, so an allele combination of IA, IA for the child is a possibility.

B. **CORRECT.** If either or both parents are heterozygous, IA, i, for type A blood, an allele combination of IA, i for the child is a possibility.

C. Allele combinations for type A blood are IA, IA and IA, i, so there are no IB alleles to pass to the child for this to be a possible allele combination.

D. Allele combinations for type A blood are IA, IA and IA, i, so there are no IB alleles to pass to the child for this to be a possible allele combination.

E. **CORRECT.** If both parents are heterozygous, IA, i, for type A blood, there is an approximate 25% chance that the child will have type O blood, with an allele combination of i,i.

26. A. Bright-field is a type of light microscope.

B. Dark-field is a type of light microscope.

C. Fluorescence is a type of light microscope.

D. **CORRECT.** Electron is not a type of light microscope. This type of scope works by beaming electrons onto a specimen.

27. A. Protists can be decomposers, but they are not associated with causing skin diseases.

B. Algae are not decomposers but producers because they make their own food through photosynthesis.

C. **CORRECT.** Fungi are decomposers and are known for causing skin diseases such as ringworm and athlete's foot.

D. Viruses are not decomposers, though some viral diseases can affect the skin.

28. A. Protons and electrons are not the same size. Protons are found in the nucleus, whereas electrons surround the nucleus.

B. **CORRECT.** Protons and neutrons are found in the nucleus, whereas electrons are found orbiting the nucleus. Protons and neutrons have about the same mass, and electrons have very small amounts of mass.

C. Electrons have very small amounts of mass. It would be incorrect to say that electrons make up any significant portion of an atom's mass, and they are not found in the nucleus.

D. Protons and neutrons both have mass and can be found in the nucleus.

29. A. As heat is added to the substance, the molecules break off from one another, causing melting. This continues and eventually causes boiling and leaves the substance as a gas. Although changes of state result in density changes, the graph provides no evidence that density is increasing in this scenario.

B. As heat is added to the substance, the molecules break off from one another, causing melting. This continues and eventually causes boiling and leaves the substance as a gas.

C. **CORRECT.** As heat is added to the substance, the molecules break off from one another, causing melting. This continues and eventually causes boiling and leaves the substance as a gas.

D. As heat is added to the substance, the molecules break off from one another, causing melting. This continues and eventually causes boiling and leaves the substance as a gas. The graph does not show the maintenance of constant temperature.

30. A. **CORRECT.** Ionic compounds form when an electron from a metal is donated to a nonmetal atom. This donation causes ions to be formed, which are attracted to one another, and form ionic bonds. Sodium is a metal, and chloride is a nonmetal.

B. Carbon and oxygen are both nonmetals, which form covalent rather than ionic bonds. They have fairly high ionization energies and electron affinities. Carbon monoxide (CO) is a molecule.

C. $C_6H_{12}O_6$ is a molecule containing carbon, hydrogen, and oxygen, all of which readily share electrons to form covalent bonds. They all have fairly high ionization energies and similar electron affinities.

D. H_2O is a molecule with covalent, not ionic, bonds. Although oxygen has a higher electronegativity than hydrogen, they have similar ionization energies, and oxygen does not completely take the shared electron.

31. A. Density depends on the mass divided by volume. Because both containers are of equal size, the volume does not change. As there is a difference in the masses of the substances, they cannot have the same density.

B. Density depends on the mass divided by volume. Because both containers are of equal size, the volume does not change. The first substance is less dense because it has less mass in the same amount of volume.

C. **CORRECT.** Looking at the substances in the same containers, the first is less dense. Density depends on the mass divided by volume. Because both containers are of equal size, the volume does not change. The second substance has more particles and, thus, more mass, making it denser than the first substance.

D. Density depends on the mass divided by volume. Because both containers are of equal size, the volume does not change. The second substance is denser because it has more mass in the same amount of volume.

32. A. **CORRECT.** A mole is a unit that corresponds to 6.022×10^{23} particles of anything; using it preserves the correct relationship between all substances in the equation.

B. Since each element has a different atomic mass and we sum the atomic masses to get masses of compounds, grams will not preserve the correct ratio of each substance.

C. All of the substances in the reaction contain atoms, but they are compounds, and the coefficients are multipliers of the entire compound, not individual atoms.

D. All substances in this reaction are ionic compounds, not molecules.

33. Molarity is calculated by dividing the moles of solute by the total liters of solution.

Molarity (M) = moles of solute / liters of solution

M = 0.02 mol / (200 mL / 1000)

M = 0.02 mol / 0.2 mL = 0.1 M

34. A. Decreasing the pressure lowers the probability the reactants will come in contact with each other, which decreases the reaction rate.

B. Exothermic reactions slow down when the temperature is raised.

C. **CORRECT.** Catalysts lower the activation energy and increase the reaction rate.

D. Ammonia is the product of this reaction; increasing its concentration will slow the reaction down.

35. A. CH_3COOH is a weak acid, not a strong one. Additionally, the double arrow shows the reaction is reversible, not one that goes to completion.

B. Neutralization reactions produce a salt and water. This reaction produces hydronium ion ($H_3O^+<$) and acetate ion (CH_3COO^-).

C. Bronsted–Lowry acids are hydrogen ion donor. Water is accepting H^+ and is a base in this reaction.

D. **CORRECT.** Bronsted–Lowry bases are hydrogen ion acceptors. The water in this reaction is accepting an $H+$, forming H_3O^+.

36. A. **CORRECT.** A scientific control group gives reliable baseline data to compare results.

B. A scientific investigation does not begin with the premise of having a correct answer. Control groups provide reliability for the outcome of an investigation, but they do not provide a correct or incorrect answer.

C. The control group is used to determine if dependent variables are affected by manipulation of the independent variable in a scientific investigation, but it does not determine the dependent variable being measured.

D. Control groups do not function as a variable group.

37. A. A 50-mL beaker would not work to measure this small amount of liquid because the gradations on this beaker are between 5 and 10 mL.

B. **CORRECT.** A micropipette is used to measure extremely small amounts of liquids, starting at 1 microliter.

C. The gradations or marked lines on any size of graduated cylinder would be too large to measure this small amount of liquid accurately.

D. The gradations or marked lines on any size of Erlenmeyer flask would be too large to measure this small amount of liquid accurately.

38. A. The y-axis indicates enzyme activity, and the highest plot on the y-axis occurs at 40° C.

B. The activity between 20° and 30° C is increasing and not decreasing.

C. The graph shows that enzyme activity changes as temperature changes.

D. **CORRECT.** The y-axis indicates enzyme activity, and the highest plot on the y-axis occurs at 40° C.

39. A. **CORRECT.** Volume of a solid object like a brick can be found by measuring the length, width, and height and multiplying these values together. When you multiply these values together, the unit is cubed.

B. A brick is too small to be measured by a unit more than a centimeter, so a meter would not be appropriate.

C. A balance and grams would be an appropriate way to measure the mass of a brick.

D. A graduated cylinder is too small to measure a brick and is better for measuring liquids.

40. A. Daphnia can survive without caffeine, which is supported by the first trial in which no caffeine was given to the daphnia.

B. Up to the point the daphnia are no longer alive, the caffeine had been increasing their heart rates.

C. Caffeine had been increasing the heart rate, so it does have an effect.

D. **CORRECT.** The daphnia in the experiment given the most caffeine had a heart rate of 0. Organisms with a heart rate of zero are no longer alive.

41. A. Changing the substance could be interesting, but it would not help answer this experiment question.

B. Changing the organism could be interesting, but it would not help answer this experiment question.

C. **CORRECT.** To improve this experiment, the experimenter could test each condition multiple times and take the average of each trial.

D. Changes to the time could be interesting, but it would not help answer this experiment question.

42. A. The number of minutes before collecting heart beats is the same for each trial, making it a constant variable.

B. The amount of caffeine is the independent variable.

C. **CORRECT.** The number of heart beats is the observed condition that is responding to the amount of caffeine given to the daphnia.

D. The type of organism used remained the same and is a constant variable.

43. A. The data provided only gives results for one type of organism.

   B. The data provided only gives results for one type of organism.

   C. **CORRECT.** According the data, the daphnia's heart rate was increased when given caffeine. For example, a daphnia given no caffeine had a heart rate of 180 beats per minute, but the daphnia given 1 mg of caffeine had an increased heart rate of 207 beats per minute. The daphnia that was given 2 mg of caffeine had a heart rate of 0, meaning it is no longer alive. This does not necessarily mean the caffeine decreased the heart rate because there is no pattern of this seen in the data. See S.4.4 for related information.

   D. According the data, the daphnia's heart rate was increased when given caffeine not decreased. The daphnia that was given 2 mg of caffeine had a heart rate of 0, meaning it is no longer alive. This does not necessarily mean the caffeine decreased the heart rate because there is no pattern of this seen in the data.

44. A. **CORRECT.** Maintaining a constant temperature requires a balance between entry and exit of energy.

   B. Photosynthesis requires a small, albeit vital, proportion of incoming solar energy.

   C. If the energy emitted by nuclear reactions exceeded energy loss by radiation, this excess of energy would raise the Earth's temperature when combined with incoming solar radiation.

   D. Entry of radiant energy does not explain the loss of energy that must occur to keep temperatures in equilibrium.

Unit 4: English and Language Usage

The 8 lessons in this unit cover the tasks from the ATI TEAS test plan for the English and Language Usage section. These are focused on assessment of knowledge and understanding of English language and are organized into three chapters:

- Conventions of standard English

- Knowledge of language

- Vocabulary acquisition

Each lesson introduces knowledge, skills, and abilities relevant to the corresponding English and Language Usage test plan task and provides an overview of some essential topics, along with specific examples to highlight important concepts. Practice questions at the end of each lesson will allow you to test your knowledge of select concepts. In addition, there are key terms included at the end of the chapter, followed by a practice English and Language Usage quiz. This quiz includes the same number of questions as the English and Language Usage section on the ATI TEAS and matches the test plan task allocations (shown below). The quiz will give you a good idea of the number and types of questions you will encounter. Keep in mind that these lessons are a great starting point and guide to your studies, but they are not an exhaustive review of all concepts that might be tested in the English and Language Usage unit of the ATI TEAS. You should use other sources (textbooks, online resources, etc.) for additional study and practice in areas that you have not mastered.

There are 33 scored English and Language Usage items on the TEAS. These are divided as shown below. In addition, there will be four unscored pretest items that can be in any of these categories.

Section	Number of scored questions
Conventions of standard English	12
Knowledge of language	11
Using language and vocabulary to express ideas in writing	10

Conventions of Standard English

E.1.1 — Use conventions of standard English spelling

Correct spelling is important to clear written communication. For example, what is the difference between aural and oral? Not much if you are saying them out loud, but there is a big difference if you are reading them. A prescription might direct you to administer a medication in the ear (aurally) or the mouth (orally). Using **homophones** and **homographs** correctly is essential to reading and writing accurately. You also need to know common spelling rules, such as those for forming **plurals**, and the exceptions to those rules. Being able to identify incorrectly spelled words in your writing and correcting them will help you communicate your ideas more effectively.

SPELLING RULES

One of the most common spelling rules is taught by the mnemonic "'i' before 'e' except after 'c' or when sounding like 'a' as in 'neighbor' and 'weigh.'" This rhyme helps you remember the rule. It states the rule as well as exceptions to it. There are many more spelling rules that you could learn, but it is best to master the most common ones and to know some common exceptions to those rules. Here are four rules you should know for the TEAS.

Objectives

This objective includes, but is not limited to, the following examples of knowledge, skills, and abilities.

- Apply common rules for English spelling (e.g., using i before e, dropping the final e, changing the final y to i, doubling a final consonant).

- Identify common words that are exceptions to common rules for English spelling (e.g., receive, vein, height, protein, neither).

- Identify plural form of common words found in the English language.

- Differentiate between correctly and incorrectly used homophones/homographs such as their/they're, its/it's.

"i" Before "e"

This rule is well known, but it has plenty of exceptions.

"I" Before "E"	Except After "C"	Sounding Like "A"	Exceptions
believe	ceiling	beige	codeine
hygiene	conceit	rein	leisure
friend	receive	sleigh	caffeine

homophones. Words that sound the same, such as "new" and "knew," but have different meanings.

homographs. Words that are spelled the same, such as "bass" (a fish) and "bass" (a musical instrument), but have different meanings and may be pronounced differently.

plural. More than one item.

Drop the Final "e"

When adding a suffix to a word that ends in "e," drop the "e" if the suffix begins with a vowel. Keep the "e" before a suffix beginning with a consonant.

Drop the "E" Before a Vowel	Keep the "E" Before a Consonant	Exceptions
believe + able = believable	nice + ly = nicely	notice + able = noticeable
advise + ing = advising	amaze + ment = amazement	argue + ment = argument
guide + ance = guidance	rude + ness = rudeness	courage + ous = courageous

Double the Final Consonant

In a verb ending in a consonant, double the final consonant when a single vowel precedes the final consonant and the last syllable of the word is stressed after the ending is added. For words of two or more syllables, if the last syllable of the original word is stressed and a single vowel precedes the final consonant before adding the suffix, double the final consonant. For example, in the word prefer, which is pronounced preFER with the stress placed on FER, the "r" would be doubled when adding a suffix: preferred, preferring. If the last syllable of a multisyllable word is unstressed, do not double the final consonant. Never double "w," "x," or "y," and be aware of exceptions to this rule.

Double the Consonant	Do Not Double the Consonant	Exceptions: Both Forms Correct
blur + r + ing = blurring	bleed + ing = bleeding	traveling, travelling
plan + n + er = planner	plow + ed = plowed	canceled, cancelled
begin + n + ing = beginning	despair + ing = despairing	modeled, modelled

Change the Final "y" to "i"

When adding a suffix to a word ending in "y" preceded by a consonant, change the "y" to "i" and add the suffix. Do not change the "y" if the suffix begins with "i."

Change the "Y" to "I" Following a Consonant	Do Not Change the "Y" Following a Vowel	Do Not Change If the Suffix Begins With "I"	Exceptions
beauty + ful = beautiful	day + s = days	cry + ing = crying	shy + ly = shyly
worry + ed = worried	obey + ed = obeyed	worry + ing = worrying	day + ly = daily
supply + er = supplier	relay + s = relays	supply + ing = supplying	memory + ize = memorize

Rules for Plurals

You should also understand the rules for constructing plurals. Here are some rules to keep in mind.

- For regular plurals, you only need to add "–s." Examples: apple/apples, car/cars, nurse/nurses.

- Add "–es" for words ending in "–ch," "–s," "–sh," "–x," or "–z." Examples: dash/dashes, lunch/lunches, boss/bosses.

- Change to "–ves" for some words ending in "–f" or "–fe." Examples: elf/elves, life/lives, self/selves. Exceptions: chief/chiefs, proof/proofs.

IDENTIFYING HOMOPHONES AND HOMOGRAPHS

Use **context** to identify homophones, or words that are pronounced the same but are spelled differently. You also need to correctly use homographs, which are words that are spelled the same but have different meanings and may be pronounced differently or be used as different **parts of speech**. Here is just a small set of examples often found on the TEAS.

Homophones	Homographs
to/too/two	bow: to bend at the waist (v); the front of a boat (n); a decoration (n); something that shoots arrows (n)
its/it's	fair: reasonable (adj); an appearance (n); an exhibition (n)
lead/led	lead: to show the way (v); a metal (n)
bare/bear	perfect: flawless (adj); to make flawless (v)
their/there/they're	tear: to rip something (v); water from the eye (n)

Practice Problems

Read the sample and answer the following question.

The explorers traveled across the desert, and it seemed that it's heat would stop their progress.

1. Which of the following corrects an error in the sentence above?

    A. "Desert" should be "dessert."

    B. "It's" should be "its."

    C. "Seemed" should be "seamed."

    D. "Their" should be "they're."

Read the sample and answer the following question.

The explorers became thirstier and their vision blurred as they traveled farther across the arid desert and tryed to make their way to the oasis.

2. Which of the following corrects a misspelling in the sentence above?

    A. "Blurred" should be "blured."

    B. "Thirstier" should be "thirstyer."

    C. "Their" should be "they're."

    D. "Tryed" should be "tried."

3. Which of the following are spelled correctly, showing an exception to a spelling rule? (Select all that apply.)

    A. recieve

    B. beleive

    C. codeine

    D. feirce

    E. changeable

4. Which of the following uses the "double the consonant" rule correctly?

    A. "bleed" to "bleedding"

    B. "vomit" to "vomitted"

    C. "refer" to "referring"

    D. "plow" to "plowwed"

5. Perform a search and locate two more spelling rules that can support your writing. Write each rule, and then give an example of a word using that rule.

---

context. Surrounding words or ideas within a sentence or passage that affect the meaning of a word and influence how it is understood.

parts of speech. Eight categories for classifying words: adjective, adverb, conjunction, interjection, noun, preposition, pronoun, and verb.

E.1.2 — Use conventions of standard English punctuation

Punctuation is like a system of road signs for written language. Punctuation directs the reader how to read a sentence correctly. Mastering punctuation allows you to read and write with clarity. To successfully answer questions about punctuation for the TEAS exam, you will need to study the rules for **commas** and **quotation marks**. There are many great websites to reference for rules on using punctuation, but be sure to distinguish between established punctuation rules and matters of opinion. The following concepts are likely to be tested.

COMMAS

The comma is used for many purposes, from dividing items in a series to indicating pauses in the flow of a sentence. You will need to be careful to distinguish between rules and preferences. For example, the serial comma, also known as the **Oxford comma**, is the comma before the "and" in a simple series of items. It is preferred in many forms of writing but not all. Questions on the TEAS address rules, not preferences, so the omission of a serial comma would not be considered an error. Using a comma without a **conjunction** to separate two **independent clauses**, however, is the kind of error that you will need to recognize on the TEAS.

Here are some rules to follow regarding the use of commas:

- Place a comma before a conjunction in a **compound sentence**.

- Place a comma after an introductory **phrase** or clause.

- Place a comma before and after dependent phrases and clauses or around nonessential elements that interrupt the main clause of a sentence.

- Place commas after items in a series. The comma before the "and" in a series is a preference.

- Place a comma between two or more **coordinate adjectives** describing the same noun. (Adjectives are coordinate, or equal, if they can be used in a different order and still make sense. You can test if adjectives are coordinate by using the word "and" between the adjectives. If "and" works, they are coordinate adjectives.)

> ## Objectives
>
> This objective includes, but is not limited to, the following examples of knowledge, skills, and abilities.
>
> - Use of the comma to clarify meaning (e.g., in compound sentences, after introductory elements, with dependent phrases and clauses, around nonessential elements, in a series, and with adjectives).
>
> - Use direct quotations and indirect quotations following standard conventions.

---

comma. Punctuation mark used to separate parts of sentences.

Oxford comma. The comma before the "and" in a simple series of items.

conjunction. A connecting word.

independent clause. A group of words that includes a subject and predicate and can stand alone as a complete sentence because it expresses a complete thought.

compound sentence. Sentence that contains at least two independent clauses.

phrase. A group of words that work together as a unit.

coordinate adjectives. Two equally weighted adjectives that describe the same noun and require a comma between them.

INDIRECT QUOTATIONS

An indirect quotation is when a writer paraphrases what another person has written or said. If a writer relays an idea in their own words, it does not need quotation marks. However, the writer must cite the source of the idea.

DIRECT QUOTATIONS

A direct quotation indicates that the words within the quotation marks are exactly what someone else has written or stated. The exact words must be placed within quotation marks, with the end mark within the quotation marks. A comma is used after the phrase introducing the person who is being quoted, before the opening quotation mark. For example: Scientist Albert Einstein said, "Education is that which remains when one has forgotten everything he learned in school." If the sentence identifies the person after the quotation, the comma is placed inside the end quotation mark. For example: "Education is that which remains when one has forgotten everything he learned in school," Albert Einstein said. If a writer uses someone else's words without quotation marks, this practice is called plagiarism.

SENTENCE PUNCTUATION PATTERNS

Different sentence types use specific punctuation. To understand the sentence types, it is necessary to know the difference between independent clauses and **dependent clauses**. An independent clause has a **subject** and a verb. It can stand on its own as a sentence. A dependent clause lacks a subject and cannot stand on its own.

- A **simple sentence** contains one idea or independent clause and uses only an end mark.

- A **complex sentence** has an independent clause and a dependent clause. Use a comma following an introductory subordinate clause to separate it from the independent clause. You do not need a comma if the subordinate clause follows the independent clause.

- A compound sentence has two independent clauses. Use a comma before the conjunction that joins the clauses. Use a semicolon between two related independent clauses. Use a semicolon before a **transition word** that connects two independent clauses and a comma after a transition.

---

dependent clause. A group of words that includes a subject and verb but cannot stand alone as a complete sentence because it does not express a complete thought.

subject. The main noun of a sentence that is doing or being.

simple sentence. Sentence that contains only one idea or independent clause and uses only an end mark.

complex sentence. Sentence that contains an independent clause and a dependent clause.

transition words. Words that link or introduce ideas.

Punctuation Examples

Punctuation can indicate the type of sentence and how to read the sentence. Consider the commas in the following sentences.

> *I have been lifting weights for over a year, and I finally set a new maximum bench press.*

The comma in this sentence indicates that what follows will be a second independent clause rather than a dependent clause.

> *When I went to the gym, I found it was closed.*

The comma in this sentence separates an introductory dependent clause from the independent clause.

Commas help you identify independent and dependent clauses and interpret how they build compound and complex sentences. You will also need to recognize how to use quotation marks, **apostrophes**, **end marks**, and other punctuation correctly.

The following example uses a variety of punctuation to convey meaning.

> *"It's not easy to increase your bench press," she announced. "You've probably heard that there are many different theories for the best approach!"*

This example demonstrates a number of concepts. Quotation marks are used for the direct quotation, and a comma is used before the closed quote to indicate that there is additional text in the sentence. An apostrophe is used for a contraction. An **exclamation mark** is used to indicate both the end of the sentence and strong feeling.

Any concrete rule regarding punctuation is fair game for this task on the TEAS, so be sure to brush up using a variety of sources.

---

apostrophe. Punctuation mark that denotes possessive case or omission of letters. article. Word ("a," "an," or "the") that refers to a noun.

end marks. Punctuation marks that end sentences: period, question mark, and exclamation mark.

exclamation mark. End mark that denotes strong feeling.

Practice Problems

1. Which of the following are correctly punctuated compound sentences? (Select all that apply.)

   A. I've decided to run a 5K race, but running a long race requires training.

   B. I plan on taking two rest days per week and this will help me avoid injury.

   C. I'll run long distances on the weekend, and rest on the following day.

   D. Running a 5K race would be a great accomplishment, and exercise will improve my health.

2. Which of the following uses correct punctuation for a quotation?

   A. "A good laugh and a long run," she said. "Are the two best cures for anything."

   B. "A good laugh and a long run," she said, "are the two best cures for anything."

   C. "A good laugh and a long run are the two best cures for anything." she said.

   D. "A good laugh and a long run are the two best cures for anything," She said.

3. Which of the following uses a correct punctuation pattern for a complex sentence?

   A. Although I enjoy running I would never want to run a marathon.

   B. Although I enjoy running, I would never want to run a marathon.

   C. Although, I enjoy running I would never want to run a marathon

   D. Although I enjoy running I would never want to run, a marathon.

4. Which sentence uses commas correctly to clarify the meaning of the sentence?

   A. In order to begin training as a long-distance runner, you will need high-quality shoes, socks, and running clothes.

   B. In order to begin training as a long-distance runner you will need high-quality shoes, socks, and running clothes.

   C. In order to begin training as a long-distance runner, you will need high-quality shoes socks, and running clothes.

   D. In order to begin training as a long-distance runner you will need high-quality shoes socks and running clothes.

5. Which of the following uses commas correctly?

   A. Several dark ominous clouds formed in the sky about halfway through our run.

   B. Several dark, ominous clouds formed in the sky about halfway through our run.

   C. Several dark, ominous, clouds formed in the sky about halfway through our run.

   D. Several, dark, ominous, clouds formed in the sky about halfway through our run.

E.1.3 — Use correct sentence structures

A sentence is a set of words ordered to express a complete thought. For this TEAS task, you will need to be familiar with different types of sentences and how they are built using sentence parts, including subjects, *predicates*, phrases, and clauses. You will also need to know the parts of speech and how they function within sentences.

CLAUSES, PHRASES, AND SENTENCES TYPES

A good way to enhance your understanding of sentence construction is to practice identifying clauses, phrases, and sentence types. There are plenty of online resources available with information on identifying sentences and opportunities for practice.

A clause is a word group that contains a subject and a verb.

An independent clause contains a subject and a predicate that contains a verb and states something about the subject. An independent clause can stand on its own as a sentence because it expresses a complete thought.

> *I am studying. (subject = I; predicate = am studying)*

A dependent clause begins with a subordinating word such as "although," "because," or "since" and cannot stand on its own because it does not finish a complete thought.

> *Although I feel confident in my skills . . .*

A phrase is a group of words that does not have a subject or a verb and functions as a single part of speech.

> *. . . for my TEAS exam.*

Attaching the dependent clause and the phrase to the independent clause forms the following sentence:

> *Although I feel confident in my skills, I am studying for my TEAS exam.*

Objectives

This objective includes, but is not limited to, the following examples of knowledge, skills, and abilities.

- Use correct sentence types (e.g., simple, compound, and complex sentences).

- Combine dependent and independent clauses correctly when prompted.

- Distinguish the eight parts of speech—noun, pronoun, verb, adjective, adverb, preposition, conjunction, interjection—and understand how they function to create meaning.

- Create coherent sentences using sentence parts correctly (e.g., subject, predicate, object, indirect object, complement).

---

predicate. The part of a sentence that explains what the subject does or is like.

The previous example is a complex sentence. There are four types of sentences.

1. A simple sentence contains one independent clause.

   Charlie studies every day.

2. A complex sentence contains an independent clause and one or more dependent clauses.

   Charlie studies every day because he wants to get good grades.

3. A compound sentence contains two or more independent clauses joined by a coordinating conjunction, such as "and," "but," "or," "for," or "so," or by a semicolon.

   Charlie studies every day, and he turns in his homework on time.

4. A compound-complex sentence contains two or more independent clauses and one or more dependent clauses.

   Because Charlie studies every day and turns in his homework on time, he is passing all his classes, and he will graduate with honors.

PARTS OF SPEECH

The term "parts of speech" refers to how words are classified in sentences. There are generally considered to be eight parts of speech: **nouns**, **pronouns**, **verbs**, **adjectives**, **adverbs**, **prepositions**, conjunctions, and **interjections**.

- Nouns are people, places, objects, and ideas: brother, school, computer, philosophy.
- Pronouns take the place of nouns: she, he, they, we.
- Verbs are action words: walk, grasps, questioned.
- Adjectives describe or modify nouns: frozen, ridiculous, excitable.
- Adverbs describe or modify adjectives, verbs, or other adverbs: easily, quickly, triumphantly.
- Prepositions describe the relationships between other words: before, according to, since.
- Conjunctions are connecting words: and, so, but.
- Interjections represent short bursts of emotion: Hey! Ouch! Yay!

noun. A person, place, thing, or idea.

pronoun. A word that takes the place of a noun.

verb. A word that describes an action or state of being.

adjective. Word or phrase that describes or modifies a noun.

adverb. Word or phrase that describes or modifies an adjective, verb, or other adverb.

preposition. A word that describes relationships between other words.

interjection. A word or phrase that represents a short burst of emotion.

SUBJECTS, PREDICATES, AND OTHER SENTENCE PARTS

A complete sentence contains a subject and predicate. The simple subject is a noun (or noun substitute, such as a pronoun), and the complete subject includes the noun and all its **complements** and **modifiers**. The simple predicate is a verb, and the complete predicate includes the verb and all its complements and modifiers.

A modifier is a word or phrase that makes the meaning of other words more specific, such as in "green shirt." "Green" is an adjective that modifies, or gives more information about, "shirt."

The term "complement" describes words that are needed to complete a thought in a sentence. Complements usually cannot be removed from a sentence without changing the meaning of the sentence. For example, in the sentence "Math is fun," "Math" is the subject, "is" constitutes the simple predicate, and "fun" is a complement because it completes the sentence, which would not make sense without it.

Direct objects and **indirect objects** are also important parts of sentence structure. A direct object receives the action of the sentence. For example, in the sentence "She kicked the ball," "She" is the subject, "kicked" is the verb, and "ball" is the direct object because it is what is being kicked. You can usually figure out the direct object by asking "what?" as in "She kicked what?" "Ball" is the answer, so it is the direct object. An indirect object expresses to whom or to what the action was done, such as in the sentence "He left me a ticket at the information desk." For whom was the ticket left? Me!

Next, consider this example:

> *The eager, enthusiastic child told the teacher his story in an excited voice.*

The simple subject is the noun "child." The complete subject includes the article "the" and the modifiers "eager" and "enthusiastic": "the eager, enthusiastic child." The simple predicate is the verb "told." The complete predicate includes the indirect object "the teacher," the direct object "his story," and the prepositional phrase "in an excited voice," which serves as a modifier.

Some sentences contain complements instead of objects, as in this example:

> *She seemed happy with the result.*

The subject is "She," and the complete predicate is "seemed happy with the result," which contains the verb "seemed," the complement "happy," and the prepositional phrase "with the result."

---

complement. Sentence part that gives more information about a subject or object.

modifier. A word or group of words that provides description for another word.

object/direct object. A word or group of words that receives the action of a verb.

indirect object. The person or thing to whom or which something is done.

SENTENCE DIAGRAMMING

Another way to enhance your understanding of sentence construction and the parts of speech is to practice diagramming sentences. There are plenty of online resources available with information on diagramming sentences and opportunities for practice. Key rules for diagramming include:

- The key sentence parts of subject, verb, and object are written in a line. They are separated by vertical lines.

- The modifiers of each of these sentence parts extend below them on slanted lines.

- In the case of the prepositional phrase, the preposition extends from the word it modifies and then introduces the prepositional object with its modifiers.

Here is just one example of how to diagram a sentence.

The agile surfer rode that wave with expert balance.

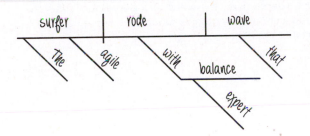

The subject "surfer," verb "rode," and object "wave" are on the straight line separated by vertical lines. "The" and "agile" modify "surfer." "That" modifies "wave." "With" is the preposition, and "balance" is the object of the preposition. "Expert" modifies "balance."

Practice Problems

1. Which of the following examples is a compound-complex sentence?

   A. The large amusement park was packed with people, and they had all come for the opening of a new roller coaster.

   B. Although the weather forecast called for rain, people came to the park to ride the roller coaster.

   C. Just as the roller coaster was about to open, the crowd looked to the cloudy sky, and a wonderful sight appeared.

   D. The sun came out and was surrounded by a rainbow that brought gasps of awe from the crowd.

Read the sample and answer the following question.

The new building gives students more spaces to study.

2. Which of the following is the simple subject in the sentence above?

   A. building

   B. gives

   C. students

   D. spaces

3. Which of the following are dependent clauses? (Select all that apply.)

   A. Swimming is a great form of exercise.

   B. Even though swimming can be difficult.

   C. There are four main swimming strokes to learn.

   D. Including the backstroke and the sidestroke.

   E. Although learning to swim is time-consuming, everyone should do it.

4. Diagram the following sentence: The parents served their children fresh vegetables.

5. Use a dependent clause and an independent clause to write a complex sentence about one of your hobbies or favorite activities.

Knowledge of Language

E.2.1 — Use grammar to enhance clarity in writing

Clear communication in writing requires a common understanding between the writer and reader. Grammar helps build that understanding. Grammar is the set of rules and conventions that allow writers to convey ideas effectively. This TEAS task requires you to recognize both correct and incorrect use of grammar, as well as precise versus ambiguous language. To prepare for this task, take note of reading passages you encounter that are unclear. Ask yourself why the passage is unclear and how it could be made more effective. Does the passage use correct grammar and precise **diction**? How would you change the passage to improve its clarity?

In this TEAS task, you will be asked to make judgments regarding the clarity of sentences and reading passages using your knowledge of grammar. The following are conventions that you should know and be able to use.

Objectives

This objective includes, but is not limited to, the following examples of knowledge, skills, and abilities.

- Use complete sentences appropriately.

- Use transition words—such as but, and, next, however, and therefore—to clarify relationships.

- Use past, present, and future tenses appropriately.

- Use precise diction or punctuation to convey mood or tone.

- Revise a text to eliminate language that does not adequately convey the nuance of meaning.

- Revise sentences that impede a reader's understanding.

COMPLETE SENTENCES

The most fundamental element in grammar is the sentence. A sentence conveys a complete thought. A complete sentence must have a subject and a predicate that communicates something about the subject—its state of being or its action. Predicates must contain a verb. For this task, you will need to be able to recognize complete sentences. You will also need to recognize incomplete sentences, or **fragments**, which are missing a subject or predicate. Study these examples.

> *We are going to eat breakfast.*

This is a complete sentence because it has a subject ("we"), has a predicate ("are going"), and expresses a complete thought.

> *Thinking about my weekend.*

This is a fragment because it lacks a subject. It does not state who is doing the action of thinking about the weekend.

---

diction. The style of writing determined by word choice.

fragment. An incomplete sentence.

Sometimes, sentences can be hard to recognize. The subject often comes at the beginning of a sentence, but questions do not usually follow this pattern. The predicate can be broken up by the subject, as in this example:

> Can I borrow your pencil?

This is a sentence because it has a subject ("I"), has a predicate ("can borrow"), and expresses a complete thought.

Do not be fooled by an *imperative sentence*, or a command, instruction, or request with an implied or understood subject. Consider this example:

> Finish your homework!

This is a complete sentence because it has an understood subject ("you"), has a predicate ("finish"), and expresses a complete thought.

TRANSITIONS

Transition words and phrases are used to connect ideas and clarify the relationship between ideas. You should be able to identify appropriate transitions based on context and to recognize when a transition word is misused or another word is needed for clarity. This table provides examples of the types of transitions and specific transition words and phrases.

Transition Type	Examples	Transition Type	Examples
Agreement	correspondingly, equally important, in the same way	Examples	like, including, in other words, for example
Opposition	but, although, however, conversely	Conclusion	after all, in short, altogether, ultimately
Cause	if, unless, in order to, in the event that	Chronology	before, after, in the meantime, suddenly
Effect	therefore, consequently, accordingly, as a result	Location	here, there, wherever, adjacent to

TENSE

Tense refers to when an action occurs. The basic tenses are past, present, and future, but tense can also capture whether an action is complete. An action can be *progressive*, meaning incomplete, or *perfect*, meaning complete. You will need to be able to recognize and correct the inappropriate use of tense, including inappropriate shifts in tense within a sentence or passage. The chart provides an example of how verbs indicate time.

	Past	Present	Future
Simple	walked	walks	will walk
Progressive	was walking	is walking	will be walking
Perfect	had walked	has walked	will have walked

imperative sentence. A complete sentence that conveys a command, instruction, or request and has the implied or understood subject "you."

tense. Refers to when an action occurs: past, present, or future.

progressive. A verb tense indicating that the action described is currently happening.

perfective. A verb tense indicating that the action described has been completed.

DICTION

Word choice, or diction, and punctuation are also important elements of clear communication. Different words create different **moods** (feeling or atmosphere) or **tones** (attitude). Mood includes how writing makes the reader feel. The mood can be mysterious, cheerful, or somber, for example. "Tone" is a term used to describe the author's or the narrator's attitude toward the subject. The tone can be **formal**, sarcastic, or earnest, for example. Punctuation can be used to express meaning as well. Exclamation marks, for instance, are often used to express excitement or surprise.

You will need to be able to identify which word choices are best for a given context. For example, the words "inaudible," "discreet," and "soft" are **synonyms** for "quiet." Which synonym might appropriately replace "quiet" in the sentence below?

> *Florence enjoys camping because she loves how quiet nature can be.*

Now consider how replacing the **period** with an exclamation mark changes the nature of this sentence.

> *Florence enjoys camping because she loves how quiet nature can be!*

The exclamation is inappropriate because the idea of emotion contradicts the appreciation of quiet described in the sentence.

RUN-ON SENTENCES

You will also be asked to revise sentences that impede a reader's understanding. This task includes identifying and correcting **run-on sentences**. A run-on sentence is a sentence that has too many ideas to be clearly understood. Here is an example:

> *The story had a thrilling ending the plot was built with suspense.*

This is a run-on sentence due to the lack of a conjunction or appropriate punctuation. The two ideas ("the story had a thrilling ending" and "the plot was built with suspense") are complete thoughts that must be separated to be correct.

> *The story had a thrilling ending because the plot was built with suspense.*

As you read, consider whether sentences can be rewritten to make them clear to the reader. Sometimes, simply replacing an ambiguous pronoun or adding a conjunction is all that is needed to fix a sentence so that readers can clearly understand its meaning.

---

mood. How the elements in a text, such as word choice, make the reader feel.

tone. An author's implied or explicit attitude toward a topic.

formal. A style that follows conventional rules.

synonyms. Words with identical or similar meanings.

period. End mark that denotes the end of a standard sentence.

run-on sentence. A sentence with extra parts that are not joined properly by the correct conjunction or punctuation.

OTHER CONVENTIONS

There are a number of other grammar conventions that you will need to apply, such as **subject-verb agreement** and **pronoun-antecedent agreement**. For this task, any grammar rule is fair game, so be sure to review a number of grammar resources.

Practice Problems

1. Which of the following is a sentence fragment?

   A. Let's hike to a glacier!

   B. According to many experts in Alaska.

   C. Hiking is a great activity for your health.

   D. Maria loves to hike and enjoys going to new places.

Read the sample and answer the following question.

Maria was unable to complete her 10-mile hike, _____ she had trained for several months.

2. Which of the following transition words or phrases best completes the sentence?

   A. although

   B. in other words

   C. accordingly

   D. meanwhile

Read the sample and answer the following question.

Maria loved to travel, and no advice about safety is going to keep her from taking a trek across Alaska.

3. Which of the following grammar errors appears in the sentence?

   A. Inappropriate transition word choice

   B. Tense disagreement

   C. Poor diction

   D. Ambiguous word choice

Read the sample and answer the following question.

Navigating the vast wilderness of Denali National Park in Alaska requires that hikers have equipment that can determine their location and other things.

4. Which of the following words in the above sentence is an example of ambiguous language?

   A. navigating

   B. requires

   C. hikers

   D. things

5. Practice analyzing diction by reading a passage from your favorite book or a magazine article that appeals to you. Evaluate the author's word choice as you read. Choose a sentence that uses precise diction, and write the sentence below. Explain how two of the words in the sentence enhance the clarity of the sentence.

---

subject-verb agreement. Matching like numbers of subjects and verbs: singular with singular, plural with plural.

pronoun-antecedent agreement. Matching like numbers of pronouns and their antecedents: singular with singular, plural with plural.

E.2.2 — Evaluate if language meets the needs of an audience for a provided rhetorical context

Experienced writers choose language that suits their purpose for writing and their intended audience. The purpose and intended audience are two elements of the rhetorical context for a particular writing task. Other elements include the setting or occasion for writing, the **genre** (referring to texts that share common characteristics), and the topic. For example, research papers written for academics require formal language. Text messages written for family and friends typically contain **informal** language such as **slang** (words and phrases shared only among a specific group of people) and **colloquialisms** (everyday or ordinary language). In this TEAS task, you will evaluate language and match it to the correct purpose and audience.

IDENTIFYING A NARRATOR'S SETTING OR SCENARIO

One task on the TEAS is to identify an occasion or setting for writing, or the genre or type of publication, by analyzing the language used. In order to evaluate the language in a passage and determine the appropriate scenario or context, look for keywords and phrases that can help you identify the purpose or the intended audience. When you are reading these passages, ask yourself the following questions.

- Is the author using language or conventions that seem specific to a certain genre or type of writing?

- What is the author's purpose for writing?

- What is the setting or occasion for writing?

- Who is the intended audience?

- What is the author's style? Does the author address the audience in a formal way, or does the author use informal language?

- What is the author's tone or attitude toward the topic? Is the language serious and neutral, or does the author use humor, satire (mocking hypotheticals), or sarcasm (verbal irony)?

- What is the author's **register** or degree of formality? Does the author use informal slang and colloquialisms? Does the author use technical **jargon** and abbreviations, indicating that the author is writing to professional and workplace colleagues?

Objectives

This objective includes, but is not limited to, the following examples of knowledge, skills, and abilities.

- Identify the narrator's setting/situation from given information.

- Revise language for style (e.g., formal, informal) to fit a scenario.

- Revise language for tone (e.g., satiric, ironic, humorous) to fit a scenario given several short passages.

- Revise language for register (e.g., informal slang, colloquialisms, jargon, formal language for the workplace or used among professionals) to fit a scenario given several short passages.

- Revise language to meet the needs of culturally-diverse audiences.

---

genre. A group of related writings or other media.

informal. A style that is relaxed and unofficial.

slang. Informal language usually tied to a specific group of people.

colloquialism. An informal word or phrase.

register. Degree of formality in a text.

jargon. Words used in a specific profession or discipline.

REVISING LANGUAGE FOR STYLE, TONE, AND REGISTER FORMAL LANGUAGE

Certain genres of writing—research papers, business communications, journalism, scientific and medical writing, and other academic writing—have conventions that go beyond simple grammar. The style of these genres is generally formal. Writers use sentence structures, words, and phrases that meet the expectations of their audience. Formal writing often has longer sentences, uses the third-person point of view, and uses a neutral tone and vocabulary in an appropriate register, or degree of formality.

Tone in formal writing is generally serious and neutral. It is usually not ironic, satirical, or humorous. For instance, a scientific paper should use neutral language and tone in reporting data because an objective approach is expected. Most business communications, journalism, and other academic writing are similarly neutral and serious.

The register of the language can vary. In business and professional communications, acronyms and jargon (CEO, B2B) are often used without explanation because the audience knows and understands certain terms. Journalistic reporting is expected to address the "who, what, why, when, and where" of a news story efficiently. While these conventions can change over time, you can identify the style, tone, and register that will help you identify the intended audience for a given piece of writing. Formal genres you will be asked to identify include business letters, speeches, textbook articles, science reports, news stories, and essays.

INFORMAL LANGUAGE

Informal writing has specific conventions, too. It is often closer to speech, typically featuring shorter sentences, the use of the first-person "I" or **second-person** "you," and more variety in tone and vocabulary.

A text message is a good example of informal written language. You would not expect a text message from a friend to open with a formal salutation such as "Dear Emily," but depending on the friend, you might expect the text to have an informal tone and include irony, sarcasm, or humor. You would also expect the register to be informal and include slang and colloquialisms, such as "Hey" and "Let's link up." Slang and colloquialisms can make a piece of writing feel more conversational and intimate. They can also help create a mood or atmosphere that captures a time and place, and provide otherwise unstated information about the time and place in which the communication originated. Consider the following examples.

Decade	Slang	Meaning
1920s	all wet	incorrect or ineffective
	bee's knees	extraordinary person, place, or thing
	a bucket	a car
1960s	cool	hip or very good
	bug out	to leave
	a gas	a good time
2000s	bling	something fancy
	bounce	leave
	throw shade	publicly criticize

second person. A narrative mode that addresses the reader as "you."

Literary works and narratives, such as novels and short fiction, often use informal language to create a feeling of realism.

REVISING INFORMAL AND FORMAL LANGUAGE

You will be asked to recognize formal and informal language on the TEAS and to identify an appropriate style, tone, and register for a particular situation. Consider these examples. Which version is appropriate for a college paper?

Original

> *Give little kiddos a snack after school or they'll get hangry.*

Revision

> *School-aged children need snacks after school because they are often hungry and tired.*

Both sentences are grammatically correct; however, the original is an informal sentence that uses colloquial language, slang, and humor. It would likely be used in speech. The revision is a formal sentence and is appropriate for a college paper about young children.

Here are two more examples.

Original

> *Hey professor! I was absent yesterday. Did I miss anything?*

Revision

> *Dear Professor: I was absent from class yesterday. I checked the syllabus and saw that I missed peer review. Is there a way I can make it up?*

Both messages to the professor are grammatically correct; however, the original is written in an informal style and uses an informal tone. The revision is appropriately formal for communicating with an instructor.

REVISING LANGUAGE FOR CULTURALLY DIVERSE AUDIENCES

Biased language excludes or demeans people based on gender, sex, sexual orientation, age, ethnicity, social class, or other physical or mental traits. Biased language also reinforces negative stereotypes about groups of people.

Some words that were once considered neutral are now considered gender-biased, such as "mankind," "businessman," and "policeman." Increasingly, these words are being replaced by gender-neutral terms such as "humanity," "businessperson," and "police officer." Consider these examples:

Gender-biased

Man-made fibers have improved fabrics for clothing.

Revised

Synthetic fibers have improved fabrics for clothing.

In addition, the pronouns "he," "his," and "him" were traditionally used as the gender-neutral pronouns in English. They are now much less common. Consider these examples:

Gender-biased

A dentist should explain procedures to his patients.

Revised

Dentists should explain procedures to their patients.

Finally, be aware of labels and stereotypes that can insult members of the intended audience. Use labels that put people first: "a person who has cancer" instead of "cancer victim"; "a person who uses a wheelchair" instead of "wheelchair-bound." Revise language that reinforces potentially harmful stereotypes about entire groups of people, such as teenagers, elderly people, girls, boys, same-sex couples, and so on.

Practice Problems

Read the sample and answer the following question.

Our organization's vertical synergy positions us to produce a quality proposal by EOD.

1. Which of the following publications would most likely contain this sentence?

    A. Business memo

    B. Scientific journal

    C. Literary work

    D. Motivational speech

2. Which of the following sentences contains informal language?

    A. Many people are unaware of the variety of ways they can enhance the privacy settings on their mobile devices.

    B. A recent study found that using a passcode is more secure than using a swipe pattern to unlock a mobile phone.

    C. Security experts advise users to write down their serial numbers in case their phones are ever lost or stolen.

    D. Having a blinged-out phone case can make your phone a target for theft, so stick with something plain.

3. Which of the following sentences would indicate that the setting is the United States in the 1920s?

    A. Many people were able to endure the Blitz by the Germans during World War II.

    B. The film critics praised the new actor as the bee's knees, but the film itself was all wet.

    C. You could feel the tension in the air as the gunslinger entered the room to confront his enemies.

    D. She was a cool cat who had a new hit that she was about to introduce at a gig in Chicago.

Read the sample and answer the following question.

Communication skills are important to success in any profession, but effective communication takes practice. First, decide upon the key message you want to convey in clear, straightforward language. Engage your listener by asking questions and soliciting feedback. Then, take time to listen carefully and respond to your listener's ideas. The best communicators are the best listeners. If you have not been understood, think of ways to put your ideas in other words, or use examples to make your thoughts more clear to others.

4. Which of the following sentences uses language that fits the style of the passage?

    A. In addition, maintain eye contact to build credibility and show your listener that you care.

    B. Speakers who bounce from topic to topic can make their listeners feel like they have whiplash.

    C. Talking with your homeskillet will be boss if you cool your jets and really focus on your listener.

    D. Speakers who maintain eye contact with listeners have higher rates of success in communicating their message.

5. Perform an internet search for examples of each of the following and make a list of three conventions or rules for each genre or type of writing.

    A. Business letter

    B. News article

    C. Essay

E.2.3 — Develop a well-organized paragraph

KNOWLEDGE OF LANGUAGE

A sentence expresses a complete thought or idea. A paragraph organizes related sentences into a coherent message on a particular topic. In this TEAS task, you will identify the conventions of paragraph development, including the use of *topic sentences*, *supporting details*, transitions, and conclusions. You will also analyze paragraphs to identify where revision is required, where extraneous or irrelevant information is introduced, and where more information may be needed.

PARTS OF A PARAGRAPH

A paragraph focuses on and explores one main idea. A paragraph can be as short as a single sentence, but most ideas require more explanation. First, the topic sentence introduces the main idea. Subsequent sentences provide supporting details, or information that expands on the main idea introduced in the topic sentence. Supporting details provide facts, descriptions, definitions, or other information to support the main idea. A paragraph ends with a conclusion, which sums up the main idea. Just as transitions (such as conjunctions) are used to show how ideas within a sentence are related, so, too, are transitions used to show the relationship between sentences within a paragraph.

Consider how the following example uses a clear paragraph structure to explain one way to improve your phone photography.

Topic sentence	To improve the quality of photographs taken with your phone, you can learn to use the gridlines setting for better balance and contrast.
Supporting details	When you switch to "grid on" in your settings, the lines of a grid will appear in your viewfinder. There will be nine boxes. According to a photographic theory, you should place the focal points of your image in the intersections or along the grid lines. Seeing the grid will help you decide how to balance the images in the photographs that you take. The lines will also help you keep the images level.
Conclusion	By using this tool, your phone photographs will become more visually interesting, especially if you also use a few strategies for lighting.

Notice in this example how transitions are used to show the connection between ideas. The word "also" in the last sentence of the supporting details section shows that this idea is a continuation or additional example. The phrase "By using this tool" in the conclusion links back to the main idea of the paragraph: using the gridlines.

> ### Objectives
>
> This objective includes, but is not limited to, the following examples of knowledge, skills, and abilities.
>
> - Use the parts of a paragraph to convey meaning, including topic sentence, supporting details, transitions, and conclusion.
>
> - Arrange information in an order (e.g., chronological, cause/effect) best suited to the purpose of the paragraph.
>
> - Identify information that is relevant and irrelevant.
>
> - Identify where more information/development is needed.

---

topic sentence. The sentence that summarizes the main idea of a text or paragraph.

supporting detail. Information that supports the main idea by answering who, what, where, when, or why.

LOGICAL ORDER IN PARAGRAPHS

Search online for "text structures," and you will find that there are many ways to organize sentences within a paragraph. The key to an effective paragraph is to present information in a logical way. Paragraphs are often organized in chronological order, which presents events according to the order in which they happen. Sequential order, a type of chronological order, shows events that happen one after another in a fixed pattern, as in the previous example. This structure is an appropriate choice for a text that describes a procedure, such as how to use a certain function on a camera, one step at a time.

Consider the intent of your paragraph to find the most logical organization. If you are exploring cause–and–effect relationships, for instance, you might want to begin with an event and then discuss how this event causes other things to happen. Other common ways to organize a paragraph are by introducing a problem and then discussing solutions and presenting ideas in the order of importance. For this TEAS task, you will be asked to discern the sequence of information in a paragraph by putting it in a logical order.

IDENTIFYING UNNECESSARY AND OMITTED INFORMATION

Supporting details are essential building blocks of a paragraph, but not all details are equal. Details that do not support the main idea of a paragraph—even if they are interesting—should sometimes be omitted. Ask yourself, "Does this sentence support the main idea?" If the answer is "no," delete it or move it to a paragraph where it fits better.

Some paragraphs suffer from the opposite problem: important information is missing. Sometimes it is a transition that is missing—a word, phrase, or sentence that helps the reader make the connection to the main idea. Other times, there are too few supporting details, so that the paragraph seems to jump from one main idea to another. Sometimes, it can be a concluding sentence that is missing, so that readers do not have a clear understanding of the point. If the paragraph causes you to think, "What is the point?" it is probably in need of additional information.

Practice Problems

1. Which of the following are key parts of a paragraph? (Select all that apply.)

   A. Sources

   B. Topic sentence

   C. Supporting details

   D. Introductory phrase

   E. Opposition

2. Which of the following examples would most likely act as a transition sentence?

   A. When you tap on the screen to refocus, a sun icon appears.

   B. Manually tapping on the subject of your photo adjusts the focus of the camera and also adjusts the exposure.

   C. Another phone camera feature that can improve your photography is manually setting exposure times.

   D. If you make the sun icon brighter, this will increase the light exposure of the photo.

3. Reorder the sentences below into the best chronological sequence to construct a paragraph.

   1. By the time I returned home from vacation, I was starting to get excited about the new courses I would be taking.

   2. I headed to my final exam with a mixture of fear and confidence. I could not wait for the exam to be over so I could take a break from my studies.

   3. The exam was difficult, but by keeping to my study schedule, I was well prepared.

   4. As soon as I completed my exam, our family headed to my grandmother's home for the holiday.

Read the sample and answer the following question.

You might also want to improve your phone photography by setting the focus on your phone camera. Most people do not realize that the automatic focus setting of most phone cameras is on the foreground of the image in the view-finder. Most people do not bother to read the instruction manual of their phone. This can be a problem if the subject of your photograph is centered or in the background. It is also a problem if there is not a single subject for a photograph. Luckily, you can change the focus feature on your phone camera easily. Open your camera application and simply tap on the screen where you want to sharpen the view. A square icon will appear on your screen. The focus of your photo will be the image inside the icon.

4. Which of the following sentences contains information that does not belong in the paragraph?

   A. You might also want to improve your phone photography by setting the focus on your phone camera.

   B. Open your camera application, and simply tap on the screen where you want to sharpen the view.

   C. Most people do not bother to read the instruction manual of their phone.

   D. It is also a problem if there is not a single subject for a photograph.

5. Write a paragraph about an experience you had with photography. Use the following table to organize your ideas.

Topic sentence	
Supporting details	
Conclusion	

Vocabulary Acquisition

E.3.1 — Apply basic knowledge of the elements of the writing process to communicate effectively

Writing is a process that involves several steps, including **drafting** and revision. Sometimes these steps move quickly, but sometimes they can prove to be challenging. Thankfully, there are plenty of tools and resources available to assist writers in the process. Given a writing task, what steps do writers take? How do they determine their ideas? How do they organize information? This TEAS task will require you to be familiar with the writing process and the strategies that writers use during that process.

Objectives

This objective includes, but is not limited to, the following examples of knowledge, skills, and abilities.

- Identify steps necessary to complete a writing task.
- Identify when citation is needed.

STEPS IN THE WRITING PROCESS

There might be nearly as many writing processes as there are writers, but in its basic form, the process consists of five steps: prewriting, writing, conferencing, revision, and editing. These steps are not necessarily distinct and often overlap, and each writer will approach them in their own way. However, there are elements of each step about which you should be knowledgeable.

Prewriting

Prewriting includes all the tasks that a writer must complete before starting to draft. Prewriting tasks include understanding the purpose for writing, finding a topic, generating ideas, gathering information from sources, crafting a tentative thesis statement, and making an organization plan. Writers use a variety of techniques during prewriting. For example, some writers use **brainstorming** techniques such as **stream-of-consciousness writing** or **mind mapping** to generate ideas about possible topics.

---

draft. An unfinished version of a text.

brainstorming. Discussing as a group to create an idea or solve a problem.

stream-of-consciousness writing. A narrative device that mimics interior monologue.

mind mapping. Visually diagramming ideas around a central concept.

Writers can also use tree diagrams or outlines to organize their ideas, such as the following partial outline for a paper on effective time management:

II. *Using a Monthly Schedule*

   A. *Visualizing the month as a whole*

   B. *Mapping important deadlines and appointments*

   C. *Setting time to accomplish tasks to meet deadlines*

III. *Establishing Priorities*

   A. *Determining which tasks are urgent*

   B. *Estimating the time needed for each task*

   C. *Determining the resources needed for each task*

Some writing assignments require informal or formal research. For example, the informal research for a personal essay might consist of talking to a friend or family member to recall the details of a memory or experience. A research paper usually requires the writer to consult primary and/or secondary sources that the writer will need to cite within the finished paper.

Writing

During the writing step of the writing process, often called drafting, the writer drafts the paragraphs of the piece of writing (the introduction, body paragraphs, and conclusion). Each paragraph has a main point and is developed with examples, details, and information. Any information borrowed from research sources is cited in the text of the paper, and the sources are listed in a bibliography at the end of the paper.

Conferencing, Revising, and Editing

When you have a finished draft, it is time for feedback. This feedback, from peers or writing tutors, will help you gauge how well your intention matches your execution and give you ideas about elements that you might change to improve the draft. Revising and editing are also important steps in the writing process. Writers differ in how they draft and revise. Revision involves large-scale changes, while editing focuses more on sentence-level changes. Large-scale changes include revising the thesis statement, rewriting and rearranging paragraphs, and adding evidence to support main points and transitional sentences to connect ideas. Sentence-level editing includes careful review of word choice, grammar, punctuation, capital letters, and spelling, followed by proofreading.

NEEDED CITATIONS

Any material borrowed from research sources and used in a piece of writing must be **cited** in the text of the paper, and the sources must be listed in a bibliography at the end of the paper. Borrowed material includes quotations, visuals, and other media taken directly from a source, as well as ideas, data, and information that the writer has paraphrased or summarized. There are different documentation styles used to cite sources, including the guidelines of the Modern Language Association (MLA) and the American Psychological Association (APA). In this TEAS task, you will need to identify when a citation is needed.

---

citation. A strictly formatted line of text that provides a source reference.

Practice Problems

1. Which of the following is an example of prewriting?

   A. Citing sources

   B. Brainstorming

   C. Proofreading

   D. Editing

2. If all the following tasks are used in writing, which of the following would likely occur last?

   A. Researching potential sources

   B. Mapping possible topics and subtopics

   C. Developing an organizational outline

   D. Editing and proofreading

3. Malik is writing a research paper on a national park near his home. He has consulted several reliable sources, created an outline to plan his paper, written a rough draft, and revised his draft. Which of the followings elements of the writing process does Malik need to add?

   A. Citing sources

   B. Finding a topic

   C. Developing a writing plan

   D. Brainstorming

4. Which of the following situations requires a source citation?

   A. The author is stating their own ideas.

   B. The author thinks that the ideas described are important.

   C. The author is describing the setting of a story.

   D. The author is quoting another writer's words.

5. Locate an article about how to revise writing. Organize the ideas in the article into an outline with one to three main points. Then write subordinate ideas below each main point. Consider using these ideas when you are revising your next piece of writing.

E.3.2 — Determine the meaning of words by analyzing word parts

The English language can be a lot like social networking: knowing one word (or person) easily leads you to countless others. That connection is especially evident when you familiarize yourself with the common **affixes**, bases, and **roots** that are used to build English words. Adding an affix to a base or root word forms a new word with a new meaning. A "root" is the primary form of a word, while a "base" can stand alone with its own meaning. Words that are **derived** from the same root words are called "cognates." Affixes consist of **prefixes**, which are added to the beginning of base or root words, and **suffixes**, which are added to the end.

Many English words come from Greek and Latin roots. Knowing common roots and affixes can help you determine the meanings of unfamiliar words. For this TEAS task, you will use your knowledge of word parts to determine the meanings of words.

PREFIXES

The meanings of many prefixes will be familiar. For instance, the prefix re– means "again." Adding re– to the base word do creates "redo," meaning "to do again." The prefix un– means "not." Adding the prefix un– to the base word happy creates "unhappy," which means "not happy." Prefixes do not change a word's part of speech. If a prefix is added to a verb, the new word will also be a verb. "Do" and "redo" are both verbs; "happy" and "unhappy" are both adjectives.

Some common prefixes are shown in the following chart.

Prefix	Meaning	Example	Example Meaning
anti-	against	anti-apartheid	against separation of groups
dis-	apart; having a reversing influence	discredit	to harm someone's good reputation
dys-	bad; difficult	dysfunction	failure to function or work properly
hyper-	over; in excess	hyperactive	overly active
hypo-	under; too little	hypotension	less tension than normal
inter-	between	interstellar	between the stars
intra-	within or through	intravenous	within or through the veins
mid-	indicating a middle part, point, time, or position	Midwestern	in the middle of an area considered west

affix. Letters placed at the beginning or end of a word or word part to modify its meaning.

root. A word part to which an affix can be attached.

derivation. Determining the origin of a word.

prefix. An affix that appears at the beginning of a word.

suffix. An affix that appears at the end of a word.

Prefix	Meaning	Example	Example Meaning
mis-	badly; wrongly; incorrectly	misinterpret	to interpret incorrectly
non-	not	nonfiction	a text that is not fiction
out-	greater; longer; better	outperform	to perform better than someone else
over-	too much; above	oversleep	to sleep too much
		overhang	to hang over or extend outward
pre-	before	preorder	to place an order before something
sub-	less than; under	subset	part of a whole
super-	more than; above	superhuman	greater than the usual capacity of humans

SUFFIXES

Suffixes, which are added to the ends of words, come in two forms: **inflectional** and **derivational**. Inflectional suffixes do not change the essential meaning of a word. Instead, they express different aspects of a word, such as tense or number. A plural is often formed by adding –s or –es, for example. Adding –ed to a present–tense verb makes it past tense; adding –ing creates the verb used for the progressive aspect of a tense, as in the sentence "We are going." As another example, adding the suffixes –er or –est to a base word creates the comparative and superlative versions, which reveal the differences between the items these words describe, as in "faster" and "fastest" or "brighter" and "brightest." The base word happy becomes "happier" or "happiest."

You will also want to be familiar with derivational suffixes, or those that form new words with new meanings when added to a base or root word. These suffixes often change the part of speech. The following chart contains suffixes often seen on the TEAS exam.

Suffix	Meaning	Example	Example Meaning
-ate	to cause to be	pollen, n. → pollinate, v.	to cause to be fertilized
-ful	having the characteristic of	regret, n. → regretful, adj.	having the feeling of regret
-ic	having the characteristic or form of	melody, n. → melodic, adj.	having a pleasing sound or melody
-ize	to cause or show to be	character, n. → characterize, v.	to show the features of something
-ness	having the quality or being in the state of	kind, adj. → kindness, n.	having the quality of being kind
-ology	the study of	Greek root **anthropo**, meaning "man" → anthropology, n.	the study of human beings
-ous	having the characteristic of	pore, n. → porous, adj.	having spaces or pores within a substance
-tion, -ation	the act of	demonstrate, v. → demonstration, n.	the act of demonstrating something

inflectional suffix. A suffix that does not change the essential meaning of a word when added to it.

derivational suffix. A suffix that forms a new word with a new meaning when added.

DETERMINING WORD MEANING

If you come across an unfamiliar word, break it apart into its base or root and affixes. Think about the meanings of any affixes. You might not know the exact meaning of a given word, but if you note the prefix anti-, you can decipher that it is against whatever the base or root is. So, an anti-inflammatory drug is one that is against inflammation. Knowing that the prefix dys- means "bad" or "difficult" can help you know that the meaning of "dystrophy" is "a disorder in which tissues and organs perform poorly or waste away." Suffixes can also be used to discern word meanings. The suffix -ous means that something has the characteristic of whatever the base or root word is. So, something that is advantageous has advantages. The suffix -ful means "full of," so someone who is spiteful is full of spite.

Sometimes a base or root word will have more than one affix.

The word "unconsciousness" breaks into several parts:

> *unconsciousness = un- (not) + conscious + -ness (state of)*

The base word conscious comes from the Latin root meaning "knowing" or "aware," so "unconsciousness" means "the state of not being aware."

Another example is the word "mistrustful." A person who is trustful is full of trust; a person who is mistrustful is full of mistrust, or the lack of trust.

COMBINING AFFIXES WITH ROOT WORDS

Just as you can determine word meaning by breaking a word into its base or root and its affixes, so too can you use your knowledge of affixes to build words. You cannot add any affix to any base or root to create a new word, but understanding how to use affixes can help you enhance your vocabulary. Instead of saying that someone does something in a way that they are unaware of, for instance, you can say that they do something unconsciously. Or instead of saying that someone does not trust you, you can say that they are distrustful.

These are just a few of the many affixes and base or root words that are used to build English words. Becoming familiar with a range of affixes and roots—particularly those used commonly in medical settings—should help you succeed on this TEAS task.

Practice Problems

1. In which of the following options does the suffix create a word that is a different part of speech from the base word? (Select all that apply.)

   A. Goodness

   B. Demonstrated

   C. Shinier

   D. Writes

   E. Lifelike

2. Based on an examination of the word parts, which of the following means "to breathe too quickly or too much"?

   A. Hypoventilate

   B. Hyperventilate

   C. Superventilate

   D. Interventilate

3. Based on an examination of the word parts, which of the following means "to stop doing something"?

   A. Continuation

   B. Continuous

   C. Discontinue

   D. Anticontinue

4. Using your knowledge of word parts, which of the following means "the act of judging beforehand"?

   A. Judged

   B. Judicious

   C. Postjudgment

   D. Prejudgment

5. Perform an internet search for "medical roots, prefixes, and suffixes" and choose a reliable website that ends in ".edu" or a dictionary website. Choose five medical roots that are unfamiliar to you. Write each root, its meaning, and an example of its use.

English Key Terms

adjective. Word or phrase that describes or modifies a noun.

adverb. Word or phrase that describes or modifies an adjective, verb, or other adverb.

affix. Letters placed at the beginning or end of a word or word part to modify its meaning.

apostrophe. Punctuation mark that denotes possessive case or omission of letters. article. Word ("a," "an," or "the") that refers to a noun.

brainstorming. Discussing as a group to create an idea or solve a problem.

citation. A strictly formatted line of text that provides a source reference.

colloquialism. An informal word or phrase.

comma. Punctuation mark used to separate parts of sentences.

complement. Sentence part that gives more information about a subject or object.

complex sentence. Sentence that contains an independent clause and a dependent clause.

compound sentence. Sentence that contains at least two independent clauses.

conjunction. A connecting word.

context. Surrounding words or ideas within a sentence or passage that affect the meaning of a word and influence how it is understood.

coordinate adjectives. Two equally weighted adjectives that describe the same noun and require a comma between them.

dependent clause. A group of words that includes a subject and verb but cannot stand alone as a complete sentence because it does not express a complete thought.

derivation. Determining the origin of a word.

derivational suffix. A suffix that forms a new word with a new meaning when added.

diction. The style of writing determined by word choice.

draft. An unfinished version of a text.

end marks. Punctuation marks that end sentences: period, question mark, and exclamation mark.

exclamation mark. End mark that denotes strong feeling.

formal. A style that follows conventional rules.

fragment. An incomplete sentence.

genre. A group of related writings or other media.

homographs. Words that are spelled the same, such as "bass" (a fish) and "bass" (a musical instrument), but have different meanings and may be pronounced differently.

homophones. Words that sound the same, such as "new" and "knew," but have different meanings.

imperative sentence. A complete sentence that conveys a command, instruction, or request and has the implied or understood subject "you."

independent clause. A group of words that includes a subject and predicate and can stand alone as a complete sentence because it expresses a complete thought.

indirect object. The person or thing to whom or which something is done.

inflection. How a word is spoken to modify its tone or meaning.

inflectional suffix. A suffix that does not change the essential meaning of a word when added to it.

informal. A style that is relaxed and unofficial.

interjection. A word or phrase that represents a short burst of emotion.

jargon. Words used in a specific profession or discipline.

mind mapping. Visually diagramming ideas around a central concept.

modifier. A word or group of words that provides description for another word.

mood. How the elements in a text, such as word choice, make the reader feel.

noun. A person, place, thing, or idea.

object/direct object. A word or group of words that receives the action of a verb.

Oxford comma. The comma before the "and" in a simple series of items.

parts of speech. Eight categories for classifying words: adjective, adverb, conjunction, interjection, noun, preposition, pronoun, and verb.

perfective. A verb tense indicating that the action described has been completed.

period. End mark that denotes the end of a standard sentence.

phrase. A group of words that work together as a unit.

plural. More than one item.

predicate. The part of a sentence that explains what the subject does or is like.

prefix. An affix that appears at the beginning of a word.

preposition. A word that describes relationships between other words.

progressive. A verb tense indicating that the action described is currently happening.

pronoun. A word that takes the place of a noun.

pronoun-antecedent agreement. Matching like numbers of pronouns and their antecedents: singular with singular, plural with plural.

quotation marks. Punctuation marks that denote spoken or other quoted text.

register. Degree of formality in a text.

root. A word part to which an affix can be attached.

run-on sentence. A sentence with extra parts that are not joined properly by the correct conjunction or punctuation.

second person. A narrative mode that addresses the reader as "you."

simple sentence. Sentence that contains only one idea or independent clause and uses only an end mark.

slang. Informal language usually tied to a specific group of people.

stream-of-consciousness writing. A narrative device that mimics interior monologue.

subject. The main noun of a sentence that is doing or being.

subject-verb agreement. Matching like numbers of subjects and verbs: singular with singular, plural with plural.

suffix. An affix that appears at the end of a word.

supporting detail. Information that supports the main idea by answering who, what, where, when, or why.

synonyms. Words with identical or similar meanings.

tense. Refers to when an action occurs: past, present, or future.

tone. An author's implied or explicit attitude toward a topic.

topic sentence. The sentence that summarizes the main idea of a text or paragraph.

transition words. Words that link or introduce ideas.

verb. A word that describes an action or state of being.

Practice Problems Answer Key

E.1.1

1. Option B is correct. "It's" is a contraction for "it is." The form should be the possessive "its," which means "belonging to it." "Its heat" means that the heat belongs to it (the desert).

   - "Desert" and "dessert" are homophones when "desert" is used as a verb meaning "to abandon." "Desert" is used correctly in the sentence, meaning "a hot, arid region."

   - "Seemed" is used correctly in the sentence, meaning "appeared."

   - The word "their" means "belonging to them." This is correct in this sentence because "their progress" means the progress belongs to them (the explorers).

2. Option D is correct. The spelling of "tryed" should be "tried" to follow the "change the final 'y' to 'i'" rule.

   - A. "Desert" is spelled correctly in the sentence. It uses the correct homophone for "desert," meaning "a hot, arid region."

   - "Thirstier" is spelled correctly in the sentence. "Thirstier" follows the "change the final 'y' to 'i'" rule: "thirsty" becomes "thirstier" when adding the suffix "–er."

   - "Their" is used correctly in the sentence. "Their," as it is used in the sentence, refers to the "way" that belongs to them— "their way."

3. Options C and E are correct.

   - "Codeine" is spelled correctly and is an exception to the "'i' before 'e'" rule.

   - "Changeable" is spelled correctly and is an exception to the "drop the final 'e'" rule.

   - "Receive" uses the rule "'i' before 'e' except after 'c.'"

   - "Believe" uses the rule "'i' before 'e.'"

   - "Fierce" uses the rule "'i' before 'e.'"

4. Option C is correct. "Referring" is spelled correctly according to the "double the consonant" rule.

   - Option A should be spelled "bleeding." This is an exception to the rule.

   - Option B should be spelled "vomited." This is an exception to the rule.

   - Option D should be spelled "plowed." This is an exception to the rule.

5. Answers will vary. Spelling rules that could be listed include:

   - Double the consonants "f," "l," and "s" at the end of one-syllable words that have just one vowel. Example: "spell."

   - Add "–es" to words ending in "–s," "–ss," "–z," "–ch," "–sh," and "–x" to make them plural. Example: "bus"/"buses"

   - Most words ending in "–f" or "–fe" change their plurals to "–ves." Example: "calf"/"–calves."

E.1.2

1. Options A and D are correct. These sentences have two independent clauses and are correctly punctuated by including a comma before the conjunction.

   - Option B has two independent clauses, so a comma should be used before the conjunction that separates the clauses.

   - Option C is not a compound sentence because there is only one subject ("I"). The comma before the "and" should not be included.

2. Option B is correct. This quotation is correctly punctuated by including a comma before the end quotation mark that leads to non-quotation text and another comma before beginning the quotation again.

   - The period in the non-quotation portion of this text divides the quotation into two fragments.

   - There should be no period before a quotation mark that is followed by additional text.

   - The first word after a quotation ("she") should not be capitalized. It does not start a new sentence.

3. Option B is correct. A comma is required after an introductory dependent clause in a complex sentence.

   - Option A is missing a comma after the introductory dependent clause.

   - Option C has misplaced the comma. It should come after the word "running."

   - Option D has misplaced the comma. It should come after the word "running."

4. Option A is correct. This sentence has a comma after an introductory phrase ending in "runner." It also has two commas to separate the items "shoes" and "socks" in a series. The comma before the "and" in the series is a preference that is correct.

- Option B is missing a comma after an introductory phrase ending in "runner."
- Option C is missing a comma after the item "shoes" to separate it from the item "socks" in a series.
- Option D is missing a comma after an introductory phrase ending in "runner" and after the item "shoes" in a series.

5. Option B is correct. The words "dark" and "ominous" are coordinate adjectives—that is, they are equal and can be used in any order—so the first adjective, "dark," needs a comma after it.

- Option A is missing a comma between the two adjectives describing "clouds."
- Option C has an extraneous comma between the second adjective and noun "clouds."
- Option D has an extraneous comma after "several," which is a noncoordinate adjective.

E.1.3

1. Option C is correct. This is a compound-complex sentence that includes two independent clauses and one dependent clause.

- Option A a compound sentence. There are two independent clauses but no dependent clause, so it is not complex.
- Option B is a complex sentence. It contains one independent clause and one dependent clause.
- Option D is a simple sentence with a compound verb.

2. Option A is correct. The simple subject is "building."

- The word "gives" is the simple predicate.
- The word "students" is the indirect object.
- The word "spaces" is the direct object.

3. Options B and D are correct. Each of these clauses begins with subordinating words and does not express a complete thought.

- Option A is an independent clause and therefore a complete sentence. The subject is "swimming," and the verb is "is."
- Option C is an independent clause and therefore a complete sentence. The subject is "there," and the verb is "are."
- Option E is a complex sentence. It contains the dependent clause "Although learning to swim is time-consuming" and the independent clause "everyone should learn to do it."

4. The following is the correct diagram of the sentence: The parents served their children fresh vegetables.

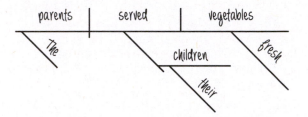

The subject "parents," verb "served," and object "vegetables" are on the straight line, separated by vertical lines. "The" modifies "parents." The indirect object is "children." "Their" modifies "children." "Fresh" modifies "vegetables."

5. Answers will vary, but sentences must contain a dependent clause and an independent clause. Example: Although I love to swim outdoors, I sometimes swim at an indoor pool.

E.2.1

1. Option B is correct. "According to many experts in Alaska" is a sentence fragment because there is no subject or verb. This group of words is an introductory phrase.

   - "Let's hike to a glacier!" is a complete sentence. It expresses a complete thought and has the implied or understood subject "we" and the verb "hike."
   - "Hiking is a great activity for your health" is a complete sentence. It expresses a complete thought and has the subject "hiking" and the predicate verb "is."
   - "Maria loves to hike and enjoys going to new places" is a complete sentence. It expresses a complete thought and has the subject "Maria" and the predicate "loves to hike and enjoys going to new places."

2. Option A is correct. The transition word "although" indicates that Maria failed despite training. This is an appropriate choice to indicate that the second idea is opposed to the first idea.

   - "In other words" is incorrect because the idea is not repeated.
   - "Accordingly" is incorrect because it indicates an effect.
   - "Meanwhile" is incorrect because it indicates events happening at the same time. The training occurred before the failure.

3. Option B is correct. The first verb is in the past tense, while the verb for the second independent clause is in the present tense. Tenses must agree.

   - Using "and" as a transition is an appropriate choice to demonstrate agreement between the ideas of loving to travel and being unable to keep her from taking a trip.
   - Poor diction is incorrect. The words selected for use in this sentence fit the context and convey a clear message.
   - Ambiguous word choice is incorrect. The words selected for use in this sentence fit the context and convey a clear message.

4. Option D is correct. The word "things" does not make clear to the reader what other equipment is needed.

   - The word "navigating" clearly describes finding a direction or location.
   - The word "requires" indicates that an item is necessary.
   - The word "hikers" describes a specific group of people.

5. Answers will vary. An example would be the following sentence and two precise terms explained.

   - Sentence: Maria decided to increase her chances of completing the hike next spring by practicing walking on ice with crampons and investing in a satellite phone.
   - Description of diction: The terms "crampons" and "satellite" are examples of precise diction that helps the reader visualize the steel equipment she will wear on her feet and the type of phone she will carry in the wilderness.

E.2.2

1. Option A is correct. This sentence contains jargon ("synergy," "EOD") that would be commonly understood within a business setting.

   - Option B does not contain scientific terms likely to be found in a scientific journal.
   - Option C would not likely be found in a novel unless that novel focused on a business setting.
   - Option D does not use persuasion to help people become motivated.

2. Option D is correct. This sentence contains the informal term "blinged-out."

   - Option A states a formal proposition that many people are unaware of ways they can enhance their privacy settings.
   - Option B describes the results of a study using formal language.
   - Option C provides formal advice.

3. Option is correct. The slang "bee's knees" and "all wet" indicates that the setting for this passage is the 1920s.

   - The references in option A are about World War II in Europe in the 1940s.
   - The reference to a gunslinger indicates that the setting for this was during the "Old West."
   - The slang from this option would be more appropriate for the 1960s or later.

4. Option A is correct. This sentence continues the informal second-person style of the passage.
   - Option B uses "bounce" and "whiplash" colloquially.
   - Option C uses the slang expressions "homeskillet," "boss," and "cool your jets."
   - Option D uses formal, third-person academic language.

5. Answers will vary. Possible conventions for each type of writing include the following examples.
   - Business letter: inside address, date, salutation, closing
   - News article: headline, byline, short sentences
   - Essay: introduction, thesis, body, conclusion

E.2.3

1. Options B and C are correct. A topic sentence is a key part of a paragraph because it reveals the subject of the entire paragraph. Supporting details provide facts, descriptions, definitions, or other information to support the main idea.
   - Not all paragraphs need a source.
   - Not all paragraphs need an introductory phrase.
   - Not all paragraphs need an opposition.

2. Option C is correct. The word "another" lets the reader know that the sentence is used to transition from one way of improving photography to a different way of improving photos.
   - Option A is describing an action, not transitioning to another idea.
   - Option B is providing a detail about the topic, not transitioning to a new topic.
   - Option D is describing a cause and effect, not transitioning to a new topic.

3. The correct order is II, III, IV, I. This chronological sequence is the most logical order for the paragraph. It starts with going to the exam, then taking the exam, then going on vacation after the exam, and, lastly, feeling ready to start new courses after the vacation.

4. Option C is correct. The paragraph is about setting the focus of a phone camera. The idea that most people do not bother to read the instruction manual of their phone is not about the focus of the camera.
   - Option A is the topic sentence of the paragraph.
   - Option B is an important detail about focusing your phone camera.
   - Option D is an important detail about focusing your phone camera.

5. Answers will vary. Sample chart/paragraph:

Topic sentence	I once owned a very expensive DSLR camera, but I have now replaced it with the camera on my new mobile phone.
Supporting details	The DSLR camera took wonderful photographs.
	I had several lenses for it, including a lens that allowed me to zoom in on objects in the distance and another that captured panoramic views.
	The camera on my new mobile phone also allows me to zoom in or take panoramic photos.
Conclusion	In my opinion, the mobile phone has replaced art with convenience.

"I once owned a very expensive DSLR camera, but I have now replaced it with the camera on my new mobile phone. The DSLR camera took wonderful photographs. I had several lenses for it, including a lens that allowed me to zoom in on objects in the distance and another that captured panoramic views. The camera on my new mobile phone also allows me to zoom in or take panoramic photos. In my opinion, the mobile phone has replaced art with convenience."

E.3.1

1. Option B is correct. Brainstorming is one way to come up with ideas before you write.
   - Citing sources occurs after a draft of a piece of writing is complete.
   - Proofreading occurs after a draft of a piece of writing is complete.
   - Editing occurs after a draft of a piece of writing is complete.

2. Option D is correct. Editing and proofreading would likely be the last step in a writing process because they occur after revision.
   - Research occurs during prewriting and during revision but before editing and proofreading.
   - Mapping possible topics and subtopics is part of prewriting.
   - Organization would occur during prewriting and sometimes during revision. This is before editing and proofreading.

3. Option A is correct. Malik needs to cite the sources he has used in his paper.

   - Finding a topic is a prewriting task. Malik has already written and revised a draft of his paper.
   - Developing a writing plan is a prewriting task.
   - Brainstorming is a prewriting task.

4. Option D is correct. Quoting a source, whether published or unpublished, requires inclusion of a citation.

   - Authors do not need to use citations for their own ideas.
   - The need for citation is not related to emphasis.
   - Fictional events do not require citation.

5. Answers will vary. Below is an example taken from an outline of a research paper on revision.

   Strategies for Revision

   I. Reading the Paper Out Loud

   a. Notice whether each paragraph has a clear main point.

   b. Decide whether each paragraph is developed with enough supporting information.

   c. Listen for grammatical errors.

   II. Peer Editing

   a. Ask a friend to read and comment on a draft.

   b. Talk over the strengths of the paper.

E.3.2

1. Options A and E are correct. The suffix "-ness" changes the base adjective "good" to a noun indicating the quality of being good. The suffix "-like" changes the base noun "life" to an adjective.

   - The suffix "-ed" does not change the part of speech. It changes the tense of the verb.
   - The suffix "-er" does not change the part of speech. It creates a comparative and superlative version of the adjective.
   - The suffix "-s" does not change the part of speech. It changes the tense of the verb.

2. Option B is correct. The prefix "hyper-" means "more than or too much."

   - The prefix "hypo-" means "less than or too little."
   - The prefix "super-" means "beyond."
   - The prefix "inter-" means "between."

3. Option C is correct. The prefix "dis-" means "not."

   - The suffix "-ation" means "the state of."
   - The suffix "-ous" means "to have the quality of."
   - The prefix "anti-" means "the opposite of."

4. Option D is correct. The prefix "pre-" means "before." The suffix "ment" means "the act of."

   - Option A is the past tense of "judge."
   - Option B means "the quality of making good decisions."
   - The prefix "post-" means "after."

5. Answers will vary. Examples of medical roots and their meanings include the following.

   - "Derma" means "skin." A dermatologist is a doctor of the skin.
   - "Kardia" means "heart." She suffered a cardiac arrest.
   - "Osteon" means "bone." My aunt is being treated for osteoarthritis.
   - "Pepsis" means "digestion." He is being treated for a peptic ulcer.
   - "Trauma" means "wound." The pair work in the trauma center at the emergency room.

English Unit Quiz

They're going to lead the group through the park because it's trails can be confusing.

1. Which of the following corrects a spelling error in the sentence?
   A. "They're" should be "Their."
   B. "Lead" should be "led."
   C. "Through" should be "threw."
   D. "It's" should be "its."

2. Which of the following words correctly follows the spelling rule to drop the final "e"?
   A. Excitment
   B. Movable
   C. Likness
   D. Tracable

3. Which of the following statements is correct?
   A. The plural of "self" is "selfs."
   B. The plural of "dash" is "dashs."
   C. The plural of "elf" is "elves."
   D. The plural of "church" is "churchs."

4. Which of the following is a complex sentence?
   A. We waited for more than 2 hours.
   B. Although the line was long, it moved rather quickly.
   C. The line was short for me, but it was much longer when I left.
   D. She looked for the shortest checkout line; she did not have much time to waste.

That street runs parallel to Main Street on the other side of the park.

5. Which of the following words in the sentence modifies the simple subject?
   A. That
   B. Parallel
   C. Main
   D. Other

6. Which of the following sentences uses correct punctuation?
   A. The ice skater trained by lifting weights doing box jumps, and stretching to increase flexibility.
   B. The ice skater trained by lifting, weights doing, box jumps and stretching to increase flexibility.
   C. The ice skater trained by lifting weights, doing box jumps, and stretching to increase flexibility.
   D. The ice skater trained by lifting, weights doing, box jumps and stretching, to increase flexibility.

7. Which of the following correctly uses punctuation?
   A. "The movie had an interesting plot." she said. "However, the lack of action made the movie seem too long."
   B. "The movie had an interesting plot", she said. "However, the lack of action made the movie seem too long."
   C. "The movie had an interesting plot, she said." "However, the lack of action made the movie seem too long."
   D. "The movie had an interesting plot," she said. "However, the lack of action made the movie seem too long."

8. Which of the following sentences uses correct punctuation?
   A. Subir and Aisha wanted to play in the snow over the weekend but the warm weather ruined their plans.
   B. Subir and Aisha wanted to play in the snow over the weekend, but the warm weather ruined their plans.
   C. Subir and Aisha wanted to play in the snow over the weekend but, the warm weather ruined their plans.
   D. Subir and Aisha wanted to play in the snow over the weekend, but, the warm weather ruined their plans.

> *Running for at least 30 minutes three times per week is a great way to get exercise and to stay healthy.*

9. Which of the following words is the simple subject of the sentence?

   A. Running

   B. Minutes

   C. Way

   D. Exercise

10. Which of the following sentences contains a dependent clause? (Select all that apply.)

    A. Many students go to college because they want to enter a professional field.

    B. The wildfire spread quickly and forced people to evacuate in the middle of the night.

    C. Even though the twin sisters look alike, they have different personalities, styles, and interests.

    D. Some people argue that social media makes people lonelier, but other people point out that it gives people a sense of community.

    E. During the football game, the crowd went wild whenever the home team scored.

11. Which of the following sentences is correctly punctuated?

    A. When students first enter my pottery class; they are often intimidated by the equipment in the room.

    B. The first lesson in this introductory class requires mastery of safety methods; so that I can ensure the protection of all students.

    C. Throughout the semester, students have opportunities to use any of the equipment; in fact, they are encouraged to try everything at least once.

    D. Any pottery studio will include a lot of the same equipment; a wedging table, a spray booth, and a ball mill.

12. Which of the following is a compound sentence?

    A. I needed to give my dog a bath after he rolled in the mud.

    B. She wanted to make cookies but she didn't have any sugar.

    C. They went to the museum before meeting us for lunch.

    D. We didn't go to the concert because of the rain.

    E. Despite donating four boxes of old toys, Keegan still had stuff in her room.

13. Which of the following words from the sentence should be revised to clarify ambiguous language?

    A. Boxes

    B. Toys

    C. Stuff

    D. Room

> *_____ Gareth cooked and enjoyed a wonderful meal, he cleaned and put away the dishes.*

14. Which of the following transition words best completes the sentence?

    A. But

    B. After

    C. In addition

    D. Altogether

(1) My friends love to dance.

(2) Gwendolyn is a professionally trained ballet dancer who is well versed in classical, neoclassical, and contemporary ballet.

(3) Timothy recently learned how to line dance, but he also attended a dance academy for several years.

(4) Jarvis has some groovy moves on the dance floor and loves to create his own music.

(5) Marta is a member of her university's dance squad, and the team just won a national tournament.

15. Which sentence in the paragraph contains informal language?

A. Sentence 2

B. Sentence 3

C. Sentence 4

D. Sentence 5

16. Which of the following is an example of a topic sentence?

A. Giraffes are the tallest animals in the world.

B. Great white sharks have about 3,000 teeth.

C. Cheetahs can run at a speed of about to 60 miles per hour.

D. The tongue of a blue whale can weigh as much as an elephant.

I. Finally, my mother was able to drop me off at school, just before the bell rang.

II. We worked together to replace the flat with the spare tire that was in the trunk.

III. Then we had some more trouble as we discovered that my mother's car had a flat tire.

IV. This morning, we woke up to realize that the storm overnight had knocked out the power at our house.

17. Which of the following options shows the correct chronological or time sequence for the sentences above?

A. III, II, I, IV

B. III, IV, I, II

C. IV, II, III, I

D. IV, III, II, I

After she fell, Mikayla was sad because she realized she had ripped her favorite jeans.

18. Which of the following words would be a precise replacement for the word "sad" to convey a tone of indignation?

A. Woeful

B. Blue

C. Aggrieved

D. Brokenhearted

19. Which of the following sentences contains slang?

A. Melissa and Suzanne carpooled together to get to work today.

B. Shaquan and Janell had an exquisite dinner last night at the restaurant.

C. Joseph and Jamal had a blast last night at the dance hall.

D. Heidi and Frank are going to see a late movie tonight.

> *The congresswoman was reelected to a second term.*

20. Which of the following sentences revises the issue of gender–biased language in the above sentence? (Select all that apply.)

A. The congressperson was reelected to a second term.

B. The member of Congress was reelected to a second term.

C. The lawmaker was reelected to a second term.

D. The legislator was reelected to a second term.

E. The stateswoman was reelected to a second term.

21. Which of the following sentences is grammatically correct?

A. We had went to the concert to see our favorite band.

B. I would have come alone if no one else wants to join me.

C. I always bought a poster every time I see this band play.

D. We would enter the venue when everyone arrived.

22. In a paragraph made up of the following sentences, which sentence contains supporting details?

A. I usually wait on site any time I take my car in for an oil change, and I always bring a snack and something to read.

B. While waiting for my car at the mechanic, I was impressed by the level of hospitality in the waiting area.

C. A selection of fruit and pastries was lined up on a spotless table next to rows of bottled water.

D. I will definitely plan to leave a positive online review and visit this mechanic again the next time I need an oil change.

23. A newspaper publishes an editorial against the implementation of a proposed increase in a local tax to fund the construction of a professional sports complex. Which of the following groups is most likely the intended audience of the editorial?

A. Taxpayers

B. Sports fans

C. Business owners

D. College students

24. Based on an examination of the word parts, which of the following words means "to treat in advance"?

A. Retreat

B. Mistreat

C. Pretreat

D. Overtreat

25. A student was just assigned a research paper about pollution and needs to think about different kinds of pollution to narrow the topic for their writing. Which of the following steps of the writing process does the student need to perform?

A. Proofreading

B. Brainstorming

C. Editing

D. Revising

26. A student is finishing an essay that has been through several rounds of revisions and sentence–level editing. Which of the following steps of the writing process should the student complete next?

A. Brainstorming

B. Writing

C. Planning

D. Proofreading

Look at the definitions of Latin and Greek roots and affixes that have become part of the medical lexicon.

acanth, acantho-	thorn	hydro-	water
amyl, amylo-	starch	-itis	inflammation
cephal, cephalo-	head	kardia, cardi-	heart
cyto-, -cyte	cell	myo(-)	muscle

27. Based on an analysis of the word parts, which of the following means "swelling of the heart muscle"?

A. Amylase

B. Acanthocyte

C. Myocarditis

D. Hydrocephalus

> *Lin fell off their bicycle and injured their leg. When they went to the doctor, the doctor told them that they had a hematoma.*

28. The Greek word "haima" means "blood," and "-oma" is a suffix meaning "mass" or "tumor." Based on analysis of word parts, what is the meaning of the word "hematoma" in the sentence?

    A. A severed nerve causing loss of feeling

    B. Swelling caused by localized bleeding

    C. A broken bone

    D. A severe laceration

29. Which of the following information requires a citation in academic writing?

    A. A summary of a local urban legend

    B. A chronicle of a historical crisis

    C. A first-hand account of a community event

    D. A description of a well-known monument

30. During which of the following steps in the writing process should a writer conduct research?

    A. Prewriting

    B. Drafting

    C. Revising

    D. Editing

31. Which of the following situations exemplifies the idea that the writing process is recursive?

    A. A writer moves a paragraph from the end of an essay to the beginning, then brainstorms additional examples to illustrate and support the point of that paragraph.

    B. A writer finishes writing an essay, then runs a software program to check spelling and grammar.

    C. A writer receives a timed writing prompt, immediately begins to write the essay, then submits the essay "as is" when the time ends.

    D. A writer works with a tutor to brainstorm ideas for an essay, and then creates an outline for the essay.

32. Which of the following word parts is the root of the word "unreproducible"?

    A. Un

    B. Re

    C. Produce

    D. Ible

33. A "scope" is an instrument for viewing. Which of the following prefixes, when added to the word "scope," means "an instrument for viewing around"?

    A. Auto-

    B. Tele-

    C. Micro-

    D. Peri-

Quiz Answers

1. A. "They're," a contraction, is correct because it means "they are."
   B. "Lead" is the correct form of the verb.
   C. "Through" is correct because it means "across."
   D. **CORRECT.** The error is "it's." The possessive "its" correctly replaces the contraction "it's," which means "it is." "Its" is correct because the trail belongs to the park.

2. A. The final "e" should not be dropped when adding a suffix that begins with a consonant. The correct spelling is "excitement."
   B. **CORRECT.** "Movable" is correct. The final "e" should be dropped when adding a suffix that begins with a vowel.
   C. The final "e" should not be dropped when adding a suffix that begins with a consonant. The correct spelling is "likeness."
   D. "Traceable" is an exception to the final "e" rule. The final "e" is often kept in after the letter "c" to keep the soft consonant sound.

3. A. The correct spelling is "selves." "Self" is made plural by changing the "f" to a "v" and adding "-es" to spell "selves."
   B. The correct spelling is "dashes." Words ending in "-s," "-sh," "-ch," or "-x" form plurals by adding "-es."
   C. **CORRECT.** "Elves" correctly applies the spelling rule to change the ending "f" to a "v" and add "-es."
   D. The correct spelling is "churches." Words ending in "-s," "-sh," "-ch," or "-x" form plurals by adding "-es."

4. A. This option is a simple sentence.
   B. **CORRECT.** This option contains both a dependent clause ("Although the line was long") and an independent clause, ("it moved rather quickly").
   C. This option is a compound sentence that contains two independent clauses.
   D. This option is a compound sentence that contains two independent clauses.

5. A. **CORRECT.** The word "that" modifies the simple subject "street."
   B. The word "parallel" is an adverb that modifies the verb "runs."
   C. The word "Main" is part of the proper noun "Main Street."
   D. The word "other" modifies the noun "side," but that is not the subject of the sentence.

6. A. This option is missing a comma after the word "weights."
   B. This option has incorrect commas after the words "lifting" and "doing."
   C. **CORRECT.** This option is correct because it correctly punctuates the serial comma after "weights" and "jumps."
   D. This option has incorrect commas after the words "lifting," "doing," and "stretching."

7. A. This option is incorrect because it incorrectly puts a period after the word "plot."
   B. This option incorrectly puts the comma outside the closing quotation mark.
   C. This option incorrectly places the first closing quotation mark after "said."
   D. **CORRECT.** This option is correct because it correctly puts the comma inside the quotation mark following the word "plot."

8. A. This option is incorrect because it does not contain the needed comma before the coordinating conjunction "but."
   B. **CORRECT.** This option is correct because it places a comma before the coordinating conjunction "but," which joins two independent clauses.
   C. This option is incorrect because the comma should be placed before, not after, the coordinating conjunction.
   D. This option is incorrect because it places a comma on either side of the coordinating conjunction when only the comma before the coordinating conjunction is needed.

9. A. **CORRECT.** "Running" is a gerund, an -ing verb that functions as a noun and acts as the subject of the sentence.
   B. In this sentence, "minutes" is the object of a preposition, not the subject of the sentence.
   C. "Way" is a subject complement, not the subject of the sentence.
   D. In this sentence, "exercise" is the object of the infinitive phrase "to get exercise."

10. A. **CORRECT.** The dependent clause begins with the subordinating word "because": "because they want to enter a professional field."

B. This is a simple sentence consisting of one independent clause with a compound verb.

C. **CORRECT.** The dependent clause begins with the subordinating phrase "even though": "Even though the twin sisters look alike."

D. This is a compound sentence with two independent clauses joined by the conjunction "but."

E. **CORRECT.** This choice has two dependent clauses. The first dependent clause begins with the subordinating word "during": "During the football game." The second dependent clause begins with the subordinating word "whenever": "whenever the home team scored."

11. A. This sentence is not punctuated correctly. There should be a comma following the word "class" instead of a semicolon.

B. This sentence is not punctuated correctly. There should not be a semicolon following the word "methods."

C. **CORRECT.** This sentence is punctuated correctly.

D. This sentence is not punctuated correctly. There should be a colon following the word "equipment" instead of a semicolon.

12. A. This option is a complex sentence that contains both an independent clause (I needed to give my dog a bath) and a dependent clause (after he rolled in the mud).

B. **CORRECT.** This option is a compound sentence that contains two independent clauses.

C. This option is a complex sentence that contains both an independent clause (They went to the museum) and a dependent clause (before meeting us for lunch).

D. This option is a complex sentence that contains both an independent clause (We didn't go to the concert) and a dependent clause (because of the rain).

13. A. "Boxes" is a noun that has a clear meaning.

B. "Toys" is a noun that has a clear meaning.

C. **CORRECT.** "Stuff" is an ambiguous word that is inexact and unclear.

D. "Room" is a noun that has a clear meaning.

14. A. This option is incorrect because it uses an opposition transition word.

B. **CORRECT.** This option is correct because it uses a transition word that refers to chronology or time. It helps reveal and clarify the order of events: first Gareth cooked, and "after" he cooked, he cleaned and put away the dishes.

C. This option is incorrect because it uses a transition word to add an idea.

D. This option is incorrect because it uses a concluding transition word.

15. A. This sentence is written in formal language.

B. This sentence is written in formal language.

C. **CORRECT.** The word "groovy" is an example of informal language.

D. This sentence is written in formal language.

16. A. **CORRECT.** This sentence would make a good topic sentence because it states a main idea that can be supported by specific facts.

B. This sentence states a specific fact about great white sharks that could be best used as a supporting detail.

C. This sentence states a specific fact about cheetahs that could be best used as a supporting detail.

D. This sentence states a specific fact about blue whales that could be best used as a supporting detail.

17. A. This option begins after the first event of the day, which is waking up in the morning, as described in sentence IV.

B. This option begins with the flat tire incident, but the characters' day begins with sentence IV: waking up and discovering that an overnight storm has knocked out the electricity.

C. In this option, sentences III and II are in the reverse order they should be.

D. **CORRECT.** Transition words help place the sentences in correct time order from getting up "this morning" to "then" having a flat tire, then fixing it, and "finally" going to school.

18. A. This option is incorrect because "woeful" suggests mourning rather than indignation.

B. This is incorrect because "blue" suggests unhappiness rather than indignation.

C. **CORRECT.** "Aggrieved" is the most precise word because it suggests a feeling that one has been wronged or treated unfairly.

D. This is incorrect because "brokenhearted" suggests loss or rejection rather than indignation.

19. A. This sentence does not contain slang.
    B. This sentence does not contain slang.
    C. **CORRECT.** The slang phrase "had a blast" is slang for "had a fun time."
    D. This sentence does not contain slang.

20. A. **CORRECT.** "Congressperson" is a gender-neutral alternative to "congresswoman."
    B. **CORRECT.** "Member of Congress" is a gender-neutral alternative to "congresswoman."
    C. **CORRECT.** "Lawmaker" is a gender-neutral alternative to "congresswoman."
    D. **CORRECT.** "Legislator" is a gender-neutral alternative to "congresswoman."
    E. "Stateswoman" does not revise the issue of gender-biased language.

21. A. The sentence contains incorrect verb forms; the verb phrase should be "had gone" to correctly express this idea in past tense.
    B. The sentence begins with a conditional verb, which should be following by a verb in past tense. "Wants" should be "wanted."
    C. The verb tenses in this sentence are mismatched in tense, with "bought" in the past tense and "see" in the present tense. These verbs should be a consistent tense.
    D. **CORRECT.** This sentence is grammatically correct. The first verb is conditional and should be followed by a verb in past tense. "Arrived" is in past tense.

22. A. This sentence does not contain a supporting detail.
    B. This sentence does not contain a supporting detail.
    C. **CORRECT.** This sentence contains specific details that support the main idea of this paragraph.
    D. This sentence does not contain a supporting detail.

23. A. **CORRECT.** People who are likely to pay the increased tax rate are the intended audience of the editorial.
    B. Sports fans might be in favor of the increase to fund the construction of a professional sports complex, so they are not likely to be the intended audience of the editorial.
    C. Business owners are not likely to be the intended audience of the editorial.
    D. College students are not likely to be the intended audience of the editorial.

24. A. The prefix "re-" means "again," not "before."
    B. The prefix "mis-" means "badly," not "before."
    C. **CORRECT.** The prefix "pre-" means "before," so to "pretreat" means to "treat before," or "in advance."
    D. The prefix "over-" means "too much," not "before."

25. A. Proofreading is part of the editing step of the writing process.
    B. **CORRECT.** Brainstorming involves considering different aspects of a topic to help narrow the focus of a paper.
    C. Editing is the last step of the writing process.
    D. Revising is typically part of the revision step of the writing process, after conferencing, or peer review.

26. A. Brainstorming is typically done during the prewriting stage of the writing process.
    B. The student has already written and revised the essay.
    C. The student has already planned, drafted, received feedback on, and revised the essay.
    D. **CORRECT.** Proofreading is the last step in the editing stage of the writing process.

27. A. The affix "amylo-" is derived from a Greek root that means "starch."
    B. The affix "acantho-" is derived from a Greek root meaning "thorn" and is used in English to refer to the spine. The affix "-cyte" means "cell."
    C. **CORRECT.** The affix "cardi-" comes from the Greek root "kardia," meaning "heart." The affix "myo-"comes from the Latin word for "muscle." The affix "-itis" means inflammation or swelling. So "myocarditis" is the word for "swelling of the heart muscle."
    D. The affix "hydro-" means "water," and the Latinized root "cephal" comes from the Greek word "kephale," meaning "head."

28. A. The root "hema" is derived from the Greek word "haima," meaning "blood," and the suffix "-oma" means "mass or tumor." These word parts do not combine to mean "a severed nerve."

B. **CORRECT.** The root "hema" is derived from the Greek word "haima," meaning "blood," and the suffix "-oma" means "mass or tumor." A hematoma is a mass of blood, or swelling caused by bleeding.

C. The root "hema" is derived from the Greek word "haima," meaning "blood," and the suffix "-oma" means "mass or tumor." These word parts do not combine to mean "a broken bone."

D. The root "hema" is derived from the Greek word "haima," meaning "blood," and the suffix "-oma means "mass or tumor." These word parts do not combine to mean "a severe laceration."

29. A. This information is considered common knowledge and does not require a citation.

B. **CORRECT.** This information requires outside research and verification; therefore, this information requires a citation.

C. The author is the authority in this instance and no additional citation is required.

D. This information is considered common knowledge and does not require a citation.

30. A. **CORRECT.** During the prewriting stage, a writer should gather any information, including outside research, that is necessary.

B. During the drafting stage, the writer puts ideas into sentences and paragraphs with the aim of expressing ideas fully and making connections between ideas.

C. During the revising stage, the writer develops, clarifies, and organizes the writing that occurred in the drafting stage.

D. During the editing stage, the writer reviews the writing to ensure correct spelling, grammar, and mechanics.

31. A. **CORRECT.** This scenario indicates that revision led the writer to return to prewriting and drafting, which are steps that occur earlier in the writing process.

B. These steps are linear and adjacent in the writing process.

C. This scenario offers no opportunity to return to an earlier step in the writing process.

D. These steps are linear and adjacent in the writing process.

32. A. "Un-" is a prefix.

B. "Re-" is a prefix.

C. **CORRECT.** "Produce" is a root word.

D. "-ible" is a suffix.

33. A. "Auto-" means "self."

B. "Tele-" means "far."

C. "Micro-" means "small."

D. **CORRECT.** "Peri-" means "around or about"; a periscope is an instrument used to view a surrounding area.

Comprehensive Practice Test

The following practice test matches the ATI TEAS test plan and is composed of questions that have usage data from previous administrations. This data enables ATI to provide the table below that you can use to determine your predicted preparedness*. To ensure the most accurate prediction of your preparedness level, be sure to:

- Take each section in the order in which they are presented. You must complete and score yourself on all four sections.

- Record your responses on a piece of paper and use the answer key to grade your responses after you've completed all four sections. The total number of questions you answered correctly determines your score range for the table below (e.g., 50 total correct answers equals "Basic" preparedness level).

- Time yourself using the following time limits:
  - Reading – 55 min
  - Mathematics – 57 min
  - Science – 60 min
  - English and Language Usage – 37 min

- As much as possible, replicate the proctored testing environment, including:
  - Do not refer to notes or use outside resources other than scrap paper.
  - Do not communicate with others during testing.
  - Do not use electronic devices other than a four-function calculator.
  - Allow yourself a 10-min break after the Mathematics section.

Score Range (total correct answers)	Predicted ATI TEAS Preparedness Level	Academic Preparedness Level Definition
0 to 48	Developmental	Developmental scores generally indicate a very low level of overall academic preparedness necessary to support learning of health sciences-related content. Students at this level will require additional preparation for most objectives assessed on ATI TEAS.
49 to 79	Basic	Basic scores generally indicate a low level of overall academic preparedness necessary to support learning of health sciences-related content. Students at this level are likely to require additional preparation for many objectives assessed on ATI TEAS.
80 to 115	Proficient	Proficient scores generally indicate a moderate level of overall academic preparedness necessary to support learning of health sciences-related content. Students at this level can require additional preparation for some objectives assessed on ATI TEAS.
116 to 136	Advanced	Advanced scores generally indicate a high level of overall academic preparedness necessary to support learning of health sciences-related content. Students at this level are not likely to require additional preparation for the objectives assessed on ATI TEAS.
137 to 150	Exemplary	Exemplary scores generally indicate a very high level of overall academic preparedness necessary to support learning of health sciences-related content. Students at this level are not likely to require additional preparation for the objectives assessed on ATI TEAS.

SUBSCORE COMPARISON TABLE

If your overall score prediction indicates that you would benefit from additional study before taking the proctored TEAS exam, an indication of your relative strengths and weaknesses on the four subscore areas of the test may help you to effectively focus your study efforts.

The table below accounts for variations in difficulty among the sections of the test and can be used to determine which of your section scores indicates the greatest need for additional study.

Directions

Find and circle the number of questions you answered correctly in each content area. Which circled score is in the lowest row of the table? We recommend that you start your studying there!

Reading	Mathematics	Science	English
		47	
	32		
			24
47			
		46	
	31		
46			
		45	
			23
	30		
		44	
45			
		43	
			22
	29		
		42	
44			
		41	
	28		
			21
		40	
43			
		39	
	27		
		38	
42			
			20
		37	
	26		
41			
		36	
	25		
		35	
			19
40			
		34	
	24		

Reading	Mathematics	Science	English
		33	
39			
			18
		32	
	23		
38			
		31	
		30	
37			
			17
	22		
		29	
36			
	21		
		28	
			16
35			
		27	
	20		
		26	
34			
			15
	19		
		25	
33			
		24	
	18		
32			
			14
		23	
31			
		22	
	17		
			13
		21	
30			
		16	

Reading	Mathematics	Science	English
		20	
29			
			12
		19	
	15		
28			
		18	
27			
	14		
			11
		17	
26			
		16	
	13		
25			
			10
		15	
24			
	12		
		14	
23			
			9
	11		
		13	
22			
		12	
21			
			8
	10		
20			
		11	
	9		
19			
			7
		10	
18			
	8		
		9	

Reading	Mathematics	Science	English
17			
			6
16			
		8	
	7		
15			
			5
		7	
14			
	6		
13			
		6	
			4
12			
	5		
		5	
11			
10			
			3
	4		
		4	
9			
8			
		3	
	3		
			2
7			
6			
		2	
5			
	2		
4			
			1
3			
		1	
	1		
2			
			0
1			

Practice Test Questions

READING

Bards

Storytellers known as bards were an important element in sustaining Celtic civilization. They were trained at barding schools where they learned hundreds of poems and different styles of verse. Some bards trained for up to 7 years. In addition to singing memorized poems, they composed poems of their own to celebrate important events or commemorate fallen leaders. Many scholars believe that the bards of Brittany, a region in northwest France, and those of Wales created and passed on the legends of King Arthur and the Knights of the Round Table. Without the oral traditions, these stories would have been lost.

1. Which of the following supporting details best reinforces the argument presented in the first sentence that bards sustained Celtic civilization?

    A. Bards were specially trained at barding schools.

    B. Bards trained for as long as 7 years and learned different styles of verse.

    C. In addition to singing memorized poems, bards would compose poems of their own.

    D. Poems written by bards celebrated important events and commemorated fallen leaders.

2. Which of the following best rephrases the topic of the passage?

    A. The events that led to sustaining Celtic civilization

    B. The history and purpose of bards

    C. The importance of the King Arthur legends

    D. The purpose of barding schools

3. Which of the following is the main purpose of the passage?

    A. To inform

    B. To persuade

    C. To entertain

    D. To analyze

Locavores

In school, students are taught that carnivores are meat-eating animals, herbivores are plant-consuming animals, and omnivores eat everything. Now, add "locavore" to this list. A locavore is a person who strives to maintain a diet out of locally grown food. Typically, this would include food produced within a 100-mile radius. At a time when there are growing concerns over the safety of our food supply, more and more people are turning to nearby sources of food — whether organic or grown with chemicals — and liking it.

Today, it is common for food products to travel 1,500 "food miles" from a large corporate farm to a consumer's dinner plate. It is entirely possible that some of the produce found at a grocery store in Kansas was grown and harvested in California. This system has evolved to suit Industrial scale production and distribution instead of taste or nutrition. This development has led to the worrisome situation in which the average consumer has little chance of knowing where or how the food they buy was grown or raised.

There are a number of local alternatives to industrial food, and the variety is growing. Farmers markets are located in nearly every city and town. Some markets operate throughout the year, offering the produce that thrives in the local environment. The organic food movement is thriving to the point that it is the fastest growing sector in the overall food industry, and organic producers often sell their products at local grocery stores. A third alternative is CSA, or community-supported agriculture. A CSA is a subscription service that individuals can purchase from local farms. A subscriber is typically given a weekly supply of whatever the farm produces. Increasingly, it is possible for us to become more and more locavorous.

4. Which of the following is a logical conclusion based on the passage?

   A. People are becoming locavores to avoid food grown with chemicals.

   B. Organic foods are grown within 100 miles of where they are sold.

   C. An increasing number of consumers want to know where their food is grown.

   D. Farmers markets provide a greater diversity of food products than grocery stores.

5. Which of the following is an opinion stated in the passage?

   A. It is worrisome that the average consumer does not know where or how most food is grown or raised.

   B. It is entirely possible that some of the produce found in a grocery store in Kansas was grown and harvested in California.

   C. Some food products travel 1,500 "food miles" from a large corporate farm to a consumer's dinner plate.

   D. Farmers markets offer produce that thrives in the local environment.

6. Which of the following is the author's primary argument in the passage?

   A. Consumers should primarily eat organically grown food.

   B. Consumers should take the time to learn where all of their food is produced.

   C. Subscribing to a CSA will promote a healthy diet and support local farmers.

   D. Consuming locally grown food is a viable and beneficial alternative.

7. Which of the following inferences can be drawn from the passage?

   A. Large industrial farms are causing local farms to go out of business.

   B. Organic foods are comprised of fruits and vegetables but not meats and dairy.

   C. Locavores prefer to consume a vegetarian or vegan diet based on local produce.

   D. Industrial scale food production and distribution can affect the quality of foods.

8. Which of the following sentences from the passage supports the claim made in the final sentence of the passage?

   A. A locavore is a person who strives to maintain a diet out of locally grown food.

   B. Today, it is common for food products to travel 1,500 "food miles" from a large corporate farm to a consumer's dinner plate.

   C. There are a number of local alternatives to industrial food, and the variety is growing.

   D. It is entirely possible that some of the produce found at a grocery store in Kansas was grown and harvested in California.

The Nearings

Among those who subscribe to self-sufficiency and moving back to the land, Helen and Scott Nearing are a legendary couple. Together, the Nearings exemplified the notion of the good life by living simply in a rural setting.

Scott (1883-1983) came from a wealthy Pennsylvania coal mining family, and Helen Knothe Nearing (1904-1995) was the daughter of an intellectual Ridgewood, New Jersey family. Together, they would travel a path very far away from their rather conventional beginnings. By the time he was in his early 20s, Scott had taken to social activism, speaking out against the unsafe working conditions in the Pennsylvania coal mines. Helen spent a brief period working in a factory before meeting Scott and leaving behind the creature comforts of her former lifestyle.

The two met first in 1921 and again in 1928, and were together from that point. In 1932, they left New York City for rural southern Vermont, where they developed a self-sufficient lifestyle and philosophy. They divided their waking hours into three 4-hour blocks: "bread labor," which was work for food, shelter, fuel, etc.; civic work, such as community service; and recreational or professional pursuits, economics research for Scott and music for Helen. Until 1952, their bread labor in Vermont was primarily maple products; after 1952, when they moved to Maine, it was blueberries. They were prolific builders of stone and concrete structures, completing 21 in all, and all by hand. Because they were cult figures of a sort, they often had the willing help of enthusiastic young volunteers who made the pilgrimage to New England.

The two authored many books, the most famous of which is Living the Good Life (1954). This and other titles by the Nearings are credited with spurring the "back to the land" movement in the 1960s.

9. Which of the following is a logical conclusion based on the passage?

   A. The Nearings' writings were their most influential contribution to the culture.

   B. Community service was an example of "bread labor" as defined by the Nearings.

   C. The Nearings inherited their philosophy from the "back to the land" movement.

   D. The Nearings followed in their parents' footsteps in embracing a rural lifestyle.

10. Scott Nearing was likely involved in which of the following activities the year Helen was born?

    A. Writing Living the Good Life

    B. Harvesting blueberries

    C. Speaking against unsafe coal mines

    D. Building concrete structures by hand

11. Which of the following is a key part of the Nearings' philosophy of a self-sufficient lifestyle?

    A. Dividing time into 4-hour blocks to accomplish goals

    B. Social activism against factory work

    C. Writing books, like Living the Good Life

    D. Moving from New York City to Vermont

12. Which of the following activities might the Nearings have practiced during their civic work based on the passage?

    A. Campaigning to increase coal mining in their area

    B. Shopping for lavish home furnishings

    C. Fundraising for factories that make processed food

    D. Teaching a class on baking bread

13. Which of the following sentences contains an opinion?

    A. In 1932, they left New York City for rural southern Vermont, where they developed a self-sufficient lifestyle and philosophy.

    B. By the time he was in his early 20s, Scott had taken to social activism, speaking out against the unsafe working conditions in the Pennsylvania coal mines.

    C. Together, the Nearings exemplified the notion of the good life by living simply in a rural setting.

    D. The two authored many books, the most famous of which is Living the Good Life (1954).

Multiple Intelligences

In the late 1970s, the directors of the Bernard Van Leer Foundation invited a team of professors from Harvard University's Graduate School of Education to respond to a daunting challenge: Discover a way for every human being to develop to their maximum potential. Out of this collaboration of dozens of esteemed professionals came the theory of multiple intelligences (MI).

In 1983, Howard Gardner, a project team member, published Frames of Mind, which sets out the theory in some detail. In this book, Gardner posits that traditional notions of intelligence, which are largely based on I.Q. testing, do not sufficiently address the range of cerebral engagement. In short, various types of intelligence should be considered because different minds have different strengths. For too long, our notion of intelligence has been too narrow.

Originally, Gardner identified seven areas of human intelligence: verbal-linguistic, musical, logical-mathematical, visual-spatial, bodily-kinesthetic, interpersonal, and intra-personal. A short time later, Gardner added an eighth intelligence: naturalistic.

Traditional school curriculum in Western culture has heavily emphasized learning through the verbal-linguistic and logical-mathematical intelligences. This has, according to Gardner, left many students poorly served by our educational system. Gifts in other areas of intelligence, such as the arts, should be identified and encouraged as well. Also, different method-ologies of conveying information should be used to engage the distinct strengths of students with varying types of intelligence.

Gardner and others, like author Thomas Armstrong, Ph.D., have done much to cause the American educational establishment to rethink the way children learn in school. Many universities include courses about multiple intelligences, and teachers are often encouraged to use the theory of MI in planning their lessons. The result of this re-evaluation of intelligence has begun to transform the way teachers teach.

14. Which of the following is a supporting detail of the author's main idea in the passage?

   A. In this book, Gardner posits that traditional notions of intelligence, which are largely based on I.Q. testing, do not sufficiently address the range of cerebral engagement.

   B. Traditional notions of intelligence have limited the achievement of many students.

   C. Traditional school curriculum in Western culture has heavily emphasized learning through the verbal-linguistic and logical-mathematical intelligences.

   D. Researchers who developed the theory of multiple intelligences have had an effect on education.

15. Which of the following is a logical conclusion based on the passage?

   A. Howard Gardner, at the time of the study, had multiple intelligences.

   B. I.Q. testing focuses mainly on verbal-linguistic and mathematical-logical skills.

   C. Most teachers prefer to use traditional teaching methods in the classroom.

   D. Multiple intelligence principles are excluded from school curricula because they are difficult to test.

16. Which of the following statements best rephrases the key point of Howard Gardner's theory of multiple intelligences as described in the passage?

   A. Verbal-linguistic and logical-mathematical are the two most important types of multiple intelligences.

   B. Cerebral engagement is unrelated to I.Q. testing.

   C. Traditional school curriculum accommodates multiple types of intelligence.

   D. Understanding intelligence effectively requires taking into account overall cerebral engagement.

17. Which of the following changes is appropriate for a teacher who wants to address the theory of MI?

   A. Replacing a history slide show with memori-zation of names and dates

   B. Replacing written book reports with multi-media collaborations among students

   C. Encouraging more girls to enroll in upper-level mathematics courses

   D. Encouraging classroom competition by using flash card games

18. Which of the following students would most likely benefit the most from an educational system that incorporates MI into its curriculum?

A. A student who draws intricate portraits on their notebook

B. A student who excels at taking notes during lectures

C. A student who likes to take part in spelling bees

D. A student who reads at a higher level than their classmates

National Pastime

Baseball has long been known as "the national pastime." Does the name still fit? While baseball's contribution to U.S. culture dates back to the early part of the 19th century, football seems to have supplanted baseball in the U.S. imagination. For instance, in 2007, the top 10 sports broadcasts in television ratings were all games from the National Football League. Meanwhile, participation in youth baseball has fallen, and Major League Baseball teams are now composed of nearly 30% foreign-born players. While the criteria for the status of national pastime are elusive, football fans can make a persuasive argument that there is a new national pastime in the U.S.

19. Which of the following is a supporting detail of the author's main idea?

A. Baseball has long been known as "the national pastime."

B. Baseball's contribution to American culture dates back to the early part of the 19th century.

C. Football fans can make a compelling case that there is a new "national pastime" in America.

D. The top 10 sports broadcasts in television ratings were all games from the National Football League.

20. Which of the following is the author's main purpose in the passage?

A. To argue that football should be considered America's "national pastime"

B. To inform readers about the historical association between baseball and American culture

C. To persuade readers that America should revive the popularity of baseball

D. To express feelings about the importance of football in American culture

A nursery has exactly seven types of flowers: 1, 2, 3, 4, 5, 6, and 7. Choose five different types of flowers to plant in a garden, using the following guidelines:

If type 1 is chosen, type 5 cannot be chosen.

If type 3 is chosen, type 5 must be chosen.

If type 2 is chosen, type 6 must be chosen.

21. Which of the following combinations of flowers corresponds with the directions?

A. 2, 3, 4, 5, 6

B. 1, 2, 3, 6, 7

C. 2, 3, 4, 5, 7

D. 1, 4, 5, 6, 7

> *Draw a horizontal line. From the midpoint of this line, draw a perpendicular line extending upward. Write the letter "A" at each end of the horizontal line and the letter "Z" at the end of the vertical line. Rotate the drawing 90 degrees clockwise.*

22. Which of the following drawings correctly corresponds with the directions?

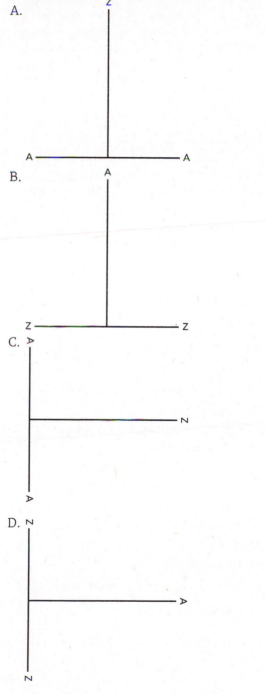

Job Announcement

DD&P Industries is seeking motivated individuals to fill entry-level call center positions.

DD&P is an industry leader in the manufacture and servicing of medical equipment. We are committed to providing excellent customer service and dedicated to hiring individuals with excellent communication skills.

DD&P offers flexible work schedules with daytime, evening, weekend, and holiday shifts. We offer competitive pay and benefits packages, including medical/dental, 401(k), and profit sharing (after a year of employment).

Compensation: Hourly

Responsibilities:

- Providing professional customer service for calls regarding products and services

- Understanding and communicating product and service information

- Routing calls to appropriate sources

- Handling customer complaints

Qualifications:

- Good communication skills

- Ability to type 60 wpm

- Working knowledge of basic PC applications (Word, Outlook, etc.)

- Previous customer service experience preferred

23. Which of the following statements is a logical conclusion based on the job announcement?

   A. This position will be involved in formulating communications for marketing purposes.

   B. Applicants for this position must have previous experience in the health care industry.

   C. Applicants for this position must have effective telephone communication skills.

   D. This position includes a requirement to work on weekends and during holidays.

24. Which of the following individuals would most likely be interested in this job?

   A. A person who wants a position that provides health insurance

   B. A person who is looking for a salaried position

   C. A person who has previously managed customer service representatives

   D. A person who likes to work with and fix medical equipment

Use the chart below to answer the question.

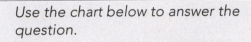

Viewership Market Analysis

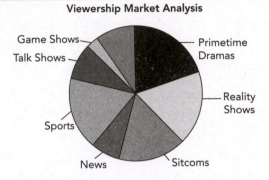

25. Which of the following television programs might an advertiser use to reach the most viewers?

   A. Game shows, talk shows, and reality shows

   B. Daytime dramas and news

   C. Sitcoms and primetime dramas

   D. Sports and talk shows

Use the drug facts label below to answer the question.

Drug Facts
Active ingredient: polymyxin B sulfate and bacitracin zinc
Purpose
....Antibiotic Ointment
Uses
Help prevent infection in cuts, scrapes, and minor burns. Relieves itching, burning, and minor irritations.
Warnings
For external use only. Do not use on children under 2 years of age unless directed by a doctor. When using this product, do not get into eyes. If contact occurs, rinse eyes thoroughly with water. Stop use ask a doctor if irritation occurs or if there is no improvement within 2 weeks. Keep out of reach of children. in case of overdose, get medical help or contact a Poison Control Center right away.
Directions
Wash the affected area and dry thoroughly. Apply a thin layer of the product over affected area four times daily or as directed by a physician. Supervise children in the use of this product. This product is not effective on scalp or nails.
Other information
Inactive ingredients cocoa butter, olive oil, and white petrolatum
Questions comments? Call 1-800-555-5555

26. Which of the following statements about this product might cause a pharmacist concern?

   A. "I used the ointment on my heat rash."

   B. "I used the ointment for an abrasion on my baby's eyelid."

   C. "I put the ointment on my 4-year-old child's knee scrape."

   D. "I put the ointment on a rash from poison ivy three times today."

Read the following before answering the question.

- *A candidate is choosing between job offers 1, 2, 3, and 4.*
- *Job 1 offers 2 weeks paid vacation per year and partial health insurance.*
- *Job 2 offers 1 week paid vacation per year and partial health insurance.*
- *Job 3 offers 2 weeks paid vacation per year and full health insurance.*
- *Job 4 offers 2 weeks paid vacation per year and full health insurance.*
- *Jobs 1 and 3 pay $5,000 more than Job 4.*
- *Job 2 pays $7,000 less than Job 4.*

27. Which of the following job offers is preferable for the candidate?

   A. 1

   B. 2

   C. 3

   D. 4

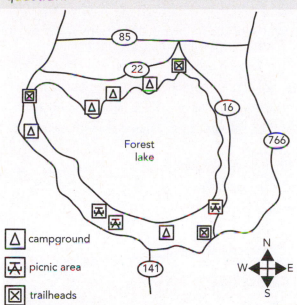

△ campground

⊞ picnic area

⊠ trailheads

N
W ◆ E
S

28. The majority of the campgrounds are located on which of the following sides of the lake?

   A. South

   B. North

   C. East

   D. West

29. Which of the following highways runs along the east coast of the lake? (Note: The numbers on the map represent highway names.)

   A. 16

   B. 22

   C. 85

   D. 141

A friend calls and says, "Before I pick you up to go to the grocery store, I have to cook breakfast, then shower, so I will see you when I'm done with those two things."

30. Of the following, when should you expect your friend to pick you up?

   A. After they shower

   B. After they go to the grocery store

   C. As soon as they hang up the phone

   D. Before breakfast

1 2 3 4 3 2 1 2 3 4

Using the number string above, replace every 1 with the letter A, every 2 with the letter B, every 3 with the letter D, and every 4 with the letter E. For letters that appear more than twice, delete the first instance of those letters. Delete the first and the last letter in the string, and replace the vowels with the letter X.

31. Which of the following letter strings corresponds with the directions above?

   A. DBXBD

   B. BXBDX

   C. XDBXBD

   D. BDXDBX

Peak Oil

Given the media coverage surrounding climate change, most people are aware of this environmental issue. One that is less well known but can become just as crucial is "peak oil." What is peak oil? Simply put, it is the point at which the world production of oil reaches its highest point and begins a steady, irreversible decline. This has been known for some time. Hubbert's Curve (1956), named for the scientist who formulated it, predicted that U.S. production would peak around 1970. He was off by 1 year. Since 1971-1972, the oil production of the United States has been gradually declining.

32. Which of the following best describes the author's purpose in the first two sentences of the passage?

   A. To argue that climate change presents a serious danger

   B. To persuade readers to take action on the issue of peak oil

   C. To introduce the subject matter by comparing it to a familiar issue

   D. To provide a definition of the term "peak oil"

33. Which of the following words would the author use to describe the issue of peak oil?

   A. Significant

   B. Confusing

   C. Reversible

   D. Avoidable

34. Which of the following statements best describes the argument made in the passage?

A. Peak oil and climate change are directly connected.

B. Increasing media coverage of peak oil will improve oil production.

C. Hubbert's Curve provides an example of a way to reverse climate change.

D. Peak oil is an important issue even if not well known.

She headed off to the track, where she hoped to make a fast dollar by betting on the races.

35. Which of the following dictionary definitions corresponds with "fast" as used in the sentence above?

A. Distinguished by rapid motion

B. Having agile mental abilities

C. Obtained with little effort

D. Characterized by wild behavior

Marsupialia (Marsupials)
- *Kangaroos*
- *Koalas*
- *Wombats*

Primates (Primates)
- *Monkeys*
- *Chimpanzees*
- *Gorillas*

Rodentia (Rodents)
- *Squirrels*
- *Mice*
- *Porcupines*

36. Using text features to determine the answer, which of the following statements is correct based on the outline above?

A. Marsupials are more similar to primates than to rodents.

B. Rodents are a subcategory of Rodentia.

C. Wombats are a subcategory of koalas.

D. Squirrels are more similar to porcupines than to monkeys.

I avoided him because he thought he had a score to settle with me.

37. Which of the following definitions is correct for "score" as used in the sentence above?

A. A scratch or mark made on a surface

B. An action that has a successful outcome

C. A grudge that one holds against another

D. The relevant facts related to a situation

Phylum Mollusca
Cephalopoda
- *Squids*
- *Octopuses*
- *Cuttlefish*

Gastropoda
- *Snails*
- *Sea Slugs*

Pelecypoda
- *Clams*
- *Mussels*
- *Oysters*

38. Using text features to determine the answer, which of the following statements is correct based on the outline above?

A. A Pelecypoda is a type of Gastropoda.

B. An octopus is a type of squid.

C. Cephalopoda is more closely related to Gastropoda than to Pelecypoda.

D. Snails are more closely related to sea slugs than to clams.

A gardener purchased lattice so they could train the grapevine along the side of the house.

39. Which of the following defines "train" as used in the sentence above?

A. To teach so as to make fit or qualified

B. To direct the growth of

C. To focus attention

D. To motivate by discipline

> "When he playfully tossed a pencil at her, she moved to bat it away angrily."
> Read the dictionary entry to answer the question.
>
> **bat**
>
> n.
>
> 1. the wooden club used in some games to hit the ball
>
> 2. any of numerous flying mammals of the order Chiroptera
>
> v.
>
> 3. to strike or hit, as if with a bat or club
>
> 4. to blink or wink

40. Which of the following definitions fits the context of the sentence?

    A. Definition 1

    B. Definition 2

    C. Definition 3

    D. Definition 4

> When she noticed the dust on her running shoes, Natalia realized she had become rather complacent about her fitness routine.

41. Which of following is the closest in meaning to "complacent" as used in the sentence above?

    A. Unconcerned

    B. Dissatisfied

    C. Confident

    D. Worried

42. Which of the following sources will be most helpful for a writer who is trying to use a greater variety of words in an article?

    A. Encyclopedia

    B. Almanac

    C. Style guide

    D. Thesaurus

YA Heroines

The heroines are in the house. In recent years, there has been a boom of young adult (YA) literature that has taken readers, and bestseller lists, by storm. Though YA novels have existed nearly as long as the novel itself, current YA novels have reinvented the genre. Now they tend to focus on the plight of a central heroine, a young girl tasked with dismantling the oppressive dystopia she lives in to save her friends and her family. The success of these stories is finally making Hollywood sit up and pay attention to the possibility of how lucrative female-led movies can be, and more female-driven films than ever are taking top spot at the box office.

43. Which of the following is the source of this passage?

    A. Young adult novel

    B. Instruction manual

    C. Book review

    D. Entertainment magazine

44. Below are several trends being discussed in the media. Which of the following trends resembles the theme of the passage's description of YA literature?

    A. More students are graduating from college in debt than ever before, and they are flooding the job market.

    B. A new cooking technique is being introduced in culinary schools across the world to great success.

    C. The percentage of people under 30 getting married has decreased greatly in the last 20 years.

    D. An automaker redesigned one of its standard models, and now it is one of their top sellers.

The Kennedy Assassination

After the assassination on November 22, 1963, a commission was formed to investigate the circumstances surrounding President Kennedy's death. The Warren Commission determined that no conspiracy was behind the assassination, but conspiracy theorists persisted in their belief that Oswald did not act alone.

45. Which of the following additional sentences would be appropriate if this passage were found in a United States history textbook?

A. The ambiguous audio recordings and flawed government investigations are proof that there was more to Kennedy's assassination than meets the eye.

B. In spite of the mystery that surrounds the President's death, one thing is clear – American politics was fundamentally changed that November day.

C. Though the nation mourned, no one mourned more than Jacqueline Kennedy.

D. The Kennedy family is still one of the most well-known political families in the United States today.

46. Based on their titles, which of the following articles would provide the most reliable information for a student who wanted to learn more about the Kennedy assassination?

A. "The Political Landscape of Cold War America, 1965-1990"

B. "The Lone Gunman: Lee Harvey Oswald, Sole Conspirator?"

C. "Did JFK Play a Part in His Own Death?"

D. "November 22, 1963: A Brief History"

47. A student is writing a research paper about the psychological effects of homework. Which of the following sources should they consult for statistical data?

A. An encyclopedia entry about the history of homework assignments

B. An academic study about hours spent on homework each night

C. A blog detailing a fellow student's experiences with homework

D. A magazine article by a teacher about the importance of daily homework

MATHEMATICS

1. Which of the following expresses 425% as a decimal?

A. 0.0425

B. 0.425

C. 4.25

D. 425

$L = 2/3k$

2. This equation is used to determine the length of crutches in inches (L) required for a person of a given height in inches (k). Which of the following statements is true?

A. Each 1/3 inch of height adds 1 inch to the crutch length.

B. Each 1 inch of height adds 1/3 inch to the crutch length.

C. Each 2 inches of height adds 3 inches to the crutch length.

D. Each 3 inches of height adds 2 inches to the crutch length.

The owner of a hot dog stand records the number of hot dogs purchased by each customer on a particular day and obtains the following data:

Number of Hot Dogs Purchased	Number of Customers
1	50
2	27
3	15
4	6
5	2

3. Which of the following is the total number of hot dogs purchased during the day?

A. 15

B. 100

C. 115

D. 183

In a neighborhood, 5% of the houses
have red mailboxes. A student
counts 60 red mailboxes in the
neighborhood.

4. Which of the following is the total number of
houses in the neighborhood?

   A. 120

   B. 300

   C. 1,200

   D. 3,000

$9 - 7\ 3/8$

5. Find the difference. Which of the following is
correct?

   A. 1 3/8

   B. 1 5/8

   C. 2 3/8

   D. 25/8

6. Which of the following is 5.4% of 35?

   A. 0.189

   B. 1.89

   C. 18.9

   D. 189

7. Which of the following fractions represents the
sum of 0.3, 0.6, 0.04, and 0.02?

   A. 3/20

   B. 24/25

   C. 25/24

   D. 3/2

$5/8 + 1\ 7/9 + 3$

8. Simplify the expression above. Which of the
following is correct?

   A. 4 29/72

   B. 4 12/17

   C. 5 7/18

   D. 5 29/72

$8\ 5/8 - 7\ 11/16$

9. Find the difference. Which of the following is
correct?

   A. 3/4

   B. 15/16

   C. 1 1/16

   D. 1 3/4

The attendance at a nursing
convention was 400 members, 75%
of whom voted for an increase in
membership dues.

10. Which of the following is the number of
members who voted for the increase?

   A. 75

   B. 100

   C. 300

   D. 325

The ratio of students who take the bus
to school to the total population of a
high school is 2:5.

11. Which of the following is the percent of students
who take the bus?

   A. 10%

   B. 20%

   C. 40%

   D. 60%

$|2x + 1| = 17$

12. Solve the equation for x. Which of the following
solution sets is correct?

   A. {8, 9}

   B. {-8, 9}

   C. {-9, -8}

   D. {-9, 8}

$5(x - 2)^2 = 125$

13. Solve the equation above for x. Which of the
following solution sets is correct?

   A. {-3, -7}

   B. {-3, 7}

   C. {3, -7}

   D. {3, 7}

> A computer is worth $1,500 at the time of purchase. After 5 years, the computer is outdated and has no monetary value.

14. Assuming the computer's value decreases at a constant rate, which of the following expressions represents the computer's value at any time (t) in years?

A. −300t + 1,500

B. −5t + 1,500

C. −300t + 5

D. −5t + 5

$(x^2 + 4x + 4) - (x^2 - 6x + 9)$

15. Simplify the expression above. Which of the following is correct?

A. 10x + 13

B. 10x − 5

C. −2x + 13

D. −2x − 5

$\sqrt{3}$, 1, 4, −0.8, −3/5

16. Which of the following lists the given values from greatest to least?

A. $\sqrt{3}$, 1, 4, −0.8, −3/5

B. 4, 1, −0.8, −3/5, $\sqrt{3}$

C. 4, $\sqrt{3}$, 1, −3/5, −0.8

D. 4, $\sqrt{3}$, 1, −0.8, −3/5

17. Which of the following expressions appropriately compares 4.67 and 4 1/3?

A. 4.67 < 4 1/3

B. 4 1/3 ≥ 4.67

C. 4.67 = 4 1/3

D. 4 1/3 < 4.67

18. Which of the following lists the values in order from least to greatest?

A. −3, −3/10, 3.3, 3

B. −3/10, −3, 3, 3.3

C. −3, −3/10, 3, 3.3

D. −3/10, 3, −3, 3.3

19. Which of the following is the volume of a rectangular box that has a height of 22.1 cm, a length of 98 cm, and a width of 54 cm? The volume of a rectangular box can be calculated by multiplying length × width × height.

A. 180,000 cm^3

B. 90,000 cm^3

C. 117,000 cm^3

D. 100,000 cm^3

20. The data from a study shows that 30 out of every 100 adults surveyed have alcohol use disorder. At this rate, in a town with 2000 adults, which of the following is how many adults would be expected to have alcohol use disorder?

A. 30

B. 300

C. 600

D. 60

21. If five gallons of paint will cover 2,000 square feet, which of the following is how many gallons of paint that would be needed to paint 30,000 square feet?

A. 15

B. 6,000

C. 400

D. 75

22. A typist can type an average of 1000 words in 15 min. At this rate, which of the following is how many words they could type in 1 hr?

A. 250

B. 15,000

C. 4,000

D. 60,000

23. The length of an envelope is 21 cm rounded to the nearest whole cm. Which of the following is the smallest possible real length of the envelope?

A. 20.5 cm

B. 20.49 cm

C. 21.44 cm

D. 20.6 cm

24. Aarav ran a distance of 5 km in 30 min. Which of the following is their speed in meters (m) per hour (h)?

A. 10,000 m/h

B. 6,000 m/h

C. 300,000 m/h

D. 150 m/h

25. The distance from Chicago, IL to St. Louis, MO is 300 miles. Which of the following is the distance in meters (m) between these two cities? (Note: 1 mile = 1.6 km)

A. 187.5 m

B. 480 m

C. 187,500 m

D. 480,000 m

In a certain city, one block equals 0.25 miles. The city's high school is 4 blocks east of a grocery store. The city's library is 6 blocks east of the grocery store. A student walks to the library after school and then walks to the grocery store a few hours later.

26. Which of the following is the number of miles this student has walked?

A. 1.5 miles

B. 2 miles

C. 2.5 miles

D. 4 miles

Use the line below to answer the question.

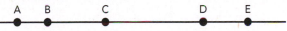

27. The distance between A and E in the graphic below represents 10 km. The distance between B and E, as well as A and D, is 8 km. If the distance between A and C is 4.5 km, which of the following is the distance between B and C?

A. 2.0 km

B. 2.5 km

C. 3.5 km

D. 6.0 km

$10° C = \underline{\hspace{1cm}} ° F$

28. Which of the following completes the equation above? (Note: ° F = [° C × 1.8] + 32)

A. −12.2

B. −1.2

C. 33.8

D. 50.0

29. A student leaves college to drive home for the weekend. Along the way they make one stop to eat lunch. They do not make any other stops. Which of the following graphs represents his trip?

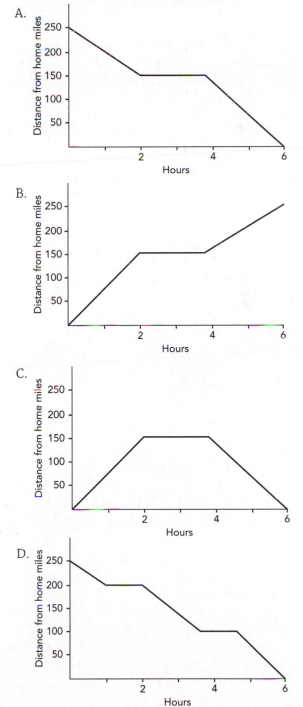

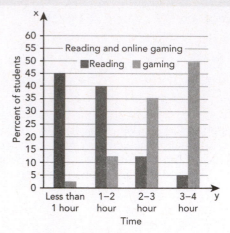

30. The bar graph shows how long teenagers in high school spend reading and online gaming. Which of the following statements is true about the bar graph?

A. Teenagers spend more time online gaming than reading.

B. For up to 1 hr, teenagers spend more time online gaming than reading.

C. Approximately twice as many teenagers spend 3 to 4 hr online gaming compared to teenagers who spend 1 to 2 hr reading.

D. About 9% of teenagers read for 3 to 4 hr.

Use the graph below to answer the question.

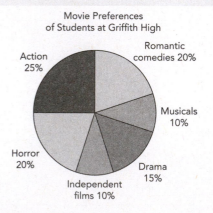

31. Which of the following statements is true about the circle graph?

A. Over half of the students prefer horror movies.

B. More students prefer romantic comedies than independent films.

C. The percent of students who prefer action is the same as the percent who prefer drama.

D. Musicals are the most popular movies among the students.

Use the scatter plot below to answer the question.

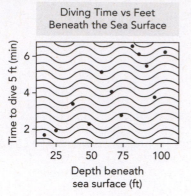

32. A group of researchers studied the relationship between the depth of a diver beneath the sea surface and the time it takes that diver to descend 5 additional feet. Which of the following statements describes the relationship between the two variables represented in the scatter plot?

A. As the depth increases, diving time decreases.

B. There is a positive correlation between depth and 5-foot diving time.

C. As the depth increases, there is no effect on diving time.

D. There is a negative correlation between depth and 5-foot diving time.

SCIENCE

1. In which of the following areas does protein breakdown begin in the human body?

   A. Mouth

   B. Stomach

   C. Small intestine

   D. Large intestine

2. Which of the following cell types is responsible for the production of soluble antibodies?

   A. Cytotoxic T cell

   B. Macrophage cell

   C. Helper T cell

   D. B cell

3. Which of the following organ systems is responsible for transporting nutrients, wastes, and other substances throughout the human body?

   A. Respiratory

   B. Immune

   C. Nervous

   D. Circulatory

4. Which of the following is characteristic of the human organism?

   A. Autotrophic with a genome stored in DNA

   B. Heterotrophic with a genome stored in DNA

   C. Autotrophic with a genome stored in RNA

   D. Heterotrophic with a genome stored in RNA

5. Which of the following is the function of the lymph nodes in mammals?

   A. Pump oxygen into tissue spaces

   B. Store extra glucose for emergencies

   C. Synthesize hemoglobin for erythrocytes

   D. Filter debris from intracellular spaces

6. The bands in muscle sarcomere are formed by actin and which of the following other proteins?

   A. Myosin

   B. Dynein

   C. Keratin

   D. Myofibril

7. Which of the following structures within a human cell is responsible for recycling the materials no longer functional or needed within the cell?

   A. Ribosome

   B. Lysosome

   C. Mitochondrion

   D. Nucleolus

8. Which of the following is the correct structure and function of the cell membrane?

   A. A double glycoprotein structure with embedded lipid bodies provides shape and rigidity to the cytoplasm.

   B. A double layer of phosphate proteins with lipid channels allows molecules to pass from the inside to the outside of cells.

   C. Nonpolar phosphate heads and polar lipid tails form a bilayer to control the transport of proteins.

   D. A phospholipid bilayer with embedded proteins regulates molecules entering and leaving cytoplasm.

9. Which of the following chemical compounds prevents the lungs from collapsing?

   A. Mucus

   B. Surfactant

   C. Enzymes

   D. Buffers

10. Which of these structures diverts food into the esophagus and prevents it from entering the lungs?

    A. Uvula

    B. Soft palate

    C. Tonsils

    D. Epiglottis

11. Which of the following terms related to the respiratory system refers to the "voice box" for sound production?

    A. Pharynx

    B. Trachea

    C. Larynx

    D. Uvula

12. Which of the following appropriately completes the below statement?

   Unlike skeletal muscle, cardiac muscle is highly resistant to lactate-mediated fatigue because cardiac muscle

   A. uses aerobic respiration in mitochondria for energy.

   B. operates with electrical energy supplied by the sinoatrial (SA) node.

   C. primarily metabolizes glucose using the fermentation pathway.

   D. does not need oxygen for the production of energy.

13. Which of the following arteries directly supplies oxygenated blood to the reproductive system?

   A. Common carotid artery

   B. Gonadal artery

   C. Femoral artery

   D. Subclavian artery

14. Which of the following options represents the chromosomal composition of a normal human zygote?

   A. 23 chromosomes

   B. 46 chromosomes

   C. 69 chromosomes

   D. 92 chromosomes

15. Which of the following produces progesterone to prepare the uterus for pregnancy?

   A. Endometrium

   B. Cervix

   C. Corpus luteum

   D. Fallopian tubes

16. Which of the following cell types provides a waterproofing function for the outer layers of skin?

   A. Melanocytes

   B. Keratinocytes

   C. Merkel cells

   D. Langerhans cells

17. Subcutaneous fat can be found in which of the following layers of the skin in the human body?

   A. Epidermis

   B. Dermis

   C. Hypodermis

   D. Dermal papillae

18. Which of the following glands primarily supplies hair shafts and skin with oily secretions?

   A. Eccrine gland

   B. Apocrine gland

   C. Sebaceous gland

   D. Ceruminous gland

19. Which of the following glands is the primary producer of insulin?

   A. Thyroid

   B. Adrenal

   C. Pituitary

   D. Pancreas

20. Type I diabetes is a disease associated with which of the following hormones?

   A. Estrogen

   B. Insulin

   C. Testosterone

   D. Thyroxine

21. Which of the following connects the kidneys to the bladder?

   A. Capillaries

   B. Ureters

   C. Urethra

   D. Arteries

22. Which of the following organs is the site of blood filtration?

   A. Kidneys

   B. Heart

   C. Lungs

   D. Brain

23. Kidneys remove which of the following from the blood?

   A. Platelets

   B. Salts

   C. Oxygen

   D. Fat

24. In which of the following parts of the body do T cells mature?

   A. Bone marrow

   B. Thymus

   C. Adrenal glands

   D. Thyroid

25. Which of the following is classified as a flat bone?

   A. Tarsal

   B. Vertebrae

   C. Rib

   D. Humerus

26. Which of the following connects two bones together?

   A. Ligament

   B. Tendon

   C. Marrow

   D. Muscle

27. Which of the following are sesamoid bones?

   A. Phalanges

   B. Patellae

   C. Scapulae

   D. Metatarsals

28. The shape of villi and microvilli facilitates which of the following?

   A. Pushing food along the intestine via ciliary motion of villi

   B. Creating barriers to food movement to increase digestion time

   C. Decreasing surface area for absorption

   D. Increasing surface area for absorption

29. A person is suddenly frightened. Which of the following reactions occurs next?

   A. Liver cells absorb glucose from the blood stream.

   B. Blood vessels supplying skeletal muscles constrict.

   C. Blood vessels supplying the intestines dilate.

   D. Liver cells release glucose into the blood stream.

30. Which of the following is an example of positive feedback?

   A. Oxytocin causes an increase in uterine muscle contractions, ultimately causing the posterior pituitary to release more oxytocin.

   B. An increase in blood glucose level causes the release of insulin, which results in the lowering of glucose levels in the blood and halting the release of insulin.

   C. A drop in body temperature causes the hypothalamus to activate warming mechanisms, which results in the increase of body temperature.

   D. An increase in blood osmolarity causes the release of ADH, which causes urine to become more concentrated and osmolarity to decrease.

31. Demyelinization results in which of the following?

   A. Inhibited detection of a stimulus at the dendrites of a nerve cell

   B. Disrupted propagation of an action potential along the axon of a nerve cell

   C. Inhibited uptake of neurotransmitters at the synapse of a nerve cell

   D. Disrupted ability of the Na+/K+ pumps to depolarize a cell

32. The nephridium in worms has a function most similar to which of the following organs in humans?

   A. Liver

   B. Spleen

   C. Lymph nodes

   D. Kidney

$Ca + H_2SO_4$

33. Which of the following statements correctly describes the product of the reaction above?

   A. Calcium sulfate

   B. Hydrogen sulfide

   C. Calcium sulfide

   D. Hydrogen sulfate

34. Which of the following classes of biomolecules can influence the rate of specific chemical reactions within the living cell?

   A. Nucleic acids

   B. Proteins

   C. Lipids

   D. Carbohydrates

35. Which of the following terms describes a sample composed of particles condensed into a small space and having vibrational, but not translational, motion?

   A. Solid

   B. Liquid

   C. Gas

   D. Plasma

36. An atom has 3 protons, 4 neutrons, and 3 electrons. Which of the following is the atom's mass number?

   A. 3

   B. 6

   C. 7

   D. 10

37. Which of the following substances will dissolve in water?

   A. CH_4

   B. CCl_4

   C. CH_3OH

   D. C_8H_{18}

On an imaginary planet called Alpha Vega, purple eyes (F) are dominant over pink eyes (f).

38. Which of the following combinations will produce only offspring with pink eyes?

   A. Ff × ff

   B. Ff × Ff

   C. FF × ff

   D. ff × ff

39. A pregnant person who is a chain smoker has just been diagnosed with lung cancer. Their biggest concern is if they have passed on the lung cancer to their child. Which of the following statements is correct regarding this situation?

   A. Children do not use their lungs until they are born, so the cancer cannot pass to the child before birth.

   B. The cancer could pass from birth parent to fetus through blood, but anticancer medications can prevent the child from developing cancer.

   C. If the pregnant parent undergoes treatment for lung cancer, both they and the child can be cured.

   D. The cancer will not be transmitted to the child.

40. In Mendelian inheritance, the dominant allele is for tall plants and the recessive allele is for short plants. Which of the following statements is correct in terms of phenotype and genotype?

   A. Tt is a phenotype that gives 50% short and 50% tall genotype.

   B. TT and Tt are both genotypes for the homozygous recessive phenotype.

   C. TT is the dominant phenotype, and tall plants is the resulting genotype.

   D. TT and Tt are both genotypes for the tall plant phenotype.

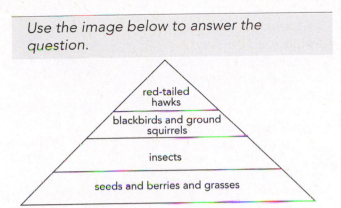

41. Which of the following appropriately completes the statement below?

Based on the scaled figure of a prairie biomass pyramid, there is a greater mass of

A. insects than seeds, berries, and grasses.

B. red-tailed hawks than blackbirds and ground squirrels.

C. seeds, berries, and grasses than insects.

D. blackbirds and ground squirrels than insects.

Two researchers note that when Weeds A and B grow next to each other, the roots of Weed A stop growing when they enter the root zone of Weed B.

Because activated charcoal is known to absorb organic compounds, the researchers apply activated charcoal to the soil around Weed B. They note that the roots of Weed A then grow into the root zone of Weed B.

42. Which of the following hypotheses is being tested by the addition of activated charcoal to the soil?

A. Weed A absorbs activated charcoal, which enhances root growth for Weed A.

B. Weed B grows best in soil that contains few organic compounds.

C. Weed A is attracted to soil that contains activated charcoal.

D. Weed B produces an organic compound that inhibits root growth for Weed A.

43. In a well-controlled experiment, researchers show that a common topical antibiotic called chloramphenicol halts a deadly fungal growth on the skin of amphibians. Which of the following is the best inference for how the antibiotic works to limit a fungal disease?

A. The antibiotic causes a mutation in the skin tissue that makes it resistant to the fungus.

B. The antibiotic acts as a physical barrier that interferes with fungal growth.

C. The antibiotic kills a bacterial partner that is essential in the fungal infection.

D. The antibiotic activates white blood cell production in amphibians.

44. Which of the following appropriately completes the statement below?

A defining characteristic of a scientific hypothesis is that it is

A. testable.

B. unexpected.

C. correct.

D. predictable.

45. Which of the following appropriately completes the statement below?

The use of an electron microscope would most benefit the study of

A. the structure of atoms.

B. the structure of cellular organelles.

C. the structure of skeletal joints.

D. chemical bonds in molecules.

46. Which of the following observations refutes the hypothesis that characteristics acquired during the parents' lifetime are inherited by offspring?

A. Changes in neck length in giraffe populations are due to genetic mutations.

B. Finches that live on different sources of food become unable to mate with one another after many generations.

C. Peppered moths turn from gray to white or black depending on the color of the tree bark on which they live.

D. Primates that have been taught sign language pass that ability to their offspring.

47. In a population that is growing, which of the following must be true?

A. Immigrants + Births = Deaths + Emigrants

B. Emigrants + Deaths > Immigrants + Births

C. Immigrants + Births > Emigrants + Deaths

D. Emigrants + Immigrants = Births + Deaths

ENGLISH AND LANGUAGE USE

The director listens to everyone's opinions. She makes up her own mind. She informs us of her decisions.

1. Assuming that the sentences in the above passage are in chronological order, which of the following sentences correctly restates the passage?

A. Prior to making up her own mind and informing us of her decisions, the director listens to everyone's opinions.

B. Informing us of her decisions, the director listens to everyone's opinions and makes up her own mind.

C. Because she makes up her own mind and informs us of her decisions, the director listens to everyone's opinions.

D. Before listening to everyone's opinions, the director makes up her own mind and informs us of her decisions.

_____ are a power of the executive branch of the United States government.

2. Which of the following words correctly completes the sentence above?

A. Vetos

B. Vetoes

C. Vettos

D. Veitoes

He spoke quickly and tried a new method to persuade _____ to concentrate on ways to improve my company's bottom line.

3. Which of the following options correctly completes the sentence above?

A. me, he started

B. me, He started

C. me; he started

D. me; He started

The chef compiled a list that included these _____ butter, onions, peppers, and various spices.

4. Which of the following options correctly completes the sentence above?

A. groceries:

B. groceries,

C. groceries;

D. groceries

The batter argued with the umpire _____ had called her out.

5. Which of the following pronouns correctly completes the sentence above?

A. that

B. whom

C. which

D. who

Accidents do not just _____ are usually caused by a lack of attention.

6. Which of the following correctly completes the sentence above?

A. happen they

B. happen, they

C. happen; they

D. happen: they

7. Which of the following options is a complete sentence?

   A. Nominating me to serve as secretary of the club.

   B. Nominate me to serve as secretary of the club.

   C. When I am nominated to serve as secretary of the club.

   D. To be nominated to serve as secretary of the club.

On our vacation, we explored ancient architectural ruins, viewed astonishing landscapes, and visited many truely historic sites.

8. Which of the following words is misspelled in the sentence above?

   A. Ancient

   B. Viewed

   C. Truely

   D. Historic

Even in the healthiest of diets, it is permissible to indulge _____ in a favorite dessert.

9. Which of the following options is the appropriate spelling of the word that completes the sentence above?

   A. occasionally

   B. ocasionally

   C. occassionally

   D. occasionaly

In the last 6 months, more than $5 million _____ spent in this ongoing political campaign.

10. Which of the following options correctly completes the sentence above?

    A. are

    B. has been

    C. were

    D. have been

A doctor or a nurse _____ always on duty.

11. Which of the following verbs correctly completes the sentence above?

    A. are

    B. is

    C. were

    D. seem

The class is nervous about ____ first exam.

12. Which of the following options correctly completes the sentence above?

    A. they're

    B. there

    C. it's

    D. its

---

13. Which of the following sentences would likely be found in an informal letter or email?

    A. Those involved will meet with you about appropriate protocol for delivery of the message.

    B. There can be some confusion about the correct placement of the message.

    C. We really don't think there should be a bunch of odds and ends just messing up the message.

    D. A message to finalize preparation and the agenda would benefit all concerned.

Hi, I wanted to let you know that I can't make the meeting tomorrow. I know this is inconvenient but you'll do an awesome job on your own! Don't sweat it about the handouts. I'll email those to your assistant. See you soon!

14. Which of the following is the most likely audience for this passage?

    A. The president of a corporation

    B. A friend at a corporation

    C. A professor at a college

    D. A dean at a college

15. Which of the following sentences in a research paper should include a citation?

    A. This paper summarizes key aspects of supplements to support the immune system.

    B. Numerous studies have been conducted to find ways to improve the immune system.

    C. Several clinics report cases of improved immune system responses.

    D. These results are conclusive of improved immune system, according to Dr. Smith's paper.

16. Kelly is writing a research paper for class. She is keeping a list of the websites and authors from which she is gathering information to include in her paper. Which of the following elements of the writing process is Kelly performing?

    A. Preparing an outline

    B. Writing a draft

    C. Referencing sources

    D. Writing a revision

The giant panda is a rare mammal. It is easily recognizable because of its distinctive black-and-white markings. The giant panda's diet consists of bamboo stems, leaves, and shoots. It eats about 80 pounds of bamboo every day. Everyone enjoys reading about the giant panda. There are fewer than 1,000 pandas living in the wild.

17. Which of the following sentences does not belong in a well-organized paragraph?

    A. The giant panda is a rare mammal.

    B. It is easily recognizable because of its distinctive black-and-white markings.

    C. Everyone enjoys reading about the giant panda.

    D. There are fewer than 1,000 pandas living in the wild.

Soybean oil contains a high percentage of polyunsaturated fatty acids. Polyunsaturated fats are required for normal bodily functions. Dietitians recommend replacing saturated fats with polyunsaturated fatty acids.

18. Which of the following topic sentences should be added to the paragraph above?

    A. Soybeans are grown in many states.

    B. Soybeans are a good source for important fats.

    C. Soybeans are a good source of nutritional fiber.

    D. Soybeans are high in fat and should not be eaten.

The doctor's message was cryptic because of her poor handwriting.

19. Which of the following words describes the connotative meaning of the word "cryptic" as it is used in the sentence above?

    A. Rewritten

    B. Occult

    C. Illegible

    D. Terse

He typically avoided the local theater because he found its productions to be banal interpretations of over-performed plays.

20. Which of the following is the meaning of "banal" as used in the sentence above?

    A. Confusing

    B. Ostentatious

    C. Bland

    D. Practiced

> *The doctor prescribed physical therapy so that the muscles in the athlete's injured leg would not atrophy while she was healing.*

21. Which of the following phrases is an antonym for the word "atrophy" as used in the sentence above?

    A. Become infected

    B. Increase in size

    C. Weaken gradually

    D. Injure through over-exertion

22. Based on the two parts of the word "circumlocution," which of the following definitions is correct?

    A. Meandering expedition

    B. Roundabout way of speaking

    C. Type of geometrical pattern

    D. Remote destination

23. A can of chemicals has the word "antidote" on the label providing information and directions. Which of the following is the definition of "antidote" in this context?

    A. An ingredient that is present in the chemicals

    B. A contraindication for the use of the chemicals

    C. An appropriate place to store the chemicals when not in use

    D. A substance that counteracts the effects of the chemicals

> *The client was diagnosed as having dysesthesia.*

24. Which of the following is the definition of "dysesthesia" in this context?

    A. Pleasant reaction to touch

    B. Painful reaction to touch

    C. Normal reaction to touch

    D. No reaction to touch

Practice Test Answers

READING

1. A. While this is mentioned in the passage, it does not provide the best support for the argument that bards were an important element in sustaining Celtic civilization.

   B. While this is mentioned in the passage, it does not provide the best support for the argument that bards were an important element in sustaining Celtic civilization.

   C. While this is mentioned in the passage, it does not provide the best support for the argument that bards were an important element in sustaining Celtic civilization.

   D. **CORRECT.** This detail regarding bards' involvement in passing on information about events and people best supports the idea that bards were an important element in sustaining Celtic civilization.

2. A. While the passage mentions the bard's importance in sustaining Celtic civilization, the topic of the passage is the history and purpose of bards.

   B. **CORRECT.** The passage explains the place, purpose, and historical significance of bards and the oral traditions they practiced.

   C. The passage discusses the role of bards in passing on the legends of King Arthur, but this is a supporting detail.

   D. The passage discusses the purpose of barding schools to train bards, but this is a supporting detail.

3. A. **CORRECT.** The passage provides general information about the history and purpose of bards in Celtic culture.

   B. The passage is not attempting to make a persuasive argument but is providing general information about bards.

   C. The passage is not a narrative intended to entertain, but a collection of facts about bards in Celtic culture.

   D. The passage is providing general historical information about bards and does not make critical judgments about bards.

4. A. The last sentence of the first paragraph indicates that local food can be grown with or without chemicals.

   B. The definition of organic foods is based on growing methods rather than distribution proximity.

   C. **CORRECT.** The passage indicates that there is an increasing number of people buying local food and that one of the benefits of buying local food is knowing where it is grown. Therefore, it is a logical conclusion that more consumers want to know where their food is grown.

   D. There is no information in the passage to indicate that farmers markets provide a greater diversity of food products than grocery stores.

5. A. **CORRECT.** The notion of what is worrisome is subjective and implies an opinion.

   B. The information in this statement can be factually verified and is not an opinion.

   C. The information in this statement can be factually verified and is not an opinion.

   D. The information in this statement can be factually verified and is not an opinion.

6. A. The passage focuses on locally, not organically, grown food.

   B. While the author indicates that it is worrisome when people do not know where their food comes from, this is a supporting detail rather than the author's primary purpose.

   C. This could be inferred from the passage, but it is not the author's primary purpose.

   D. **CORRECT.** The passage supports the two ideas stated in this option: that locally grown food is more available now and that consuming locally grown food is beneficial.

7. A. While this might be true, there is no information in the passage that supports this inference.

   B. This is not true, and there is no information in the passage that supports this inference.

   C. There is no information in the passage that supports this inference.

   D. **CORRECT.** The third sentence in the second paragraph implies that taste and nutrition are less important than the requirements of industrial food production, which include the use of preservatives and altered harvesting and processing practices.

8. A. This is the definition of locavore, but doesn't tell us how we can become more locavorous.

   B. This is a description of why some people might want to become a locavore, but does not tell us how to do it.

   C. **CORRECT.** This explains how we can start avoiding industrial food and become more like a locavore.

   D. This tells us more about the problem of trying to "eat local," but does not tell us how to do it.

9. A. **CORRECT.** While many people visited the Nearings to follow their example, it is a logical conclusion that the Nearings' writings were available to a larger number of people and continue to be available. Also, the last sentence states that their books were credited with spurring the "back to the land" movement.

   B. Community service was considered by the Nearings to be civic work, not bread labor.

   C. The passage indicates that the Nearings developed their own philosophy and that they preceded the "back to the land" movement.

   D. There is nothing in the passage to indicate that the Nearings' parents came from a rural lifestyle.

10. A. Helen was born in 1904. Scott wrote this book with Helen in 1954.

    B. Helen was born in 1904. Blueberries were part of the Nearings' "bread labor" in the years after 1952.

    C. **CORRECT.** Helen was born in 1904. In 1904, Scott would have been 21 years old. The passage states that he was involved in social activism about unsafe working conditions in the coal minds during his early 20s.

    D. Helen was born in 1904. The Nearings began work on building stone and concrete buildings by hand sometime after they met in 1928.

11. A. **CORRECT.** This division of time is the heart of the philosophy that the Nearings pioneered, because it is what allowed them to be self-sufficient.

    B. This was a part of Scott Nearing's life in his early twenties and was not necessarily a part of his philosophy as stated in the text.

    C. Writing books about their self-sufficient lifestyle was a part of the Nearings' lives. However, it was not a key part of their philosophy, as stated in the text.

    D. Moving from New York to Vermont was a part of the Nearings' lives. However, it was not a part of the Nearings' philosophy for a self-sufficient life.

12. A. Scott Nearing protested against coal mining, so he would not campaign in favor of it.

    B. The Nearings believed in a simple lifestyle, so lavish furnishings would not be a part of their home.

    C. The Nearings believed in making their own food at home, so helping to make processed food would not fit into their philosophy.

    D. **CORRECT.** The Nearings made their own food at home, so teaching others how to do this would fit into their philosophy.

13. A. This sentence contains verifiable facts that have been documented.

    B. This sentence contains verifiable facts that have been documented.

    C. **CORRECT.** The notion of what constitutes "the good life" is open to subjective interpretation.

    D. This sentence contains verifiable facts that have been documented. For instance, *Living the Good Life* can be proved to be the most famous of the Nearings' books by the number of book sales.

14. A. This statement helps determine the topic of the passage but does not support the main idea that Gardner's theory had an impact on education.

B. **CORRECT.** This statement is a supporting detail from the passage.

C. This statement helps determine the topic of the passage but does not support the main idea that Gardner's theory had an impact on education.

D. Every sentence in the passage relates to this main idea, so it is not a supporting detail.

15. A. There is nothing in the article that suggests Howard Gardner possessed multiple intelligences.

B. **CORRECT.** The second sentence of the second paragraph indicates that traditional notions of intelligence are largely based on I.Q. testing. Then, the first sentence of the fourth paragraph states that traditional school curricula emphasized learning through the verbal-linguistic and mathematical-logical intelligences.

C. There is nothing in the article to suggest that most teachers prefer to use traditional teaching methods in the classroom.

D. There is nothing in the article to suggest that multiple intelligences are excluded from school curricula because they are difficult to test.

16. A. The passage does not identify any types of multiple intelligence as more important than any other.

B. The passage does not say that cerebral engagement and I.Q. testing are unrelated. Gardner is represented as saying that I.Q. testing does not "sufficiently address the range of cerebral engagement."

C. The passage states that traditional school curriculum in Western culture focuses heavily on verbal-linguistic and logical-mathematical intelligences. This does not represent an accommodation of multiple types of intelligence.

D. **CORRECT.** The key point that the passage makes about Howard Gardner's theory of multiple intelligences is that intelligence cannot be represented by one universal score or measure, but should take into account a broader range of cerebral engagement.

17. A. This does not address the theory of MI.

B. **CORRECT.** Multimedia collaborations allow students who excel in different types of intelligence to adapt projects to their own strengths.

C. This does not address the theory of MI.

D. This does not address the theory of MI.

18. A. **CORRECT.** This student's artistic ability would more likely be identified and nurtured in an educational program that incorporates MI.

B. This student would likely excel in a traditional educational program, as well as in one that incorporates MI.

C. This student would likely excel in a traditional educational program, as well as in one that incorporates MI.

D. This student would likely excel in a traditional educational program, as well as in one that incorporates MI.

19. A. This detail does not support the main idea presented in the passage.

B. This detail does not support the main idea presented in the passage.

C. This is the main idea of the passage, rather than a supporting detail.

D. **CORRECT.** This detail supports the main idea of the passage, which is that football could be considered the new "national pastime" in America.

20. A. **CORRECT.** The author provides supporting details for the argument that football has supplanted baseball as America's "national pastime."

B. This is a supporting detail in the passage rather than the author's main purpose.

C. There are no indications in the passage that the author wants to revive the popularity of baseball.

D. The author does not express personal feelings about the importance of football in American culture.

21. A. **CORRECT.** This combination of flowers corresponds with the directions. Type 5 is chosen, but type 1 is not. Type 3 is chosen, and type 5 is included; type 2 is chosen, and type 6 is included.

    B. To conform to the directions, if type 3 is chosen, then type 5 must also be chosen. This combination is missing type 5.

    C. To conform to the directions, if type 2 is chosen, then type 6 must also be chosen. This combination is missing type 6.

    D. To conform to the directions, if type 1 is chosen, then type 5 cannot be chosen. This combination includes type 5, so it is incorrect.

22. A. This drawing does not correspond with the last step of the directions.

    B. This drawing does not correspond with the second and third steps of the directions.

    C. **CORRECT.** This drawing corresponds with all the directions, including the correct rotation of the figure and placement of the letters.

    D. This drawing does not correspond with all of the directions.

23. A. The announcement states that this is an entry-level position in the call center, so it would not include formulating communications for marketing purposes.

    B. While this company sells medical equipment, previous experience in the health care industry is not listed among the qualifications.

    C. **CORRECT.** This statement is supported by the fact that this is a call center position, which will include communicating on the telephone, and by the fact that "good communication skills" is listed among the qualifications.

    D. The announcement indicates that the company offers flexible work schedules, which include, but do not require, weekend and holiday shifts.

24. A. **CORRECT.** The announcement states that this position includes medical and dental insurance as part of the compensation package.

    B. According to the announcement, this is an hourly, not a salaried, position.

    C. Someone who has previously managed customer service representatives would most likely not want an entry-level position in a call center.

    D. While this company manufactures medical equipment, this particular position would not be involved in working with medical equipment.

25. A. According to the pie chart, game shows, talk shows, and reality shows do not reach as many viewers as sitcoms and primetime dramas.

    B. According to the pie chart, daytime dramas and news do not reach as many viewers as sitcoms and primetime dramas.

    C. **CORRECT.** The pie chart shows that the most viewers watch sitcoms and primetime dramas; therefore, advertising on these programs would reach the most viewers.

    D. According to the pie chart, sports and talk shows do not reach as many viewers as sitcoms and primetime dramas.

26. A. One of the uses listed is to treat minor burns. A heat rash is a minor burn and is treatable by this medication.

    B. **CORRECT.** The warnings on the label instruct not to use the ointment on children under 2 years of age and not to get the medicine in the eyes.

    C. One of the uses listed is to treat minor cuts and scrapes. A knee scrape is treatable by this medication. Additionally, the child is over 2 years of age, so the medication is acceptable.

    D. The label indicates that the medicine can be applied up to four times daily and can be used to treat minor itching.

27. A. Job 1 pays as much as Job 3 and has 2 weeks paid vacation, but only pays partial health insurance coverage.

    B. Job 2 only pays partial health insurance, has the lowest salary, and the least amount of vacation.

    C. **CORRECT.** Job 3 has the same amount of vacation and pays as much as Job 1, but also offers full health insurance, while Job 1 only offers partial health insurance. Additionally, Job 3 has the same benefits as Job 4, but pays $5,000 more.

    D. Job 4 offers full health insurance coverage and 2 weeks paid vacation, but pays less than the others.

28. A. The south side of the lake only has one campground.

    B. **CORRECT.** The majority of the campgrounds are on the north shore of the lake along Highway 22.

    C. There are no campgrounds on the east side of the lake.

    D. The west shore of the lake has one campground at the junction of Highway 22 and 766.

29. A. **CORRECT.** Highway 16 follows the eastern shore of the lake.

    B. Highway 22 runs along the northwestern side of the lake.

    C. Highway 85 runs across the northern side of the lake.

    D. Highway 141 is on the south side of the lake.

30. A. **CORRECT.** Your friend tells you that they have to cook breakfast and shower before they pick you up to go to the grocery store, so you can expect them to pick you up after they shower.

    B. Your friend tells you that they have to cook breakfast and shower before they pick you up to go to the grocery store, so you can expect them to pick you up before they go to the grocery store.

    C. Your friend tells you that they have to cook breakfast and shower before they pick you up to go to the grocery store, so they will not be ready to leave as soon as they hang up the phone.

    D. Your friend tells you that they have to cook breakfast and shower before they pick you up to go to the grocery store, so you can expect them to pick you up after they eat breakfast and showers.

31. A. This does not correctly follow the directions.

    B. This does not correctly follow the directions.

    C. **CORRECT.** This correctly follows the directions. Replacing every 1 with the letter A, every 2 with the letter B, every 3 with the letter D, and every 4 with the letter E results in ABDEDBABDE. The first B and D should be deleted, resulting in AEDBABDE. The first and last letters, A and E, should be deleted, leading to EDBABD. Replacing the vowels with X results in XDBXBD.

    D. This does not correctly follow the directions.

32. A. The passage does not focus on climate change, so this is not the author's primary purpose in the first two sentences.

    B. There is no explicit call to action in the passage.

    C. **CORRECT.** Readers might not be familiar with peak oil, so the author compares it to an environmental issue with which readers will be familiar. This is a method of engaging readers' interest.

    D. A definition of peak oil is not provided until the fourth sentence in the passage.

33. A. **CORRECT.** In the passage, the author compares peak oil to the widely discussed issue of climate change. The passage also states the effects of peak oil as they began in 1971 to 1972. Both the relevance and immediacy of the issue of peak oil indicate the author's view of peak oil as a significant environmental issue.

    B. The passage does not provide any information that should lead the reader to believe that the issue of peak oil is confusing.

    C. The passage states that peak oil is, by definition, the irreversible decline in possible oil production.

    D. The passage does not provide any information about plans or options for avoiding the effects of peak oil.

34. A. The passage does not make any direct connection between the issues of peak oil and climate change.

B. The passage does not make a connection to increased media coverage of peak oil and either improved or reduced oil production.

C. The passage does not make any direct connection between the issues of peak oil and climate change. Hubbert's Curve is defined in the passage as a way to understand the idea of peak oil, but it does not make any connection between this theory and climate change.

D. **CORRECT.** The passage discusses the comparative lack of general public awareness of the issue of peak oil. It goes on to provide information about reaching and passing the point of peak oil.

35. A. This definition does not fit the context of the sentence.

B. This definition does not fit the context of the sentence.

C. **CORRECT.** One of the definitions of "fast" is something that is obtained with little effort, often by unsavory means. This definition fits the context of the sentence.

D. This definition does not fit the context of the sentence.

36. A. The organization of this outline provides no information regarding the relative similarity of marsupials, primates, and rodents. All three are listed at the same level of the hierarchy.

B. Rodents is another name for Rodentia, which is indicated by the parentheses. If rodents were a subcategory of Rodentia, the term would be listed below Rodentia and indented.

C. If wombats were a subcategory of koalas, the term would be indented below koalas.

D. **CORRECT.** The outline groups squirrels with porcupines within the rodent order. Therefore, squirrels must be more similar to porcupines than to monkeys, which are within the primate order.

37. A. This definition does not fit with the context of the sentence.

B. This definition does not fit with the context of the sentence.

C. **CORRECT.** This definition fits with the context of the sentence.

D. This definition does not fit with the context of the sentence.

38. A. Pelecypoda and Gastropoda are at the same level in the outline; therefore, Pelecypoda is not a type of Gastropoda.

B. Octopuses and squids are at the same level in the outline; therefore, an octopus is not a type of squid.

C. The outline does not provide information on the degree of relation among Cephalopoda, Gastropoda, and Pelecypoda.

D. **CORRECT.** Snails and sea slugs are both within the Gastropoda class; therefore, they are more closely related than clams, which are in the Pelecypoda class.

39. A. This definition does not fit the context of the sentence, as one cannot teach a plant to make it qualified.

B. **CORRECT.** This definition is most appropriate, as the context of the sentence implies that the gardener wishes to direct the growth of the grapevine along the house.

C. This definition does not fit the context of the sentence.

D. This definition does not fit the context of the sentence, as a plant cannot be motivated.

40. A. The word in the sentence is a verb, not a noun, because it is an action she is performing.

B. The word in the sentence is a verb, not a noun, because it is an action she is performing.

C. **CORRECT.** It is possible to strike a pencil with one's hand, and this definition makes sense in the context of the sentence.

D. This definition does not make sense in the context of the sentence, as it would be impossible to "blink" a pencil away.

41. A. **CORRECT.** "Complacent" means "self-contented, smug, unconcerned."

B. This word is not the meaning of "complacent." "Dissatisfied" is the opposite of "complacent."

C. This word is not the meaning of "complacent." If Natalia were confident about her routine, her workout shoes would be in use much more.

D. This word is not the meaning of "complacent." If Natalia were worried about her routine, she would already be aware of the state of her running shoes.

42. A. An encyclopedia is a book or a set of books providing information on a range of alphabetically organized topics; it would not be the most helpful source in this situation.

B. An almanac is an annual publication containing calendar information, information about natural phenomena, and/or interesting facts; it would not be the most helpful source in this situation.

C. A style guide is a set of standards for writing that is usually specific to an organization or a purpose; it would not be the most helpful source in this situation.

D. **CORRECT.** A thesaurus is a dictionary of synonyms and antonyms, which would be helpful for a writer trying to use a greater variety of words.

43. A. This passage is about the popularity of YA novels, but it is a nonfiction piece, and novels are fictional.

B. This does not explain how to write a YA novel, or YA movie, so this does not fit.

C. Book reviews focus on just one book, and this passage refers to a type of literature in general without citing specific books.

D. **CORRECT.** Because the passage discusses two different forms of entertainment (books and movies) and has a more casual style, this is the best option.

44. A. There are more YA novels now than ever before, but that is not the focus of the passage.

B. The YA novel is not new, so this answer does not fit.

C. YA novels' success has only increased in the last 20 years, so this does not fit.

D. **CORRECT.** Because reinventing the existing genre is similar to redesigning an existing car, this answer fits best.

45. A. Conjecture by conspiracy theorists is not considered proof in an academic textbook, so a history textbook would not include it.

B. **CORRECT.** This sentence is about the big picture and the consequences after the President's death, so it would be appropriate for a history textbook.

C. This might be true, but it takes a personal look at the events of the assassination from Jacqueline Kennedy's perspective, while a history textbook would look at how the events affected the nation as a whole.

D. This might be true, but it changes focus from the assassination of Kennedy to biographical information about the family today and is unlikely to be found in a paragraph about the assassination and the Warren Commission as related to United States history.

46. A. Kennedy was killed in 1963, so this might tell a student about the after-effects, but not about the assassination.

B. Because this refers to Oswald as a conspirator, it might be about conspiracy theories and not provide objective, reliable information.

C. This article reveals in its title a bias that Kennedy brought on his own death, so it does not offer an objective view of the events.

D. **CORRECT.** This article offers historical information about the day of Kennedy's assassination, so a student can expect the main topic to be the factual events of the assassination.

47. A. This would be a good source for obtaining general information about the topic, but encyclopedias do not usually include statistical data.

B. **CORRECT.** An academic research paper about a specific subject – hours spent on homework each night – is likely to include statistical data.

C. This would be a good source for gathering anecdotal evidence or an opinion about homework, but is not likely to include statistical data.

D. This would be a good source for discovering teachers' perspectives on homework assignments, but is not likely to include statistical data.

MATHEMATICS

1. A. This is not the correct decimal placement for the numerical conversion of this percentage. 425% is 425 out of 100, which would have a value greater than 1. This decimal is 425 ten-thousandths.

    B. This is not the correct decimal placement for the numerical conversion of this percentage. 425% is 425 out of 100, which would have a value greater than 1. This decimal is 425 thousandths.

    C. **CORRECT.** When converting a percentage to the numeric equivalent, it is correct to divide by 100.

    D. This is not the correct decimal placement for the numerical conversion of this percentage. 425% is 425 out of 100, which would have a value greater than 1. This decimal is 425 whole numbers. You would need to divide 425 by 100 to convert to a decimal.

2. A. According to the equation, each 1/3 inch of height adds 2/9 inch to the crutch length.

    B. According to the equation, each 1 inch of height adds 2/3 inch to the crutch length.

    C. According to the equation, each 2 inches of height adds 1 1/3 inches to the crutch length.

    D. **CORRECT.** According to the equation, each 3 inches of height adds 2 inches to the crutch length ($2/3 \times 3 = 2$).

3. A. This is the sum of the left column of the table, not the total number of hot dogs purchased.

    B. This is the total number of customers, not the total number of hot dogs purchased.

    C. This number results from adding across the rows and then adding those totals. This is not the correct method to determine the total number of hot dogs purchased.

    D. **CORRECT.** To obtain the total number of hot dogs purchased, the numbers in the rows of the table should be multiplied and then the resulting products should be added.
    $1 \times 50 = 50$
    $2 \times 27 = 54$
    $3 \times 15 = 45$
    $4 \times 6 = 24$
    $5 \times 2 = 1050 + 54 + 45 + 24 + 10 = 183$

4. A. This is less than the actual total and represents an incorrect method for determining the total based on a percent. This results from doubling the amount of red mailboxes, or assuming that they represented 50% of the neighborhood.

    B. This is less than the actual total and represents an incorrect method for determining the total based on a percent. The amount of red mailboxes, 60, represents 5% of the total number of houses in the neighborhood. There are 20 groups of 5% in 100%, or the total number of houses. Multiplying 60 by 5 only results in 25% of the neighborhood.

    C. **CORRECT.** To determine the total number of houses, take the number of red mailboxes, 60, and divide by the numerical equivalent of the percent, 0.05. The total is 1,200 houses.

    D. This is more than the actual total and represents an incorrect method for determining the total based on a percent. This results from dividing 60 by 0.02, which would only be 2% of the houses in the neighborhood.

5. A. This represents an error in the subtraction of mixed numbers. The value 9 can be written as 8 8/8. So, 8 8/8 – 7 3/8 = 1 5/8.

    B. **CORRECT.** This expression can be rewritten as:
    9 – (7 + 3/8) =
    9 – 7 – 3/8 =
    2 – 3/8 =
    16/8 – 3/8 = 13/8 = 1 5/8

    C. This represents an error in the subtraction of mixed numbers. The value 9 can be written as 8 8/8. So, 8 8/8 – 7 3/8 = 1 5/8.

    D. This represents an error in the subtraction of mixed numbers. The value 9 can be written as 8 8/8. So, 8 8/8 – 7 3/8 = 1 5/8.

6. A. This represents incorrect placement of the decimal. The correct multiplication is 0.054 × 35.

    B. **CORRECT.** To calculate the percent of a number, multiple 35 by the decimal equivalent of 5.4%, 0.054. This product equals 1.89.

    C. This represents incorrect placement of the decimal. The correct multiplication is 0.054 × 35.

    D. This represents incorrect placement of the decimal. The correct multiplication is 0.054 × 35.

7. A. This is less than the actual amount and represents improper addition of the decimals.

   B. **CORRECT.** The total of these numbers is 0.96, which is equivalent to 96/100. This fraction can be simplified to 24/25.

   C. This is more than the actual amount and represents improper conversion from a decimal to a fraction.

   D. This is more than the actual amount and represents improper addition of the decimals.

8. A. This represents an error in simplifying a mixed number.

   B. This represents an incorrect method for adding mixed numbers.

   C. This represents an error in simplifying a mixed number.

   D. **CORRECT.** When adding mixed numbers, first find the least common denominator for the fractions. This produces the following expression.
   45/72 + 1 56/72 + 3.
   This equals 4 101/72, which can be simplified to 5 29/72.

9. A. This represents an incorrect method for subtracting mixed numbers.
   8 5/8 is equal to 7 26/16.
   So, 7 26/16 – 7 11/16 = 15/16.

   B. **CORRECT.** When subtracting mixed numbers, first find the least common denominator for the fractions. This produces the following expression:
   8 10/16 – 7 11/16.
   Since 10/16 is less than 11/16, change the mixed numbers to improper fractions and subtract.
   138/16 – 123/16 = 15/16.

   C. This represents an incorrect method for subtracting mixed numbers.
   8 5/8 is equal to 7 26/16.
   So, 7 26/16 – 7 11/16 = 15/16.

   D. This represents an incorrect method for subtracting mixed numbers.
   8 5/8 is equal to 7 26/16.
   So, 7 26/16 – 7 11/16 = 15/16.

10. A. This represents an error in determining the number of members who voted for the increase in dues.

    B. This represents an error in determining the number of members who voted for the increase in dues.

    C. **CORRECT.** To find the number of members who voted for the increase in dues, take the total number (400) and multiply by the numerical equivalent of 75% (0.75). This equals 300.

    D. This represents an error in determining the number of members who voted for the increase in dues.

11. A. This represents a misinterpretation of the ratio.

    B. This represents an improper method for converting this ratio to a percent.

    C. **CORRECT.** To convert from a ratio to percent, divide the first number, 2, by the second number, 5. This equals 0.4, which is the equivalent of 40%.

    D. This represents an improper method for converting this ratio to a percent.

12. A. These numbers do not both make the equation true.

    B. These numbers do not both make the equation true.

    C. These numbers do not both make the equation true.

    D. **CORRECT.** Both of these numbers can be substituted for x to make the equation true.

13. A. This is not the correct solution set.

    B. **CORRECT.** Either of these numbers makes the equation true:
    $(x - 2)^2 = 125/5$
    $(x - 2)^2 = 25$
    $x = 7$ or $x = -3$

    C. This is not the correct solution set.

    D. This is not the correct solution set.

14. A. **CORRECT.** The value of the computer at the time of purchase was $1,500. Five years later, the computer's value was $0. This means the computer's value decreased by $1,500/5 or $300 each year.

B. This expression does not yield a value of $0 after t = 5 years.

C. This expression does not yield an initial value (t = 0 years) of $1,500, nor a value of $0 after t = 5 years.

D. This expression does not yield an initial value (t = 0 years) of $1,500.

15. A. This represents an error in simplifying the expression. This is the result of adding the 4 and 9, rather than subtracting and finding the difference.

B. **CORRECT.**
$(x^2 + 4x + 4) - (x^2 - 6x + 9) =$
$x^2 + 4x + 4 - x^2 + 6x - 9 =$
$10x - 5$

C. This represents an error in simplifying the expression. Subtracting −6x from 4x is the same as adding 6x and 4x, resulting in a sum of 10x, rather than a difference of −2x.

D. This represents an error in simplifying the expression. Subtracting −6x from 4x is the same as adding 6x and 4x, resulting in a sum of 10x, rather than a difference of −2x.

16. A. This order is incorrect because 4 is the greatest positive number and should come first.

B. This order is incorrect because it is not in decreasing order. √3 is a positive number and would have a greater value than −0.8, −3/5, and 1.

C. **CORRECT.** This order is correct because √3 is approximately 1.7, which is between 4 and 1. The number 4 is the greatest positive, and therefore the greatest value. The value −0.8 is less than −3/5 because it is further from 0 in the negative direction.

D. This order is incorrect because it is not listed from greatest to least. In comparing the two negative numbers, −3/5 has a decimal value of −0.6. The value −0.8 is less than −3/5 because it is further from 0 in the negative direction.

17. A. 4.67 is greater than 4 1/3 (≈ 4.33), not less than.

B. 4 1/3 (≈ 4.33) is less than 4.67. It is neither greater than nor equal to 4.67.

C. 4.67 is not equal to 4 1/3 (≈ 4.33).

D. **CORRECT.** 4 1/3 (≈ 4.33) is less than 4.67.

18. A. This order is incorrect. 3.3 is greater than 3.

B. This is incorrect because −3/10 is greater than −3. With negative numbers, the closer it is to zero, the greater its value.

C. **CORRECT.** When ordering these values from least to greatest, the negative value that is the furthest from 0 should come first and the positive number that is the furthest from 0 should come at the end of the list.

D. This is incorrect because −3 is the furthest negative number from zero and has the least value; therefore, it should appear first in the list, ahead of other negative values.

19. A. This is incorrect, because it is obtained by rounding all values up instead of applying rounding rules.

B. This is incorrect, because it is obtained by rounding all values down instead of applying rounding rules.

C. This is incorrect, because it is the correct volume rounded to the nearest thousand. It is not an estimation.

D. **CORRECT.** If 22.2 is rounded to 20, 98 is rounded to 100, and 54 is rounded to 50, 20 × 100 × 50 = 100,000.

20. A. This is the numerator of the rate of alcohol use disorder.

B. This is 30% of 1000, not 30% of 2000.

C. **CORRECT.** A correctly set up proportion might look like 30 alcohol users/100 adults = x/2000 adults. Multiplying both sides by 2000 adults will give (30 alcohol users × 2000 adults)/100 adults = x. Simplifying the left side leads to x = 600 expected alcohol users.

D. Instead of multiplying the results by 20, because the new population is 20 times greater than the original survey population, this incorrect answer is found by doubling the numerator of the rate of alcohol use disorder.

21. A. The larger area is 15 times greater; therefore, the paint quantity needs to be 15 times larger.

B. This number does not take into account the number of square feet 5 gallons of paint can cover.

C. This is the number of square feet 1 gallon covers.

D. **CORRECT.** This can be calculated by 5 gallons/2,000 ft^2 × 30,000 ft^2.

22. A. The number of words per hour must be larger than the number of words in 15 min.

B. This is the product of 15 min and 1,000 words.

C. **CORRECT.**
1,000 words/15 min = x words/60 min
x = 4,000 words.
This can also be calculated by multiplying 1,000 by 4, because the time duration is 4 times longer.

D. This would be true if the typist could type 1,000 words per min.

23. A. **CORRECT.** The value 20.5 rounded to the nearest whole cm is 21 cm and is the smallest possible length.

B. The value 20.49 rounded to the nearest whole cm is 20 cm.

C. The value 21.44 rounded to the nearest whole cm would be 21 cm; however, this is the largest possible length.

D. The value 20.6 rounded to the nearest whole cm is 21 cm; however, this is greater than 20.5 cm and is not the smallest possible length.

24. A. **CORRECT.** To determine the rate per hour, 5 km per 30 min is multiplied by 2, resulting in 10 km/hr. Multiplying this by 1,000 m/km converts the units to m/hr, resulting in 10,000 m/hr.

B. This results from dividing 30 min by 5 km, finding an incorrect rate of 6 min per kilometer. This was then multiplied by 1,000 m/km, to correctly convert kilometers to meters.

C. This results from correctly converting kilometers to meters by multiplying 5 km by 1,000 m/km, resulting in 5,000 meters per half hour. This value is then multiplied by 60 min, without considering that the rate is per half-hour, and not per minute.

D. This results from multiplying 5 km by 30 min, without considering the unit conversion of kilometers to meters.

25. A. This represents an incorrect method for setting up the proportion.

B. $\dfrac{300 \text{ miles}}{1.6 \text{ km}} = \dfrac{1 \text{ mile}}{x}$

x = 480 km
The value of x is not given in the requested units.

C. This represents an incorrect method for setting up the proportion.

D. **CORRECT.**
$\dfrac{300 \text{ miles}}{1.6 \text{ km}} = \dfrac{1 \text{ mile}}{x}$

x = 480 km = 480,000 m

26. A. This distance corresponds to six blocks, which is not the correct number of blocks that the student walked.

B. **CORRECT.** The student first walks two blocks east to the library, and then walks six blocks west to the grocery store for a total of eight blocks. Eight blocks times 0.25 miles per block equals 2 miles. The street is laid out as follows:
Grocery store (4 blocks) High school (2 blocks) Library

C. This distance corresponds to 10 blocks, which is not the correct number of blocks that the student walked.

D. This distance corresponds to 16 blocks, which is not the correct number of blocks that the student walked.

27. A. Although this is the distance between A and B, as well as D and E, it is not the distance between B and C.

B. **CORRECT.** Because the distance between A and E is 10 km and the distance between B and E is 8 km, then the distance between A and B is 2 km. Because the distance between A and C is 4.5 km and the distance between A and B is 2 km, the distance between B and C must be 2.5 km.

C. Although this is the distance between C and D, it is not the distance between B and C.

D. Although this is the distance between B and D, it is not the distance between B and C.

28. A. This value does not correctly complete the equation.

B. This value does not correctly complete the equation.

C. This value does not correctly complete the equation.

D. **CORRECT.** $(10° C \times 1.8) + 32 = 18 + 32 = 50.0° F$

29. A. **CORRECT.** This graph shows that at the beginning of the trip, the student had 250 miles to travel. After 2 hr, they stopped for 2 hr. Then they finished the drive home.

B. This graph indicates that the student did not end up at home.

C. This graph indicates that the student's net distance traveled is zero miles.

D. This graph indicates two stops during the trip, which is incorrect.

30. A. **CORRECT.** The blue bars get taller as more hours apply and the red bars get smaller as more hours apply. This means teenagers spend more time online gaming than reading.

B. The opposite is true.

C. For this to be true, because 50% of teenagers spend 3 to 4 hr online gaming, 25% of teenagers would have to spend 1 to 2 hr reading. The graph shows that 40% of teenagers spend 1 to 2 hr reading.

D. About 5% of the teenagers spend 3 to 4 hr reading.

31. A. Only 20% of the students prefer horror films, which is less than half.

B. **CORRECT.** This is correct, because 20% is greater than 10%.

C. This is incorrect, because 15% is less than 25%.

D. Musicals are preferred by the smallest percent of students.

32. A. As the depth increases, diving time also increases.

B. **CORRECT.** As the depth increases, diving time also increases. A positive correlation means that as one variable increases, the other one does as well.

C. As the depth increases, diving time also increases.

D. As the depth increases, diving time also increases. A negative correlation means that as one variable increases, the other variable decreases.

SCIENCE

1. A. Carbohydrate digestion starts in the mouth, but protein breakdown does not.

B. **CORRECT.** The stomach is the first place in the digestive system in which proteinases are produced.

C. Protein breakdown continues in the small intestine, but it does not start here.

D. Protein is generally digested by the time it enters the large intestine.

2. A. Cytotoxic T cells destroy pathogens and infected cells.

B. Macrophages ingest and digest both non–self cells and dead cells.

C. Helper T cells help cytotoxic T cells and other immune cells.

D. **CORRECT.** The production of antibodies by B cells is part of the humoral response to antigens.

3. A. The respiratory system exchanges gases with the outside environment, bringing oxygen in and letting carbon dioxide out.

B. The immune system protects the body from pathogens (infectious agents) using a combination of white blood cells and antibodies.

C. The nervous system, which includes the brain, spinal cord, and peripheral nerves, controls the actions of other body systems.

D. **CORRECT.** The heart pumping blood through the arteries, capillaries, and veins provides the means of transporting substances throughout the body.

4. A. Humans consume rather than manufacture nutrient molecules.

B. **CORRECT.** Humans consume rather than manufacture nutrient molecules (heterotrophic), and human genes are encoded in DNA.

C. Humans consume rather than manufacture nutrient molecules, and human genes are encoded in DNA.

D. Human genes are encoded in DNA.

5. A. This is not a function of the lymph nodes. Oxygen diffuses to these areas from capillaries of the circulatory system.

   B. This is not a function of the lymph nodes. Glucose is stored as glycogen in the liver and muscles of mammals.

   C. This is not a function of the lymph nodes. Hemoglobin is synthesized in the red blood cells.

   D. **CORRECT.** Lymph nodes filter debris, lymphocytes, and pathogens from intracellular fluid.

6. A. **CORRECT.** Myosin contains "heads" that contact actin and pull the actin fibers together in an ATP-dependent mechanism that causes muscles to contract.

   B. Dynein is an ATP-dependent molecule that "walks" along microtubules, causing them to move, but it is not part of the sarcomere.

   C. Keratin is the fibrous protein of hair and nails and is not part of the sarcomere.

   D. Sarcomeres are located in the myofibril.

7. A. The ribosome is not involved in recycling materials that are no longer functional or needed.

   B. **CORRECT.** Lysosomes are specialized vacuoles containing digestive enzymes.

   C. Mitochondria function in cellular respiration, facilitating the production of ATP.

   D. The nucleolus functions in the assembly of ribosomes.

8. A. The double structure is not composed of glycoprotein.

   B. The double layer is not composed of phosphate proteins.

   C. The heads are polar and the tails are nonpolar; molecules pass through protein channels.

   D. **CORRECT.** The cell membrane consists of a phospholipid bilayer with polar phosphate heads, nonpolar lipid tails, and embedded proteins, which permit the movement of molecules across the membrane.

9. A. Mucin is a type of mucus produced by lung cells that absorbs water.

   B. **CORRECT.** Surfactants are lipopolysaccharides that have a hydrophobic and hydrophilic layer. They keep the lungs inflated.

   C. Enzymes are a catalytic protein and do not prevent the lungs from collapsing.

   D. Buffers maintain acid–base balance and are not involved in lung function.

10. A. The uvula is found in the back of the throat and prevents food entry into the nasal passages.

    B. The soft palate is found in the back of the buccal cavity. It helps in swallowing and prevents food entry into the nasal passages.

    C. The tonsils are made of lymphatic tissue that does not typically interfere with food movement.

    D. **CORRECT.** The epiglottis shuts off the tracheal opening, diverting food into the esophagus.

11. A. The pharynx is the muscular region at the intersection of the respiratory and digestive systems, not the voice box.

    B. The trachea is the large tube containing cartilaginous rings through which air passes into and out of the lungs.

    C. **CORRECT.** The larynx is a cartilaginous structure containing the vocal chords, which is used to generate sound.

    D. The uvula is a fleshy extension of the back of the soft palate, hanging above the throat. It does not function in the production of sound.

12. A. **CORRECT.** Aerobic respiration (oxidative respiration) is almost exclusively used by the heart. The byproducts of this type of respiration are water (H_2O) and carbon dioxide (CO_2), not lactate.

    B. The sinoatrial (SA) node, also known as the pacemaker, produces electrical impulses for heart contraction. It does not provide energy to the heart.

    C. The lactose-producing fermentation pathway operates during oxygen deprivation in the skeletal muscle. It does not primarily operate in the heart.

    D. The heart is highly sensitive to oxygen deprivation and requires a steady oxygen supply for adenosine triphosphate (ATP) production by oxidative phosphorylation during aerobic respiration.

13. A. The common carotid artery supplies oxygenated blood to the head.

B. **CORRECT.** The gonadal artery is the primary artery that supplies oxygenated blood to the gonads and male reproductive system. It is called the testicular artery in males and the ovarian artery in females.

C. The femoral artery supplies oxygenated blood to the lower limbs.

D. The subclavian artery supplies oxygenated blood to the upper limbs.

14. A. The unfertilized egg and the sperm each contain 23 chromosomes. This is the haploid chromosome number for a human.

B. **CORRECT.** The fusion of a sperm with 23 chromosomes and an egg with 23 chromosomes would result in a zygote with 46 chromosomes.

C. 69 chromosomes represent the fusion of a diploid human cell with a haploid human cell. This is not the diploid chromosome number for the average human zygote.

D. 92 chromosomes represent the fusion of two diploid human cells. This is not the chromosome number for the average human zygote.

15. A. The endometrium is the highly vascularized tissue of the uterine lining. It does not produce progesterone following ovulation.

B. The cervix is the external opening of the uterus and does not produce progesterone.

C. **CORRECT.** The corpus luteum refers to the remnant of the graafian follicle. It secretes progesterone to prepare the uterus for the pregnancy.

D. The fallopian tube carries the egg from the ovary to the uterus and does not produce progesterone.

16. A. Melanocytes are pigment cells found in lowest layer of the epidermis of skin, the basal layer. They produce melanin, a pigment that absorbs UV light. They do not provide a waterproofing function for the skin.

B. **CORRECT.** Keratinocytes contain the protein keratin. They are produced in the epidermis and migrate upwards. The tight junctions between cells prevent water entry. They eventually form a layer of dead cells on the skin surface, which produces a waterproofing effect.

C. Merkel cells are integumentary cells that work as mechanoreceptors and sense touch and pressure. They do not provide a waterproofing function for the skin.

D. Langerhans are dendritic cells of the immune system and are found in the lower layers of the epidermis. They immunologically process material that enters through the skin. They do not provide a waterproofing function for the skin.

17. A. The epidermis contains living and dead keratinocytes, melanocytes, as well as dendritic and tactile cells. It does not contain subcutaneous fat.

B. The dermis is a layer of skin that contains blood capillaries, hair shafts, nail roots, and sweat glands. It does not contain subcutaneous fat.

C. **CORRECT.** The hypodermis contains subcutaneous fat as well as deeper blood vessels.

D. Dermal papillae are wavy projections of the dermis into the epidermis that lock the two layers together. It does not contain subcutaneous fat.

18. A. Eccrine, or merocrine, glands are distributed across the surface of the skin and produce a dilute, salty sweat. They do not supply hair shafts and skin with oily secretions.

B. Apocrine glands are usually found in groin and armpits and produce sweat and scent. These glands do not supply hair shafts and skin with oily secretions.

C. **CORRECT.** Sebaceous glands produce sebum, which supplies hair shafts and skin with oily secretions.

D. Ceruminous glands produce a waxy secretion in the ear canals. Although they produce sebum, they do not primarily supply hair shafts and external skin with oily secretions.

19. A. The thyroid gland produces the thyroid hormone.

B. The adrenal glands produce cortisol and stress hormones.

C. The pituitary gland secretes hormones that control other glands.

D. **CORRECT.** The pancreas produces insulin.

20. A. Estrogen production is affected by diseases that harm the uterus and ovaries.

B. **CORRECT.** Type I diabetes is a disease that is caused by the absence of insulin.

C. Testosterone production is affected by diseases that harm the testes.

D. Thyroxine production is associated with goiters and diseases that affect the thyroid gland.

21. A. Capillaries connect veins to arteries.

B. **CORRECT.** Ureters connect the kidney to the bladder.

C. The urethra connect the bladder to the outside of the body.

D. Arteries carry blood away from the heart.

22. A. **CORRECT.** The kidneys filter blood.

B. The heart pumps blood but does not filter it.

C. The lung oxygenates blood but does not filter it.

D. Some drugs can cross the blood–brain barrier, but it does not actually filter the blood.

23. A. Platelets are removed by the spleen and liver.

B. **CORRECT.** Salts are removed by the kidneys.

C. Oxygen is used in every cell in the body, not filtered by the kidneys.

D. Fat in the blood is taken up by cells or metabolized in the liver.

24. A. T cells are produced in the bone marrow, but they are not matured there. B cells are matured in the bone marrow.

B. **CORRECT.** The thymus is the location of maturation for T cells.

C. Adrenal glands produce several hormones, but they do not produce parts of the immune system.

D. The thyroid produces the thyroid hormone.

25. A. The tarsal is a short bone.

B. The vertebrae are irregular bones.

C. **CORRECT.** The rib is a flat bone.

D. The humerus is a long bone.

26. A. **CORRECT.** Ligaments connect bones together.

B. Tendons connect muscle to bones.

C. Marrow is inside the bone and does not connect to other bones.

D. Muscle is not typically a connective tissue.

27. A. Phalanges are long bones because their length is greater than their width.

B. **CORRECT.** Patellae are sesamoid bones, which develop in response to strain. Patellae are also considered short bones.

C. Scapulae are flat bones because they do not have a bone marrow cavity.

D. Metatarsals are long bones because their length is greater than their width.

28. A. Movement of food is aided by smooth muscle contractions, not by villi projections.

B. Movement of food is aided by smooth muscle contractions, not impeded by villi projections.

C. The folds increase the surface area, allowing more nutrients to be absorbed and delivered to the blood stream.

D. **CORRECT.** The folds increase the surface area, allowing more nutrients to be absorbed and delivered to the blood stream.

29. A. Epinephrine causes liver cells to break down glycogen, which causes an increase in sugar in the blood stream, not the absorption of sugar from the blood.

B. Epinephrine causes blood vessels supplying skeletal muscles to dilate, which increases blood flow to muscle cells.

C. Epinephrine causes blood vessels supplying the intestines to constrict, restricting blood flow to the organs of the digestive system.

D. **CORRECT.** Epinephrine causes liver cells to break down glycogen, which causes an increase in sugar in the blood stream.

30. A. **CORRECT.** When a response reinforces a stimulus, causing an even greater response, positive feedback is occurring.

 B. This is an example of negative feedback. The response of lower glucose levels reduces the initial stimulus and stops the pancreas from releasing insulin.

 C. This is an example of negative feedback. The response of increasing body temperature reduces the initial stimulus and stops the hypothalamus from activating warming mechanisms.

 D. This is an example of negative feedback. An osmolarity increase causes a response that decreases osmolarity and reduces the release of ADH.

31. A. The myelin sheath does not directly affect the reception of a stimulus at the dendrites.

 B. **CORRECT.** The myelin sheath, which is a lipid-based structure, insulates the axon, allowing rapid electrical conduction of the action potential down the axon. Deterioration of the myelin sheath disrupts this process.

 C. The myelin sheath covers the axon and does not function in the reabsorption of neurotransmitters.

 D. Na+/K+ pumps still function even if the myelin sheath has deteriorated.

32. A. Liver cells make bile and help regulate blood sugar levels. They do not contain collecting tubules used to collect and concentrate filtrate.

 B. The spleen functions to remove old, fragmented red blood cells and pathogens from the blood. Spleen cells do not contain collecting tubules used to collect and concentrate filtrate.

 C. The lymph nodes filter out pathogens from interstitial fluid (lymph). The cells of the lymph nodes do not contain collecting tubules used to collect and concentrate filtrate.

 D. **CORRECT.** Nephridia in segmented worms operate similarly to the nephron of the kidneys. Nephrons in the kidneys contain a collecting tubule that aids in urine production.

33. A. **CORRECT.** Calcium and sulfuric acid react to produce calcium sulfate and hydrogen gas.

 B. Hydrogen sulfide is not produced by this reaction. Hydrogen sulfide is produced by iron sulfide reacting with hydrochloric acid.

 C. Calcium sulfide is not produced by this reaction. Calcium sulfate can be reduced to calcium sulfide using carbon.

 D. Hydrogen sulfate is not produced by this reaction. Hydrogen sulfate (bisulfate ion) is the conjugate base of sulfuric acid.

34. A. These contain genetic information for the synthesis of proteins.

 B. **CORRECT.** Some proteins fold into shapes that allow them to function as biochemical catalysts or enzymes within a cell.

 C. These molecules, which repel water, function in cellular membranes and in the storage of excess energy.

 D. These "sugar and starch" molecules function in energy input and storage, as well as in some structural capacities.

35. A. **CORRECT.** Solids have little space between particles, and the particles vibrate within a fixed lattice structure.

 B. Liquid particles move about in a fluid manner due to translational motion.

 C. Gas particles are widely separated by empty space and move about randomly due to translational motion.

 D. Atoms in a plasma state move so rapidly that their electrons separate from the rest of the atom; it is as fluid as a gas.

36. A. This is the atomic number of the atom, not its mass.

 B. The sum of protons and electrons in an atom is not the atomic mass number.

 C. **CORRECT.** The mass of an atom is the sum of protons and neutrons in its nucleus.

 D. The sum of protons, neutrons, and electrons is not the atomic mass number.

37. A. CH$_4$ is a nonpolar molecule. Because water molecules are polar, water does not act as a solvent for nonpolar molecules.

   B. CCl$_4$ is a nonpolar molecule. Because water molecules are polar, water does not act as a solvent for nonpolar molecules.

   C. **CORRECT.** CH$_3$OH is a polar molecule, because oxygen is highly electronegative and draws electrons towards itself. Because water molecules are polar, water acts as a solvent for polar molecules.

   D. Octane is a nonpolar molecule. Because water molecules are polar, water does not act as a solvent for nonpolar molecules.

38. A. Because the F is dominant, half the offspring will have purple eyes.

   B. Because the F is dominant, three quarters of the offspring will have purple eyes.

   C. Because the F is dominant, all the offspring will have purple eyes.

   D. **CORRECT.** Because there is no F, all the offspring will have pink eyes.

39. A. Somatic mutations, such as lung cancer, are not passed on in this manner.

   B. Somatic mutations, such as lung cancer, are not transmitted through the blood.

   C. Somatic mutations, such as lung cancer, are not passed on in this manner. The child does not require treatment for lung cancer.

   D. **CORRECT.** Only germline mutations are transmitted, so the lung cancer, a somatic mutation, will not be passed to the child.

40. A. The use of the terms phenotype and genotype is incorrect. Phenotype refers to physical attributes, and genotype refers to genetic makeup.

   B. TT and Tt both code for dominant phenotypes. Phenotype refers to physical attributes, and genotype refers to genetic makeup.

   C. The use of the terms phenotype and genotype is incorrect. Phenotype refers to physical attributes, and genotype refers to genetic makeup.

   D. **CORRECT.** The T allele is dominant and encodes the tall plant phenotype, and it requires only one dominant allele to express the dominant trait.

41. A. According to the pyramid, there is a greater mass of seeds, berries, and grasses than insects.

   B. According to the pyramid, there is a greater mass of blackbirds and ground squirrels than red-tailed hawks.

   C. **CORRECT.** In a biomass pyramid, the greater mass is at the lower levels. According to the pyramid, there is a greater mass of seeds, berries, and grasses than insects.

   D. According to the pyramid, there is a greater mass of insects than blackbirds and ground squirrels.

42. A. This is not the hypothesis being tested.

   B. This is not the hypothesis being tested.

   C. This is not the hypothesis being tested.

   D. **CORRECT.** Because activated charcoal is known to absorb organic compounds, its use indicates that the hypothesis being tested is that Weed B produces an organic compound that inhibits root growth for Weed A.

43. A. Mutations occur in DNA, and antibiotics do not cause mutations in DNA.

   B. Antibiotics work on cellular action rather than by creating a physical barrier.

   C. **CORRECT.** If an essential bacterial partner is killed by the antibiotic, then the disease-causing potential will be reduced. This is the best inference.

   D. White blood cell production is increased by infection, not by antibiotics.

44. A. **CORRECT.** A testable and falsifiable hypothesis is the hallmark of scientific investigation. Experiments can only be used to accept or discard hypotheses.

   B. Unexpected experimental results lead to the formulation of new, different hypotheses. However, this is not a defining principle of scientific hypotheses.

   C. A scientific hypothesis will either be supported or refuted by the evidence, but it is never considered correct or incorrect.

   D. Only some scientific predictions are supported by evidence; other predictions are refuted by testing.

45. A. Electron wavelength in electron microscopy is of the same order of magnitude as the size of an atom. This is too small to visualize because electron waves cannot resolve particles that are of the same order of magnitude.

B. **CORRECT.** Electron microscopy has significantly improved the ability to see and understand the workings of these organelles, because electron wavelengths are short enough to resolve the structure of organelles, which are around 100 times larger than the wavelengths of an electron.

C. The structure of skeletal joints can be effectively examined using an X-ray machine, rather than an electron microscope.

D. The bonds between atoms use electrons, which cannot be visualized with an electron microscope because they cannot resolve particles that are of the same order of magnitude.

46. A. **CORRECT.** The neck length of giraffes was once thought to be an acquired characteristic (due to stretching to reach food) that was passed on to offspring. Further study determined that mutations in DNA actually caused the increase in neck length, which was preferentially passed on to offspring through selection.

B. While this is an example of natural selection, it does not present any evidence that would dismiss the possibility that acquired characteristics can be passed on to offspring.

C. While this is an example of natural selection, it does not present any evidence that would dismiss the possibility that acquired characteristics can be passed on to offspring.

D. This observation would support, not refute, the hypothesis that acquired characteristics are passed on to offspring. Inherited aptitude is a better indicator of learning language than parental training.

47. A. This equation describes a stable population.

B. This equation describes a decrease in population.

C. **CORRECT.** If immigration (people joining a population) and births are greater than emigration (people leaving a population) and deaths, then the population will grow.

D. This equation describes a stable population.

ENGLISH AND LANGUAGE USE

1. A. **CORRECT.** This construction reflects the same chronology of the original passage, with the director listening to everyone's opinions before making up her mind and informing people of her decisions.

B. This sentence construction implies that the director is simultaneously informing people of her decisions while listening to everyone's opinions and making up her own mind, which does not reflect the order of events in the passage.

C. The word "because" implies a cause-and-effect relationship that is not evident in the original passage.

D. This construction does not reflect the chronology of the original passage.

2. A. When making a word plural that ends in a vowel, it is necessary to add "e" before the final "s."

B. **CORRECT.** This is the correct spelling of the plural version of "veto."

C. The plural form of "veto" is "vetoes." There is no need to double "t" when making the word plural.

D. The correct plural form of "veto" is "vetoes." The word "veto" does not require an "ei" as in the words "weigh" and "neigh", because it does not have an "a" sound.

3. A. Using a comma to separate two independent clauses in this manner is an error known as a comma splice.

B. Using a comma to separate two independent clauses is an error known as a comma splice. Also, only proper nouns are capitalized within an independent clause.

C. **CORRECT.** Using a semicolon to separate two independent clauses is appropriate, and the first word following the semicolon should not be capitalized unless it is a proper noun.

D. The first word following a semicolon should not be capitalized unless it is a proper noun.

4. A. **CORRECT.** A colon should be used to introduce a list.

B. A comma is not appropriate for introducing a list.

C. A semicolon is not appropriate for introducing a list.

D. Punctuation is required to introduce the list in this sentence.

5. A. The pronoun "that" should refer to a thing or things, rather than a person.

    B. This pronoun is in the objective case, which is incorrect in this context.

    C. The pronoun "which" should refer to a thing or things, rather than a person.

    D. **CORRECT.** The pronoun must be subjective case because it is functioning as the subject of the clause.

6. A. "Accidents do not just happen" and "they are usually caused by a lack of attention" are both independent clauses and require some form of separation. Because there is no coordinating conjunction present, such as "and," "but," or "yet," the two clauses should be separated by a semicolon.

    B. "Accidents do not just happen" and "they are usually caused by a lack of attention" are both independent clauses and require some form of separation. Because there is no coordinating conjunction present, such as "and," "but," or "yet," the two clauses should be separated by a semicolon, rather than a comma.

    C. **CORRECT.** "Accidents do not just happen" and "they are usually caused by a lack of attention" are both independent clauses and require some form of separation. Because there is no coordinating conjunction present, such as "and," "but," or "yet," the two clauses should be separated by a semicolon.

    D. "Accidents do not just happen" and "they are usually caused by a lack of attention" are both independent clauses and require some form of separation. The first independent clause is not an introductory statement; therefore, a semicolon should be used, rather than a colon.

7. A. This is not a complete sentence. A complete sentence has a subject and a verb and presents a complete thought. The pronoun "me" in this option serves as the direct object of the verb "nominating," and a subject is missing.

    B. **CORRECT.** This is a complete sentence. A complete sentence has a subject and a verb and presents a complete thought. This is an example of an imperative sentence, where the subject is the understood "you" and the verb is "nominate."

    C. This is not a complete sentence. A complete sentence has a subject and a verb and presents a complete thought. This clause does not present a complete thought, because the conjunction "when" at the beginning makes it a relative clause, which is used to modify a noun or noun phrase. The noun or noun phrase that is being modified is missing from this option.

    D. This is not a complete sentence. A complete sentence has a subject and a verb and presents a complete thought. This option is missing a subject and a verb: the phrases "to be nominated" and "to serve" are infinitives that require an auxiliary verb to function as verbs.

8. A. This is the correct spelling of the word "ancient," meaning "old." This word is a spelling exception to the rule of "I before E, except after C."

    B. This is the correct spelling of the word "viewed," meaning "to look at." "Viewed" is the past tense of the word "view."

    C. **CORRECT.** The word "truly" is an exception to the rule to drop the final e before a suffix beginning with a vowel (a, e, i, o, u), but not before a suffix beginning with a consonant. The silent "e" is sometimes dropped before a suffix beginning with a consonant when another vowel comes before the "e."

    D. This is the correct spelling for the word "historic," meaning "significant."

9. A. **CORRECT.** When adding "–ly" to a word ending in "–al," keep the original "l" and add "ly." When forming an adverb, an "–ly" is added to an adjective without changing the original spelling of the word, except in cases where the root word ends "e" or "y." These exceptions do not apply to the word occasional.

    B. There is no need to remove a letter "c" from "occasional" when adding an "ly." The addition of a suffix to a root word rarely changes the spelling of the root, except in cases where the root word ends "e" or "y." These exceptions do not apply to the word "occasional".

    C. There is no need to insert an additional "s" into the word "occasional" when adding an "–ly." The addition of a suffix to a root word rarely changes the spelling of the root, except in cases where the root word ends "e" or "y." These exceptions do not apply to the word "occasional".

    D. This spelling does not follow the rule for adding "–ly" to a word ending in "–al." When adding "–ly" to a word ending in "–al," keep the original "l" and add "ly."

10. A. The verb "are" is simple present tense, but the introductory phrase shows a past action.

    B. **CORRECT.** The campaign is still ongoing, so it will take a present tense verb. However, the verb also refers to a complete action—namely, the amount collected to date—so it will take the perfect aspect of present tense: "has been spent." The subject is an indeterminate amount of money, "more than $5 million," which serves as a collective noun that takes a singular verb.

    C. The verb "were" is past tense and plural, both of which are incorrect for the context of this sentence.

    D. Using "have been" is incorrect for the context of this sentence. When the subject of the verb phrase is plural, using "have been" is appropriate; however, an indeterminate amount of money, such as "more than 5 million," serves as a collective noun and takes a singular verb.

11. A. This verb is in the plural form, which does not agree with the singular subject.

    B. **CORRECT.** This verb is in the singular form, which agrees with the singular subject. The word "or" in the phrase "A doctor or a nurse" makes the subject singular.

    C. This verb is in the plural form, which does not agree with the singular subject.

    D. This verb is in the plural form, which does not agree with the singular subject.

12. A. The subject of the sentence is "the class," which is singular, and the plural "they" would not be an appropriate pronoun. Additionally, the pronoun should be possessive, whereas "they're" is a contraction of the phrase "they are."

    B. The subject of the sentence is "the class," which is singular and requires a singular pronoun. The adverb "there," denoting a place or position, would not be appropriate.

    C. While it is true that the subject of the sentence is "the class," which is singular and requires the singular pronoun "it," the pronoun must also be possessive. "It's" is a contraction of the phrase "it is."

    D. **CORRECT.** The subject of the sentence is "the class," which is singular and requires the singular pronoun "it." Additionally, the pronoun should be possessive. "It" is an exception to the usual grammar rule to add an "apostrophe s" to indicate possession, and is instead written as "its."

13. A. The tone and language in this sentence are formal and appropriate for a business letter.

    B. The tone and language in this sentence are formal and appropriate for a business letter.

    C. **CORRECT.** The use of the word "really" and the contraction "don't" indicates that the letter is informal. Contractions should be spelled as two separate words (i.e., do not) in a formal letter. The use of the phrase "bunch of odds and ends just messing up the message" is colloquial and indicates informal writing.

    D. The tone and language in this sentence are formal and appropriate for a business letter.

14. A. This passage is informal and is not appropriate for a president of a corporation.

B. **CORRECT.** This passage is informal and is appropriate for a close colleague at work. The use of the informal greeting "Hi"; the use of contractions, such as "can't," "you'll," and "don't"; the use of exclamation points; and the use of informal phrases, such as "don't sweat it," are all indicative of informal language.

C. This passage is informal and is not appropriate for a professor at a college.

D. This passage is informal and is not appropriate for a dean at a college.

15. A. This sentence does not require a citation. It summarizes the purpose of the paper.

B. This sentence does not require a citation. It is a general statement introducing a supporting detail of the paper.

C. This sentence does not require a citation. It is a general statement introducing a supporting detail of the paper.

D. This sentence does require a citation. It refers to a specific point from Dr. Smith's research and requires a citation for their work.

16. A. Kelly is not preparing an outline. An outline is an organizational tool used to create a summary of the key points and supporting details that will be included in a paper.

B. Kelly is not writing a draft. During this stage, the writer collects ideas and begins to write.

C. **CORRECT.** Kelly is referencing sources found on the internet. Keeping a list of these references will enable her to include citations for each source.

D. Kelly is not writing a revision. This is the final element of the writing process, where the writer rereads a completed draft of the paper and makes any necessary changes.

17. A. This is the topic sentence and introduces the topic of the paragraph.

B. This sentence is a supporting detail about the topic sentence.

C. **CORRECT.** This sentence does not belong in this paragraph. It is an opinion that does not support the topic sentence about the rarity of giant pandas.

D. This sentence is a supporting detail about the topic sentence.

18. A. This sentence does not introduce the topic of soybeans and fats.

B. **CORRECT.** This sentence establishes soybeans and fats as the topic of the paragraph.

C. This sentence does not introduce the topic of soybeans and fats.

D. This sentence gives the opposite information of the supporting sentences.

19. A. "Rewritten" does not fit the context of the sentence.

B. While "occult" is a synonym for "cryptic," it does not fit the context of the sentence.

C. **CORRECT.** The context clue "because of her poor handwriting" suggests that "illegible" is the correct connotation for this context.

D. "Terse" is a synonym for "brief" or "concise"; it does not fit the context of the sentence.

20. A. Confusing is not a synonym for banal.

B. Ostentatious is not a synonym for banal.

C. **CORRECT.** Bland is a synonym for banal, and it fits the context of the sentence because it makes sense that one would avoid bland plays.

D. Practiced is not a synonym for banal.

21. A. The phrase "become infected" is not an antonym for atrophy.

B. **CORRECT.** Atrophy means "to waste away," so this is an appropriate antonym.

C. The phrase "weaken gradually" is not an antonym for atrophy.

D. The phrase "injure through over-exertion" is not an antonym for atrophy.

22. A. The Latin roots "circum" and "loqui" do not combine to mean "meandering expedition."

B. **CORRECT.** The Latin root "circum" means "around," and the Latin root "loqui" means "to speak."

C. The Latin roots "circum" and "loqui" do not combine to mean "type of geometrical pattern."

D. The Latin roots "circum" and "loqui" do not combine to mean "remote destination."

23. A. The prefix "anti–" indicates opposition. Rather than referring to an ingredient in the chemicals, the word "antidote" is mostly likely referring to a substance that counteracts the effects of the chemicals.

    B. An antidote is a substance that counteracts the effects of another substance, while a contraindication is a condition or situation that prohibits the use of a substance.

    C. An antidote is a substance, not a place.

    D. **CORRECT.** An antidote is a substance that "acts against," or counteracts, the effects of another substance, such as the chemicals in the example above. The prefix "anti–" means against.

24. A. The definition of "dys–" is "difficult or painful." A client who has dysesthesia feels pain, not pleasure, when touched.

    B. **CORRECT.** The definition of "dys–" is "difficult or painful." A client who has dysesthesia feels pain when touched.

    C. The definition of "dys–" is "difficult or painful." A client who has dysesthesia does not have a normal reaction to touch.

    D. The definition of "dys–" is "difficult or painful." A client who has dysesthesia feels pain when touched.

Index

C

Canaliculi, 262

Capillaries, 169–170, 172–174, 193, 244, 262

Carbohydrates, 203, 219, 262

Cardiac muscle, 172, 180, 181, 262

Cardiovascular system, 169, 172–174, 193, 197, 262

Cartesian coordinates, 121, 122, 149

Cartilage, 262, 265

Catalysts, 240, 241, 262

Cations, 230, 235, 236, 262

Cause-and-effect relationships, 252, 255

Cell-mediated immunity, 262

Cell (plasma) membranes, 204, 205, 262

Cells

    antigen-presenting, 196, 261

    B cells, 195–197, 262

    in biological hierarchy, 203

    defined, 168, 262

    dendritic, 263

    meiosis and, 203, 207, 214, 216–217, 266

    memory, 196, 266

    mitosis and, 203, 206, 266

    nucleus of, 204–205, 220–221, 223, 267

    red blood, 173, 192, 193

    structure and function of, 204–208

    T cells, 195–197, 263, 265, 270

    white blood, 173, 196, 197

Cellular functions, 262

Central nervous system (CNS), 179–180, 189, 191, 193, 201, 262

Central tendency measures, 125, 150

Ceruminous glands, 187, 262

Cervix, 185, 191, 262

Characters, 9, 18, 33, 43–44, 48, 50

Charts

    biased information in, 25

    defined, 21, 61, 92, 149

    misleading information in, 25

    persuasive effects of, 25

    pie, 25, 121, 150

    synthesis of, 58

Chemical (enzymatic) digestion, 175–177, 264

Chemical equations, 237–238, 262

Chemical reactions, 235–242

Chemistry, 227–248

    acids and bases, 246–248

    atomic structure, 227–231

    chemical reactions, 235–242

    matter, physical properties and states of, 232–234

    solutions, properties of, 243–245

Chromatids, 207, 210, 262

Chromosomes, 206–212, 215–217, 220, 262

Chronological order, 27, 28, 41, 57, 61, 319

Chyme, 176–177, 247, 262

Circulatory system. See Cardiovascular system

Circumference, 134, 149

Citations, 31–32, 47, 301, 322, 329

Claims, 3, 31, 53–57, 61

Clarifying details, 4

Clauses, 300–302, 304–305, 329

CNS. See Central nervous system

Codons, 210, 212, 262

Coefficients, 102, 149, 237

Cognates, 324

Cohesion, 243, 263

Cohesive language, 28

Collagen, 182, 187, 201, 220, 263

Colloquialisms, 313–315, 329

Combining like terms, 103, 149

Combustion reactions, 237

Commas, 300–302, 329, 330

Commensal microorganisms, 196, 263

Common denominators, 97, 149

Communicable/infectious diseases, 222–224, 265

Dehydration reaction, 218, 219, 263

Delineation, 8, 11, 61

Dendrites, 179, 263

Dendritic cells, 263

Denominators, 91, 97, 101, 149, 150

Denotations, 35, 36, 61

Dense (compact) bone, 200, 201, 263

Density, 232, 263

Deoxyribonucleic acid (DNA), 190, 209–212, 220, 263

Deoxyribose sugar, 210, 263

Dependent clauses, 300–302, 304–305, 329

Dependent variables, 130, 149, 257, 258

Deposition, 233

Derivational suffixes, 325, 329

Derivations, 324, 329

Dermis, 187, 188, 263

Descriptive writing, 40

Details
clarifying, 4
conclusions and, 8, 9, 49
defined, 3, 61
elaborative, 4
explanatory, 4
inferences and, 8, 47, 48
irrelevant, 4
point of view and, 43
predictions and, 47, 48
supporting, 4–6, 318, 319, 330

Diabetes, 190, 197, 223, 263

Diagramming sentences, 307

Diagrams, 23, 24, 61, 322

Dialogue, 51

Diastole, 173, 263

Diction, 309, 311, 329

Diffusion, 169–170, 243–245, 263

Digestive system, 175–178, 195

Dihybrid cross, 216, 263

Dilution, 244, 263

Dimensional analysis, 138, 139, 149

Directional terminology, 166, 263

Directions, comprehension of, 11–14

Direct objects, 306, 330

Direct proportion, 114

Direct quotations, 301, 302

Direct variation, 131, 149

Disaccharides, 219

Diseases. See also specific diseases
autoimmune, 197, 262
defined, 170, 223, 263
infectious/communicable, 222–224, 265
microorganisms and, 222–225
non-infectious, 222, 223, 267

Diuretics, 263

Division, 94, 106, 149

DNA. See Deoxyribonucleic acid

Dominant traits, 214–217, 263

Drafting, 321, 322, 329

Drawing conclusions, 8–10, 29, 47, 49, 58, 252, 258

E

Eccrine sweat glands, 187, 263

Editing, 321, 322

Eggs (ova), 185, 186, 191, 267

Elaborative details, 4

Electron microscopes, 224, 263

Electrons, 224, 227–230, 235–236, 263

Elements, defined, 218, 263

Empirical evidence, 252, 263

End marks, 301, 302, 329

Endnotes, 16

Endocrine glands, 189–190, 264

Endocrine system, 186, 189–191. See also Hormones

Endoplasmic reticulum, 204–206, 269

Endothermic reactions, 240, 241, 264

English and language usage, 295–345. See also Parts of speech
evaluation for rhetorical context, 313–317
grammar conventions, 309–312
paragraph organization, 318–320

Fractions
    comparing, 100–101
    computations with, 97
    conversions involving, 92–93
    defined, 91, 149
    denominators in, 91, 97, 101, 149, 150
    numerators in, 91, 150
    ordering, 100
    reciprocals, 98, 102, 150
    rounding, 111
    simplification of, 93, 150
Fragments, 309, 329
Front-end estimations, 111, 149
FSH (follicle-stimulating hormone), 186, 191, 264
Fungi, 222–223, 264
Future tense, 28, 310

G

Gallbladder, 176, 264
Gametes, 184–185, 190, 207, 215–217, 264
Gaps in sequences, 29
Gas exchange, 169–170
Gender-biased language, 316
Genes, 209–212, 214–217, 220–221, 264
Genetic code, 221, 264
Genome, 212, 264
Genotypes, 215–216, 264
Genres, 11, 50–52, 61, 313–314, 329
Geometric quantities
    area, 106, 110, 135–136, 149
    calculation of, 133–137
    circumference, 134, 149
    length, 133–134, 150
    perimeter, 133–134, 150
    volume, 110, 136, 151
GH (growth hormone), 190, 264
Gigantism, 190, 264

Glands
    adrenal, 189, 190, 261
    ceruminous, 187, 262
    defined, 175, 264
    endocrine, 189–190, 264
    exocrine, 264
    parathyroid, 189, 268
    pineal, 189, 190, 268
    pituitary, 186, 189–191, 268
    sebaceous, 187, 269
    sweat, 187, 188, 255, 261, 263
    thymus, 189, 270
    thyroid, 189, 190, 270
Glomerulus, 193, 264
Glossaries, 16, 61
Glucagon, 176, 190, 191, 255, 264
Glucose, 176, 190–191, 193, 219, 241, 255
Glycerol, 219, 264
Glycogen, 176, 191, 219
Golgi apparatus, 204, 205, 264
Gonadotropin-releasing hormone, 186
Gonads, 264. See also Ovaries; Testes
Graduated cylinders, 250, 264
Grammar conventions, 309–312
Grams, defined, 232, 264
Graphic representations. See also Charts; Graphs
    analysis of, 21–22
    arguments strengthened with, 25
    biased information in, 25
    defined, 21, 61
    infographics, 25, 26
    interpretation of, 22–24
    misleading information in, 25

Graphs
 bar, 25, 121, 149
 biased information in, 25
 bivariate, 122, 149
 Cartesian coordinate, 121, 122
 data trends in, 128
 defined, 21, 61, 116, 149
 line, 25, 121, 150
 misleading information in, 25
 persuasive effects of, 25
 points on, 122, 150
 scatterplots, 121, 150
 synthesis of, 58
Groups, on periodic table, 228–229, 264
Growth hormone (GH), 190, 264
Growth (epiphyseal) plates, 200, 264

H

Hair follicles, 187, 264
Haversian canal, 264
Headings, 15–17, 61
Heart, 169, 172–174, 264
Helminths, 223
Helper T cells, 196, 197, 265
Hemoglobin, 173, 220, 241, 265
Heredity, 214–217
Heterozygous genotypes, 215–216, 265
Hinge joints, 200, 265
Histamines, 196, 197, 265
HIV/AIDS, 197, 223
Homeostasis, 187–193, 265
Homographs, 297, 299, 329
Homophones, 297, 299, 329
Homozygous genotypes, 215–216, 265
Hooke, Robert, 224
Hormones
 antidiuretic, 190, 261
 in blood plasma, 173
 defined, 185, 265
 in digestion, 175, 176
 epinephrine, 190, 264

 estrogen, 186, 190, 264
 follicle-stimulating, 186, 191, 264
 gonadotropin-releasing, 186
 growth, 190, 264
 inhibiting, 191, 265
 luteinizing, 186, 266
 oxytocin, 191, 267
 releasing, 191, 269
 renin, 193, 269
 steroid, 219, 270
 testosterone, 186, 270
 transport of, 172, 173
Hosts, 222, 223, 265
Hyaline cartilage, 200, 265
Hydrogen bonds, 210, 243, 265
Hydrolysis reaction, 218, 265
Hydrophilic, 176, 220, 243–244, 265
Hydrophobic, 219, 220, 243–244, 265
Hyperthyroidism, 190, 265
Hypodermis, 187, 265
Hypothalamus, 186, 189, 191, 265
Hypotheses, 257, 258, 265, 269

I

Identification
 of biases and stereotypes, 25, 31–33
 of cause-and-effect relationships, 252
 of claims and counterclaims, 53
 of clauses, 302, 304
 of cohesive language, 28
 of contradictory information, 13
 of data trends, 57
 defined, 3, 61
 of directional priorities, 12
 of evidence, 8, 32, 41, 47
 of facts vs. opinions, 33–34, 41
 of homophones and homographs, 299
 of key points, 4, 6
 of main ideas, 3, 5, 11
 of misleading information, 25
 of missing information, 13, 16, 29, 319
 of perspectives, 44, 45

R

Range, 102, 126, 150

Rate of change, 113, 115–117, 150

Rational numbers
  comparing, 100–101
  defined, 99, 150
  operations with, 94–98
  ordering, 99–100
  in real-world problems, 106

Ratios, 104, 115–117, 150

Reactants, 235, 237–241, 269

Reading skills, 1–88. See also Comprehension
  argument evaluation, 53–55
  author's purpose, evaluation of, 39–42
  compare and contrast themes, 50–52
  data evaluation and integration, 56–59
  fact vs. opinion determination, 31–34
  graphic analysis and interpretation, 21–26
  locating specific information, 15–20
  making inferences and drawing conclusions, 8–10, 29, 47–49, 58
  multi-paragraph text summaries, 3–7
  point of view, evaluation of, 43–46
  practice problem answer key, 65–70
  predictions from evidence in text, 47–49
  quiz and answer key, 71–88
  sequence interpretation, 27–30
  terminology related to, 61–63
  test item categorization, 1
  word and phrase interpretation, 35–38

Real numbers, 105–106, 150

Real-world problems, 105–120
  estimation and rounding in, 110–112
  expressions, equations, and inequalities in, 118–120
  one- or multi-step operations with real numbers, 105–106
  with percentages, 107–109
  with proportions, 113–114
  ratios and rates of change in, 115–117

Reason, defined, 16, 62

Reasoning
  assumptions based on, 8
  claims supported by, 53
  defined, 4, 62
  faulty, 31, 56
  main ideas supported by, 4
  opinions supported by, 41
  organization of, 57
  perspectives and, 45

Recessive traits, 214–217, 269

Reciprocals, 98, 102, 150

Rectum, 175, 176, 269

Recurring themes, 51

Red blood cells, 173, 192, 193

Reference planes, 166, 269

Reflexes, 269

Register, 313–315, 330

Relaxation of muscles, 173, 182, 201, 269

Releasing hormones, 191, 269

Relevant information, 15–17, 21–22, 28, 45, 56, 62

Reliability, 31, 33, 34, 44, 54, 253

Renal arteries, 192, 193, 269

Renal cortex, 192, 269

Renal medulla, 192, 269

Renal pelvis, 269

Renal veins, 192, 193, 269

Renin, 193, 269

Repeating decimals, 99, 106, 150

Rephrasing, 5, 62

Representations, 21, 62. See also Graphic representations

Reproductive system, 184–186, 195

Research, 34, 44, 45, 54, 62, 322

Residual volume, 170

Respiratory system, 168–171

Revising, 321, 322

Rhetorical context, 313–317

Rhetorical devices, 53, 54, 62

Rheumatoid arthritis, 197, 269

Ribonucleic acid (RNA), 209, 211–212, 220, 221, 269

Ribosomes, 204–205, 209–210, 212, 221, 269

Root words, 35, 62, 324–326, 330

Rough endoplasmic reticulum, 205, 206, 269

Rounding, 110–112, 150

Run-on sentences, 311, 330

S

Saliva, 175, 269

Salts, 176, 192–193, 195–196, 237, 245, 269

Sarcomeres, 182, 269

Saturated solutions, 244, 269

Scales, 21–22, 62, 113, 150, 250

Scatterplots, 121, 150

Science, 163–294. See also Anatomy and physiology; Chemistry; Life and physical sciences
   logic and evidence in, 252–254
   measurement and measurement tools, 249–251
   practice problem answer key, 273–282
   prediction of relationships in, 255–256
   quiz on, 283–294
   scientific method, 257–259
   terminology related to, 261–271
   test item categorization, 163

Scientific hypotheses, 257, 269

Scientific method, 257–259

Scrotum, 184, 269

Search engines, 19, 62

Search terms and phrases, 19, 62

Sebaceous glands, 187, 269

Secondary sources, 54, 62, 322

Second-person point of view, 32, 43, 314, 330

Semicolons, 301, 305

Seminal vesicles, 184

Sentences
   clarity of, 309
   complete, 306, 309–310
   complex, 301, 302, 305, 329
   compound, 300–302, 305, 329
   compound-complex, 305
   diagramming, 307
   editing, 322
   fragments, 309, 329
   imperative, 310, 329
   punctuation patterns in, 301–302
   run-on, 311, 330
   simple, 301, 305, 330
   structure of, 304–308
   topic, 318, 330

Sequential order, 11–12, 27–30, 62

Serial (Oxford) commas, 300, 330

Settings, 36, 37, 50

Sex cells. See Gametes

Shape of data distributions, 126, 150

Short bones, 200, 269

Sidebars, 17, 62

Signal words and phrases, 11–12, 27–29, 36

Simple sentences, 301, 305, 330

Simplification of fractions, 93, 150

SI units (Système Internationale), 249, 269. See also Metric system

Skeletal muscle, 180–182, 269

Skeletal system, 197, 199–202, 269. See also Bones

Skewness of distributions, 127

Skin, 181, 187–188, 195–196, 269. See also Integumentary system

Slang, 313–315, 330

Slope, 114, 116, 150

Small intestine, 175–177, 269

Smooth endoplasmic reticulum, 204, 206, 269

Smooth muscle, 175, 176, 180, 181, 269

Social commentary, 52, 62

Social structure, 51, 62

Solutes, 243–245, 270

T

U